Manual of Practical Audiometry

Practical Aspects of Audiology

Series Editor: Michael Martin, OBE, Royal National Institute for the Deaf, London

---

Audiology is a relatively new discipline, formed over the last 50 years. As with all new disciplines, the pace of research is high and standardisation or acceptance of agreed procedures and norms has been low. Examples of this may be seen in the work of the International Standards Organisation (ISO) which only in recent years has produced standards for basic audiometric test methods and given levels for masking signals in pure-tone audiometry.

While much is written on audiology, a great deal of the material concentrates on research aspects of the work. The aim of this series of books is to emphasise the practical aspects of audiology and to set out clearly current practice and ways in which research might be applied.

Furthermore, an international perspective will be given to the series, in order to spread the information that is available on a world-wide scale. This will bring to the attention of practitioners and students ideas and procedures that may appear novel in their own countries but which are widely used in other parts of the world. Today, audiology is an international subject, and recognition must be given to this fact in our thinking. With the move to international standardisation, particularly in instrumentation, it is essential that we are aware of the different approaches being used.

Speech Audiometry, edited by Michael Martin, Royal National Institute for the Deaf, London.

Paediatric Audiology, 0–5 Years, edited by Barry McCormick, Nottingham General Hospital, UK.

Manual of Practical Audiometry, Volume 1, edited by Stig Arlinger, Swedish Audiometry Methods Group.

Manual of Practical Audiometry, Volume 2, edited by Stig Arlinger, Swedish Audiometry Methods Group.

Cochlear Implants: A Practical Guide, edited by Huw Cooper, Royal Ear Hospital, London

Tactile Aids for the Hearing Impaired, edited by Ian Summers, University of Exeter.

Manual of Practical Audiometry
Volume 2

Edited and translated by

STIG ARLINGER
Chairman, Swedish Audiometry Methods Group (SAME)

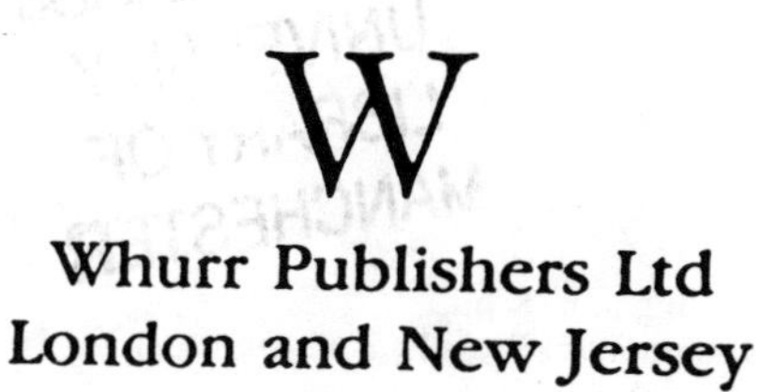

Whurr Publishers Ltd
London and New Jersey

First published 1991 by

Whurr Publishers Ltd
19b Compton Terrace
London N1 2UN
England

Reprinted 1993

British Library Cataloguing in Publication Data

Manual of practical audiometry: Vol. 2.
I. Arlinger, Stig
617.8

ISBN 1-870332-02-4

Photoset by Scribe Design, Gillingham, Kent
Printed in Great Britain by Athenaeum Press Ltd, Newcastle upon Tyne

Foreword

Last year volume 1 of the *Manual of Practical Audiometry* was published in its English language version, presenting hands-on descriptions of how to perform a variety of audiometric tests. Volume 2 is the logical complement to volume 1, its purpose being to present the physiological, psychoacoustic and acoustic background for the various test methods. Sources of error which may influence test results are discussed. The clinical applications and interpretations are other important aspects that are covered by volume 2.

Both books were produced by a Swedish working group representing a thorough professional experience in the field of audiology technicians, technical audiologists or audiological physicians. The English version follows the original one in all essential aspects, but has been adjusted to avoid specific national conditions, e.g. it omits all references to literature in Swedish.

It is the hope that volumes 1 and 2 together will find a similar use in other countries to their use in Sweden: as practical textbooks in the training of those professions for which audiometry is part of the workload – audiology technicians, audiologists, nurses, physicians, physicists, engineers etc. – and as a natural source of reference in places where measurements of hearing are carried out.

I wish to express my sincere thanks to Michael Martin, Royal National Institute for the Deaf, London, who as the general editor for the publisher's production within the field of audiology suggested the translation into English and has provided invaluable help during the work.

Stig Arlinger
Editor and Chairman of the working group
Linköping, Sweden 1990

The following were members of the working group:

Bengt Almqvist
Stig Arlinger
Lars Bergholtz
Eva Bjureus
Lena Ekström
Sten Harris
Mari Holmberg
Ingrid Lennart
Arne Leijon
Ulf Rosenhall
Inger Wikström

Contents

Foreword v

Introduction ix

Chapter 1 1

Safety aspects in audiometry

Chapter 2 4

Psychoacoustics

Chapter 3 24

Statistical aspects on measurement accuracy

Chapter 4 31

Common sources of error in audiometry

Chapter 5 40

Psychoacoustic methods with pure-tone stimuli

Pure-tone air-conduction audiometry
Pure-tone bone-conduction audiometry
Békésy audiometry
Loudness balance tests
Threshold tone decay
Sound localisation

Chapter 6 84

Psychoacoustic methods using speech stimuli

Routine speech audiometry
Distorted speech audiometry

Chapter 7 102

Audiometry in children

Chapter 8 111

Acoustic impedance audiometry

Tympanometry
Stapedius reflex thresholds
Stapedius reflex decay test
Tensor reflex test
Tubal function tests

Chapter 9 154

Electrophysiological methods

Electrocochleography
Brain-stem response audiometry
Cortical response audiometry

Chapter 10 188

Test battery for clinical evaluation

Chapter 11 202

Audiometry in schoolchildren

Chapter 12 206

Audiometry in occupational health

Chapter 13 212

Audiometry in hearing aid fitting

Hearing aid indication and prescription
Evaluation of hearing aid function on a user
Evaluation of the user's function with hearing aid

Chapter 14 227

Measurements in tinnitus evaluation

Index 235

Introduction

In volume 1 of *Manual of Practical Audiometry* the practical execution of most existing audiometric methods has been described; volume 2 is a complement to volume 1. The aim of this book is to explain the purpose of using certain methods, which factors may influence the outcome of the test and what results can be expected from test subjects with different types of hearing impairment.

The book starts with four general chapters, of which the first presents aspects of safety in audiometry. This concerns both electrical hazards for the tester and the test subject as well as acoustic hazards for the test subject. A basic chapter on psychoacoustics is well motivated by the large number of psychoacoustic test methods in use in audiometry. Statistical aspects on test accuracy and a discussion of general sources of error in audiometry also belong to these introductory chapters.

In Chapters 5–9 the five main categories of audiometric test methods, presented in volume 1, are discussed: psychoacoustic test methods using pure-tone stimulation and using speech stimulation, audiometry with children, acoustic impedance audiometry and electrophysiological tests. Within each chapter the following are discussed: the indications for the method, the physiological, psychoacoustic and acoustic background for the test method, equipment necessary, sources of error and test accuracy, and the clinical interpretation of the test results.

In the five concluding chapters various applications of audiometry are presented: clinical diagnostic evaluation, audiometric testing of schoolchildren, occupational health, the fitting of hearing aids and evaluation of tinnitus.

Chapter 1 Safety Aspects in Audiometry

Audiology is an area within the field of medical health care which makes extensive use of technical equipment. New equipment and new applications appear frequently. The use of technical equipment can involve certain risks for both patients and users, and in audiometry two types of risk are at hand: one is the risk of an electric shock to the patient or the tester by high voltage or leakage currents; the other is the risk of too high a sound level being presented to the patient, carrying the risk of acoustic trauma.

In audiological rehabilitation an additional risk exists in the possibility of harming the middle ear when making ear impressions.

Electrical Safety

The international standard IEC 601-1 (1977) provides a basis for the safety of medical electric equipment. In many countries it is adopted as a national standard. The international standard on audiometric equipment, IEC 645 (1989), refers to IEC 601 for electric safety requirements.

IEC 601-1 specifies requirements for general electromedical equipment with regard to electric shock, burns, and mechanical and other hazards. It also gives advice on installation, use, maintenance and service, and describes how to test the safety of various pieces of equipment.

A producer or distributor of electromedical equipment may verify that a unit fulfils the requirements of IEC 601 by a basic test report. This is a certificate which may be issued by the producer or by a national test institution. If a basic test report is not available, it is desirable to perform a delivery control with the corresponding tests before the equipment is put into clinical use. The basic test report verifies that a number of characteristics of importance for the safe use of the unit fulfil the requirements of IEC 601. These concern the connection to mains, ground connection and power fuses. Further, standardised colours of warning lamps and certain electric wires are checked, and also the markings on the equipment. Test units to be used in direct contact with the patient are checked for possible leakage currents. This is of particular importance in equipment for electric response audiometry, where the recording electrodes provide an electric connection to the patient with very low impedance.

Acoustic Safety

IEC 601-1 does not consider any hazard connected with the particular diagnostic procedure for which the equipment will be used. Thus, for audiometric equipment nothing is said about the possibility of causing damage to a patient's ear under test by the accidental presentation of too high a sound level. Such risks may be present also when using equipment in perfect condition and following a recommended procedure. In all suprathreshold testing, it is therefore important to evaluate the possibility of hazards in relation to the diagnostic value of the test. Accidents have been reported in stapedius reflex testing, in particular the reflex decay test, and when testing for loudness discomfort level using pure tones.

Another acoustic risk is related to equipment malfunctions not covered by IEC 601-1 (1977): an example concerns commonly found equipment where sound levels are controlled by digital electronics. Errors may occur that lead to the actual sound level being different from the indicated sound level due to an error in the electronic calibration memory of the audiometer. The revised version of the international standard for audiometers, IEC 645, specifies test methods and requirements with regard to the sensitivity of digital electronics to electric transients which might give rise to such errors.

Responsibility

The legal conditions with regard to responsibility if an accident should occur vary according to the national laws and cannot be defined in general terms. Whatever the situation, it is always recommended to consider these risks and organise the work in the clinic so as to minimise the probability of an accident occurring. Such organisation should include consideration of the safety characteristics of the equipment, including delivery control, proper training and information to staff members who will use it on patients, including how to use it and how to check its performance at regular intervals. There must be a clearly defined routine for handling a situation in which malfunction is suspected and which might imply hazard. An instruction manual in the user's language must be available. A scheme for regular service and maintenance is important. The possibility of the patient manipulating the controls of the equipment if left alone should also be considered, and rules must be formulated on how to handle such a situation should this arise.

References

IEC 601-1 (1977). *Safety of Medical Electric Equipment.* Geneva: International Electrotechnical Commission.

IEC 645 (1989). *Audiometers*. Geneva: International Electrotechnical Commission.

Chapter 2
Psychoacoustics

Psychoacoustics concerns the correlation between the acoustic characteristics of a sound and the listener's perception of it. Psychoacoustics is part of the science of psychophysics, which also deals with physical signals other than sound that may influence humans and animals via their sense organs.

Audiometry is to a large extent based on psychoacoustic test methods, i.e. methods whereby the listener has to react actively to the sound signal, e.g. by pressing a button or giving a verbal response. The requirement for active cooperation is both a strength and a weakness. The strength lies in the fact that the complete sensory system is involved. However, by a suitable choice of sound signal and listener task, the results from a stated test method may be taken to be the function of a limited part of the auditory system. The weakness is that psychoacoustic methods depend on the listener's willingness and ability to cooperate. This means that, when willingness or ability is inadequate, the test result will be influenced by this as well as by the functioning of the auditory system.

Before describing the various methods available and their advantages and limitations, a number of basic psychoacoustic quantities and concepts will be defined.

Psychoacoustic Quantities and Concepts

Threshold of hearing

This is defined as the sound level at which, under specified conditions (type of sound, method of presentation), a listener will detect 50% of presented stimuli correctly.

Hearing level (HL)

Hearing level is a measure of sound level, defined as the level in decibels (dB) above the average normal threshold of hearing for the particular sound and method of presentation, e.g. a pure tone of a certain frequency presented monaurally by means of an earphone, or bisyllabic test words, presented binaurally in a free sound field. The signal level of an audiometer is as a rule scaled in dB HL. The concept hearing level thus refers to a signal level. Sometimes it is being misused as synonymous with hearing threshold level (HTL) which is a characteristic of a listener, usually expressed in terms of dB HL.

Sensation level

Sensation level means signal level referred to the individual listener's hearing threshold level for the particular signal and manner of presentation. For example, if the hearing threshold level of a particular listener is 40 dB HL for a certain sound and this is presented at 75 dB HL in a certain test, the sensation level is 35 dB.

Loudness level

The loudness level of a sound is defined as the sound pressure level of a 1000-Hz pure tone which sounds equally loud to normal-hearing listeners. The unit is the phon. If, for example, the loudness of a particular sound equals that of a 1000-Hz tone at 76 dB sound pressure level (SPL), the loudness level of that sound is 76 phons.

A set of curves which are called equal loudness contours or isophon curves are shown in Figure 2.1. These curves relate tones of various frequencies with equal loudness. The 50-phon curve shows, for example, that a tone at 60 Hz and 67 dB SPL is as loud as a 1000-Hz tone of 50 dB SPL or a 4000-Hz tone of 42 dB SPL. This set of curves is taken from the international standard ISO 226 (1987), and is valid for binaural listening in a free sound field, i.e. when the sound is frontally incident and no reflective surfaces are present to influence the sound transmission. The bottom curve, which passes through 1000 Hz and 4 dB SPL, i.e. the 4-phon curve, represents the average normal threshold of hearing for binaural listening in a free sound field, the minimum audible field (MAF).

From a neurophysiological point of view, perception of loudness is considered to be related to the number of fibres in the auditory nerve, which are activated by the particular sound, and the impulse activity in those fibres.

Loudness

The term loudness refers to a comparison of the magnitude of a sound with that of a 1000-Hz tone at 40 dB SPL, the loudness of which is defined as 1 sone. A sound with a loudness of 20 sones is considered as 20 times louder than a sound with a loudness of 1 sone, twice as loud as a sound

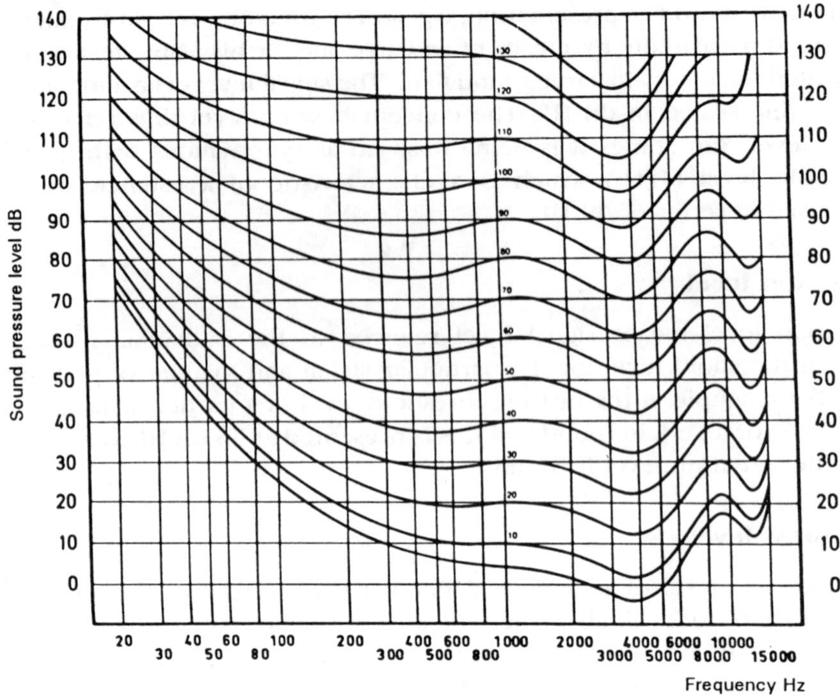

Figure 2.1 Isophon curves, connecting pure tones of different frequencies and sound pressure levels that yield equal loudness levels.

with the loudness 10 sones and half as loud as a sound having a loudness of 40 sones.

An ISO standard (ISO 131, 1979) describes these relations in detail and defines the relation between loudness and loudness level both in tabular form and as a mathematical formula.

In another ISO standard (ISO 532, 1975), two different methods are described for the calculation of the loudness level of broad band sounds of constant character, transmitted as a diffuse sound field (in a diffuse sound field the sound arrives equally from all directions). The calculations are based on measured octave or one-third octave sound pressure levels.

Pitch

Pitch is the perceptual correlate to frequency. The unit of pitch is the mel. A pure tone of frequency 1000 Hz and sound pressure level 40 dB has a pitch which is defined as 1000 mels.

Not only is the pitch of a tone determined by its frequency but it may also be influenced by its sound level. For high frequencies the pitch increases with increasing sound level. At low frequencies the opposite is found: the pitch falls when the sound level is increased. Perhaps the greatest importance of the concept of pitch concerns the relation between the pitch of various simultaneous sounds in music. Certain combinations of pitch are perceived as harmonic, and the frequency ratios in such tone combinations are then simple. Examples of such harmonic combinations are an octave with the frequency ratio 2:1, a fifth with the ratio 3:2, a major third with the ratio 5:4 and a minor third with the ratio 6:5.

The pitch of a complex tone, e.g. a tone from a musical instrument consisting of fundamental and a number of harmonics, is sometimes rather difficult to identify reliably. This is of practical importance, e.g. in tinnitus analysis, where often octave confusions can cause problems.

Neurophysiologically, the spectral pattern of a complex tone is transmitted by means of both place and time coding. Place coding means that specific fibres in the auditory nerve respond to a specific frequency range, whilst time coding means that the impulse pattern of a specific nerve fibre reflects the periodic pattern of the complex tone.

Temporal integration

This concept refers to the fact that the perception of various characteristics of a sound, e.g. loudness or pitch, is influenced by the duration of the sound. This is due to the signal analysis, which takes place at various levels in the auditory pathways, requiring a certain time. If the sound duration is too short, the analysis will not be complete and the perception consequently less clear as compared to when the duration is longer.

For the normal hearing threshold for pure tones, a tone pulse duration of less than half a second will influence the hearing threshold level. The time constant – a measure of the time required for the signal analysis – of this phenomenon is approximately 200 ms. The time dependence is such that, for shorter durations, the hearing threshold level increases by about 10 dB when the tone pulse duration is reduced by a factor of 10 (Figure 2.2). To avoid influence from temporal integration in pure-tone audiometry, pulse durations in the range 1–2 s are normally used.

The temporal integration of loudness depends on the sound level (Poulsen, 1975). At higher sound levels, the time constant decreases and is of the order of some tens of milliseconds at sound levels of around 100 dB SPL.

Temporal integration occurs also for psychoacoustic dimensions other than loudness, e.g. pitch and the ability to detect small differences or changes in pitch or loudness. Also, stapedius reflex thresholds show temporal integration. However, the temporal dependence differs from that of normal hearing thresholds (Zwicker, 1974).

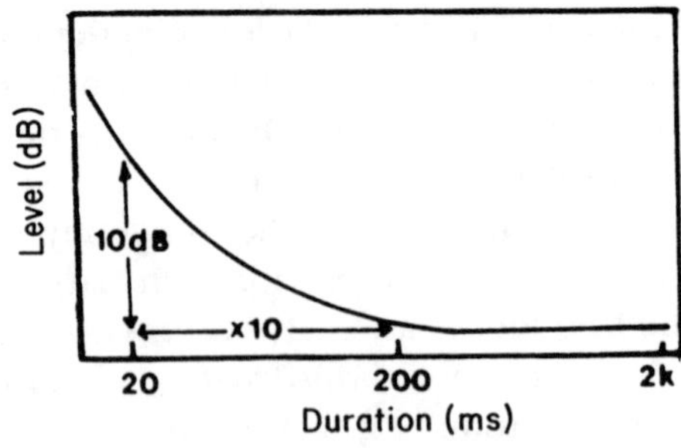

Figure 2.2 Temporal integration for the normal threshold of hearing.

Critical bandwidth

In many aspects the auditory sense organ functions as a set of bandpass filters with continuously overlapping frequency bands and with a bandwidth which is known as the critical bandwidth. When trying to detect a tone in a noisy background, the listener's attention is focused on the band in the centre of which the tone is situated. Only those parts of the background noise that are within the filter passband affect the audibility of the tone, i.e. contribute significantly to the masking of the tone. Another aspect of the critical bandwidth concept is that the loudness of a complex sound of a certain total sound pressure level remains constant as long as its bandwidth does not exceed the critical bandwidth. If its bandwidth is increased, whilst keeping its total sound level constant, its loudness will increase when its bandwidth exceeds the critical bandwidth. However, recently this critical bandwidth for loudness has been questioned by Cacace and Margolis (1985), who consider it as a misinterpretation caused by the logarithmic scale used to plot bandwidth. If, instead, the bandwidth is expressed in octaves, they find a linear relation between loudness and bandwidth of a narrow-band signal.

At low frequencies, below about 500 Hz, critical bandwidth is relatively constant at around 100 Hz. At higher frequencies, it increases with frequency. At 1000 Hz its value is about 160 Hz and at 4000 Hz about 700 Hz. From 500 Hz, critical bandwidth can be reasonably well approximated by one-third of an octave (Scharf, 1970).

Fletcher (1940), who was among the first to study the critical bandwidth, assumed that when a pure tone was barely audible in a broadband noise, the level of the noise within the critical band equalled that of the tone, i.e. the signal-to-noise ratio within the critical band was 0 dB. This assumption has later been shown to be wrong. The bandwidth obtained according to Fletcher's assumption is approximately two and a half times smaller than the critical bandwidth and is referred to as the critical ratio. The true signal-to-noise ratio for a just detectable tone in a critical bandwidth noise is −4 dB, which corresponds to the factor 2.5.

Masking

Masking means the reduction of the audibility of a sound by another sound. Usually it refers to simultaneous sounds. For narrow-band sounds, the phenomenon of masking is usually described as how the masking sound, i.e. the masker, influences another sound, i.e. the maskee, as a function of its frequency. This may be called spectral masking, and the description provides a measure of the auditory spectral resolution.

However, non-simultaneous masking also occurs. This means that a sound may influence the perception of a succeeding or a preceding sound. These phenomena are termed 'forward' and 'backward masking'; the general term 'temporal masking' may also be used. These characteristics may be used to describe the auditory temporal resolution.

The degree of masking can be specified as the change in the listener's hearing threshold for the maskee that is caused by the masker. Narrow-band sounds give rise to more masking at frequencies above the band than below, i.e. the masking effect is asymmetrical. This is the main reason why loud, low frequency noise affects speech recognition more than high frequency sounds of an equal level.

In audiometry, masking is used to make a test sound inaudible in the non-test ear when a risk of cross-hearing is present, i.e. sound reaching the inner ear of the non-test side by means of unwanted bone conduction. When the test sound is a tone, a narrow-band noise is used for masking. The IEC standard for audiometers (IEC 645, 1979) prescribes a bandwidth of between one-third and one-half of an octave. When the test sound is human speech a broad-band noise is used, filtered with regard to the frequency spectrum of the speech signal. The IEC standard prescribes a noise which is low pass filtered with a cut-off frequency of 1000 Hz and a slope of 12 dB/octave.

Psychoacoustic tuning curve (PTC)

A psychoacoustic tuning curve describes how a tone is masked by another tone as a function of the frequency difference or, more often, of the frequency ratio between the two tones. It reflects in its shape the neurophysiological tuning curves, which describe how a single nerve fibre in the auditory system reacts to tones of different frequencies. In the simplest form of PTC measurements, a small number of fixed masker frequencies above and below the test tone frequency are used. To avoid beats, the master and maskee frequencies must not have any simple relation (e.g. 1:2 or 2:3) or be very close together.

One method, sometimes used in clinical settings, makes use of masker frequencies at 43, 78, 92, 108, 123 and 148% of the test tone frequency

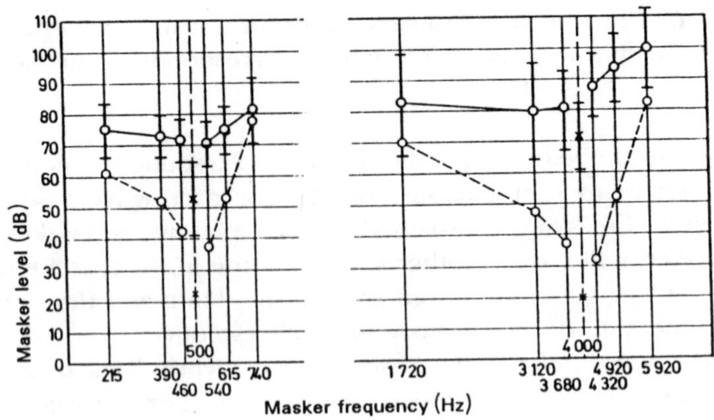

Figure 2.3 Psychoacoustic tuning curves: dashed curves are the average for normal ears and fully drawn curves are for a group of listeners with cochlear hearing loss.

(Zwicker and Schorn, 1978; Densert et al., 1986). The test tone is presented 10 dB above the hearing threshold, and for each masker frequency the masker level that barely masks the test tone is determined (Figure 2.3). Moore (1982) has shown that tuning curves determined by means of a forward masking technique show greater selectivity than those obtained by means of simultaneous masking. However, the latter technique is much simpler to apply clinically.

The determination of PTC curves for listeners with various types of hearing loss has shown that auditory frequency selectivity is often impaired in sensorineural hearing loss. This knowledge increases the understanding of the complicated and varying effects of hearing impairments (Zwicker and Schorn, 1978; Densert et al., 1986).

Non-simultaneous masking has a rather limited effect in time and forward masking usually extends at most 200 ms and backward masking 20–25 ms. If the masker duration is short, the temporal masking effects will also be shorter. One test method for determining temporal masking is gap detection. A narrow-band noise is usually used as a test signal and the purpose of the test is to determine the duration of the shortest detectable gap in the noise signal.

Difference limen (DL)

The difference limen is the smallest detectable difference in some aspect between two sounds or the smallest detectable change of a certain characteristic, e.g. sound level, tone frequency or tone pulse duration. An alternative term is 'just noticeable difference' (JND) or differential threshold. Often, the particular characteristic studied is added: difference limen for frequency or just noticeable difference for duration.

The word 'discrimination' is often used as a general term for the ability to hear such differences or changes, e.g. frequency discrimination or intensity discrimination. Often different methods are available for testing such an auditory capacity. Since they may partly make use of different physiological and psychoacoustic mechanisms, they may not yield completely comparable results. For example, frequency discrimination may be tested by means of tone pulse pairs, where the smallest detectable difference in frequency between the pulses of the pair is determined. An alternative test makes use of a frequency modulated tone, where the smallest detectable frequency variation is determined. Moore (1976) has shown that the results obtained by these two methods are not simply and perfectly correlated, and thus that the two methods are not quite comparable.

On hearing-impaired listeners a number of studies have shown abnormal test results when applying various discrimination tests (e.g. Arlinger et al., 1977; Bonding, 1979; Festen and Plomp, 1983; Moore and Glasberg, 1986). However, statistical analysis of such functional abnormalities, in relation to the hearing-impaired listeners' difficulties in recognising speech, has failed to show any simple and clear-cut correlations.

Recruitment of loudness

Recruitment of loudness, or often just recruitment, is associated with inner ear hearing impairment. It represents a steeper than normal relationship between loudness and sound level. The difference between hearing threshold level and loudness discomfort level is abnormally small, representing a compressed auditory dynamic range. Where the normal ear may have 100–120 dB between hearing threshold and loudness discomfort levels, an ear with an inner ear lesion may have as little as 20–30 dB. This implies that loudness grows five to six times faster when sound level is increased as compared to the normally hearing listener.

The recruitment phenomenon may be explained by looking at the tuning curve from fibres in the auditory nerve. In cases with inner ear lesions, the highly selective tip area of the tuning curve, representing also the highest sensitivity of the fibre, is usually lost. Thus, a high sound level is needed to reach the threshold of the fibre and give rise to stimulated activity in it. However, once there, any further increase in sound level will recruit a considerable number of additional fibres into activity, due to the shallow slopes of the tuning curves in this range (Figure 2.4).

Adaptation

Adaptation means that the reaction of the sensory organ to a constant stimulation decreases with time from an initially stronger response to a

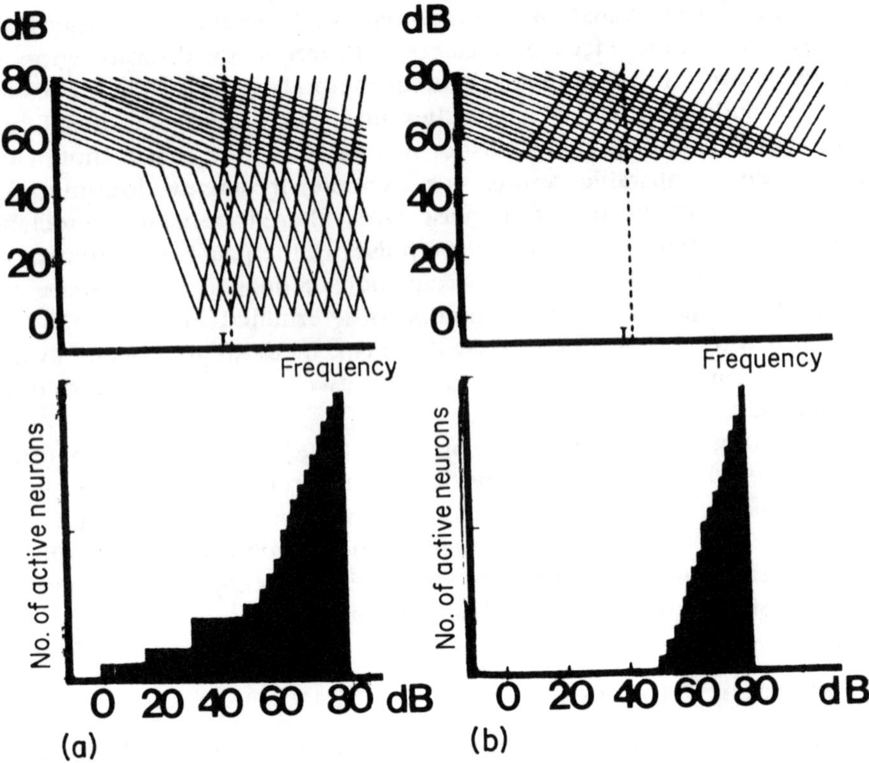

Figure 2.4 Illustration of a possible neural explanation for recruitment of loudness: (a) normal; (b) pathological.

relatively constant lower response level. Adaptation is thus a perstimulatory (i.e. during stimulation) reduction of the sensory organ response.

Physiologically, adaptation may arise in hair cells as well as nerve fibres, and is a consequence of the automatic regulatory mechanisms which give the sense organ the ability to adjust itself optimally for varying stimulation conditions.

Fatigue

According to Hood (1972), fatigue is a reduction of the sensory organ reaction which differs from adaptation in the respect that it results from a much stronger stimulation than is usually necessary for normal activity in the receptor. The most common type of auditory fatigue is called temporary threshold shift (TTS). It is described as a reversible shift in hearing thresholds after exposure to sounds of relatively high level and long duration.

However, Small (1973) offers a somewhat different definition of fatigue. He defines it as a reversible (transient) elevation of hearing threshold, caused by a preceding sound stimulation. Correspondingly, he defines adaptation as a reversible reduction of loudness, caused by a preceding sound stimulation. Thus, the difference between these two phenomena, according to Small, is the kind of effect on hearing – threshold elevation and loudness reduction, respectively – and not the difference in sound level giving rise to the effect – normal or higher than normal – as Hood suggests. Elliott and Fraser (1970) present a definition somewhere in between: adaptation is considered by them as a perstimulatory effect, which shows itself as reduced loudness of the ongoing sound, whilst fatigue is defined as a poststimulatory effect which mainly appears as elevated hearing thresholds after the fatiguing stimulation has ended. They add that adaptation studies have made use mainly of sounds of low or moderate levels, whilst fatigue studies concern the effects of stimulation at moderate to high sound levels.

Physiologically, fatigue is probably caused mainly by the hair cells in the inner ear and nerve cells becoming exhausted from the stimulation due to insufficient supplies of oxygen, energy and other factors of vital importance for the cell metabolism.

Habituation

Habituation is a phenomenon that occurs when a stimulus is repeated many times. It represents the reduced response, physiologically as well as psychologically, from repeated stimulation. Habituation is thus related to the stimulus gradually changing from being an unknown to a known sound.

Psychoacoustic Methods

Psychoacoustic methods differ with regard to the principles that govern the presentation of stimuli and the kind of responses expected from the listener (Gelfand, 1981). The listener's tasks may be described by the following concepts.

Detection

Detection is a task where the listener is required to detect the presence of a sound or of a certain characteristic of a sound. Detection is the basis for the determination of hearing threshold level, i.e. the minimum audible level of a certain sound.

Detection experiments may also be used, e.g. in studies of frequency discrimination by the ability to detect the presence of frequency modulation of a tone.

Discrimination

Discrimination represents the ability to determine the difference between two sounds, e.g. a difference in pitch between two successive tone pulses which may differ in frequency. Discrimination thus requires that the signals be detectable. In a discrimination experiment, the listener may be required to respond with the words equal/different, the first sound louder or softer than the second, the pitch of the first sound higher than that of the second sound etc.

Recognition and comprehension

Recognition means a still higher level of conscious analysis of the sound signal. The sound must not only be detected and discriminated, but also recognised so as to allow the listener to give a response that is specific for every stimulus. This is the task which is most commonly required of the listener when speech stimuli are used – the specific test words which are presented are to be recognised and repeated. Often the term 'speech discrimination' is used in clinical speech audiometry. This term is not correct; speech recognition is more correct and is the preferred term. The highest level of speech reception is comprehension or understanding which represents the ability to understand the meaning or information in a sentence.

Scaling

Scaling is a task where the listener is required to make a quantitative judgement of a certain characteristic of the test sound. Often, but not necessarily, a reference sound is used for comparison. The task may be, for example, to state how many times louder the test sound is compared to the reference sound or how many times higher the pitch is.

Psychometric functions

A psychometric function represents the probability of a certain listener's response as a function of the magnitude of the particular sound characteristic being studied. The simplest example of a psychometric function is the probability curve of a listener indicating the detection of a tone pulse as a function of the tone pulse sound level (Figure 2.5). The psychometric function is usually S-shaped in its graphical representation and may be reasonably well approximated by a cumulative normal distribution function.

Threshold

The threshold is the value of a particular sound characteristic that corresponds to a particular probability for a correct listener response.

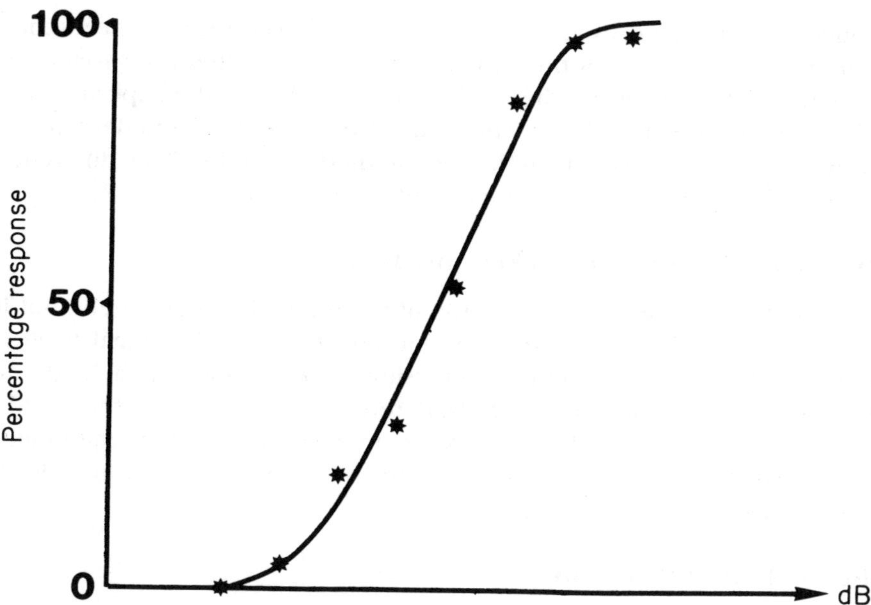

Figure 2.5 An example of a psychometric function.

Often the 50% probability value is used. In some experiments, e.g. when the probability for guessing a correct response is significant, a higher probability level is used for the threshold criterion (e.g. 70% or 75%).

Classic Methods

The method of limits

This is a classic psychoacoustic method, where stimuli are presented in series of monotonically decreasing or increasing value, in fixed steps, of the sound characteristic being studied. A series with decreasing values is stopped when the listener ceases to respond, whereas a series with increasing values is stopped when he or she begins to respond. The result is calculated as the average of a number of repeated series, which may be either a combination of increasing (ascending) and decreasing (descending) values, only increasing or only decreasing. The conventional clinical technique for the determination of hearing thresholds is based on the method of limits, using repeated series of tone pulses with ascending sound level in steps of 5 dB.

The method of adjustment

This is also based on the variation of the particular sound characteristic being studied in a regular ascending or descending manner to a certain defined type and degree of perception. However, in contrast to the method of limits, listeners control the variation themselves. Often the variation is continuous and varying starting positions, controlled by the experimenter, are used to avoid listener bias. The results from ascending and descending series often differ more than in the method of limits. The difference between these represents the uncertainty of the method.

The tracking method or Békésy method

This may be considered as a variation of the method of adjustment, but it has also some similarities with the method of limits. The signal level is controlled by the listener, either increasing or decreasing with a fixed rate of change. In its original form for the determination of hearing thresholds, the step size used was 2 dB. However, commercially available equipment normally makes use of much smaller step sizes, which makes the signal level change sound continuous.

The method of constants

This differs from the previously mentioned classic methods by not using series of stimuli with monotonically increasing or decreasing values of the sound characteristic being studied. Instead a number of predetermined values are used, assumed to be within the range of interest for the study, e.g. around the detection threshold. In a random order, a number of stimuli are presented for each predetermined value, the response to each being noted. From the results, the psychometric function can be obtained and a threshold value determined according to the threshold criterion chosen. In comparison with the previous methods, the method of constants has the advantage of providing an estimate of the guessing level. However, it has the disadvantage of requiring longer testing time since many stimuli tend to fall relatively far away from the most interesting range close to the threshold. This longer test time reduces the listener's ability to concentrate which, in turn, may reduce test reliability.

Adaptive Methods

Adaptive methods are a group of methods where direction of change, and step size in the sound characteristic being changed, are not fixed but determined according to the listener's responses. The advantage of this is that the test can be more efficiently focused on the most interesting range and less time and listener concentration is wasted on less interesting stimuli, e.g. far away from the threshold value being sought. By means of a suitable strategy for change between increase and decrease, thresholds corresponding to probabilities of detection, other than 50%, may be determined.

Simple up–down method

This is based on decreasing by one step following each response by the listener and increasing by one step following each non-response. This will result in successive stimuli moving up and down around the threshold value. After a certain number of changes of direction, the test is finished. The average of the number of changes from increasing to decreasing and from decreasing to increasing will yield the threshold value corresponding to 50% detection probability. The method shows similarity to the method of limits, but it makes use of fewer stimuli that are not very close to the threshold value.

A too-large step size will result in poor accuracy in the threshold determination. However, if the step size is too small, a large number of stimuli will be needed after each change of direction between increasing and decreasing values, resulting in longer test time and less concentrated listening. Use of the optimum step size is therefore important.

Transformed up–down methods

These make use of a somewhat different strategy to yield a threshold value corresponding to a probability level other than 50%. By using the following principle, a probability level of approximately 70% will be obtained: after each non-response, increase by one step; after a response which is followed by a non-response to an equal stimulus value, also increase by one step; after two consecutive responses to equal stimulus values, decrease by one step. This procedure is illustrated in Figure 2.6.

A large number of variations of transformed up–down methods may be devised, leading to threshold values on different probability levels (Levitt, 1978). The more complex the strategy, the more difficult the method will be to use with manual control. Therefore, computer control is normally used for such methods, their main application so far being in research rather than in clinical applications.

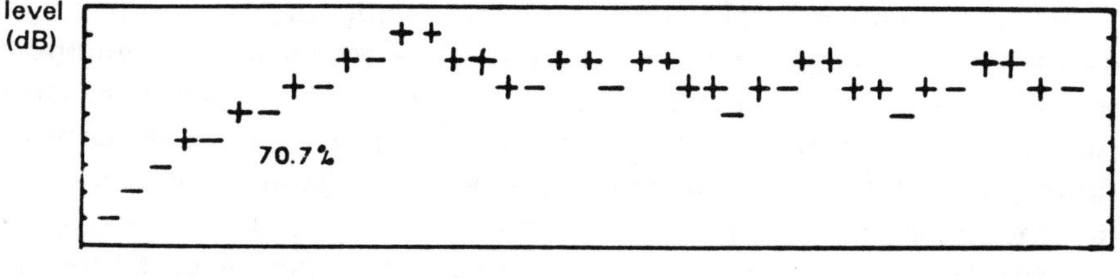

Figure 2.6 The test strategy of a transformed up–down method yielding a threshold value corresponding to approximately 70% probability of detection.

The method of maximum likelihood (MML)

This is a rather complicated method, requiring an on-line computer. After each stimulus and response, the computer calculates the most likely psychometric function according to the listener's responses to this and all previous stimuli presented.

Parameter estimation by sequential testing (PEST)

This is also a method that requires rather complex calculations on a computer. The calculations are made after each stimulus response and the results will determine what stimulus is to be presented next. In principle, step size is halved and the direction of change altered each time the listener response changes (Gelfand, 1981).

With a given requirement on test accuracy, both the PEST and MML methods will yield faster results than the classic methods. The PEST method imposes less demanding requirements on computer capacity than the MML method does.

Methods based on Detection Theory

Methods based on signal detection theory are modern test methods which, in some aspects, are similar to the classic method of constants. However, they provide the possibility of separating the listener's sensitivity from his or her subjective response criterion, i.e. how sure the listener needs to be to give a response, how disposed he or she is to guessing etc.

The theory is based on the stimulus being either present or absent during a certain time interval, which may be marked by, for example, a lamp being illuminated. The listener's response will fall into one of the following four categories: correct identification, correct rejection, false positive response and false negative response. By recording how the responses are distributed among these categories, the listener's behaviour may be described by a receiver operating curve (ROC), where the ordinate (*y* axis) represents the percentage of correctly identified stimuli, and the abscissa (*x* axis) the percentage of false positive responses. By influencing the listener's response behaviour, e.g. by the use of another set of instructions, different points on the ROC curve may be determined. Another value of the sound characteristic under study will result in a different curve, as will another test subject (Figure 2.7).

Signal detection theory is to a considerable extent based on the statistical analysis of a signal in noise (see Tanner and Sorkin, 1972; Gelfand, 1981). Practical test methods which make use of these theories may be structured in different ways. One kind which is used frequently in

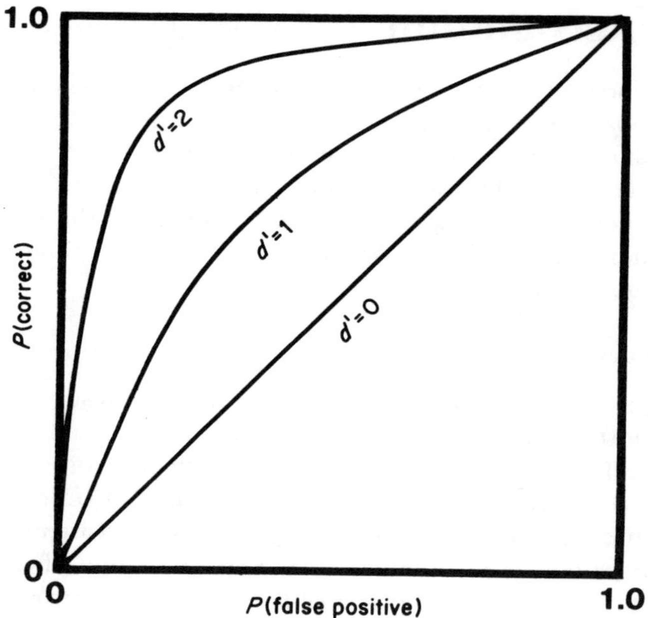

Figure 2.7 ROC curves.

psychoacoustic experiments is the 'two interval forced choice' or 'two alternative forced choice' method. Two successive time intervals are marked, usually by the illumination of lamps, and the listener has to state in which of the two intervals the signal was presented. Forced choice means that he or she has to answer either the first or the second interval; no other response, e.g. I don't know, is permitted.

Scaling Methods

In scaling, a certain characteristic of the sound signal is evaluated quantitatively. Magnitude scaling may be performed by means of a numbered scale with a certain range. This has been used, for example, in sound quality evaluation of hearing aids, where the listener may be given the task of evaluating the dimension hard–soft along a scale from 0 to 10 (Gabrielsson and Sjögren, 1979). Scaling methods have also been used in the study of tinnitus for the evaluation of degree of annoyance and effect of various treatments.

Other variations of scaling are pairwise comparisons, e.g. loudest or highest pitch, and ranking, where a series of stimuli has to be ordered in rising order with regard to some specified characteristic.

Speech Recognition

The measurement of a listener's ability to recognise speech is an important part of psychoacoustic testing. Audiologically, the purpose is to obtain a measure of the listener's ability to analyse the complex speech signal and thereby correctly identify the test words presented. In addition, speech recognition measurements have been used to describe the effect of the acoustic conditions of a room or the quality of a telephone or radio communication channel.

Speech material

Different types of speech material are used for different test purposes. Real words are most commonly used, especially when untrained listeners are being tested. The words may be presented as single words, isolated or preceded by a carrier phrase (e.g. 'Now you'll hear . . .'), or in the form of complete sentences. Common types of single words used are monosyllabic or bisyllabic (spondees). Spondees have a steeper slope of the psychometric function, describing the probability of correct recognition as a function of speech level, than monosyllabic test words because of greater redundancy in the speech material; it is easier to guess an incompletely heard bisyllabic word correctly than a monosyllabic one. Digits are used

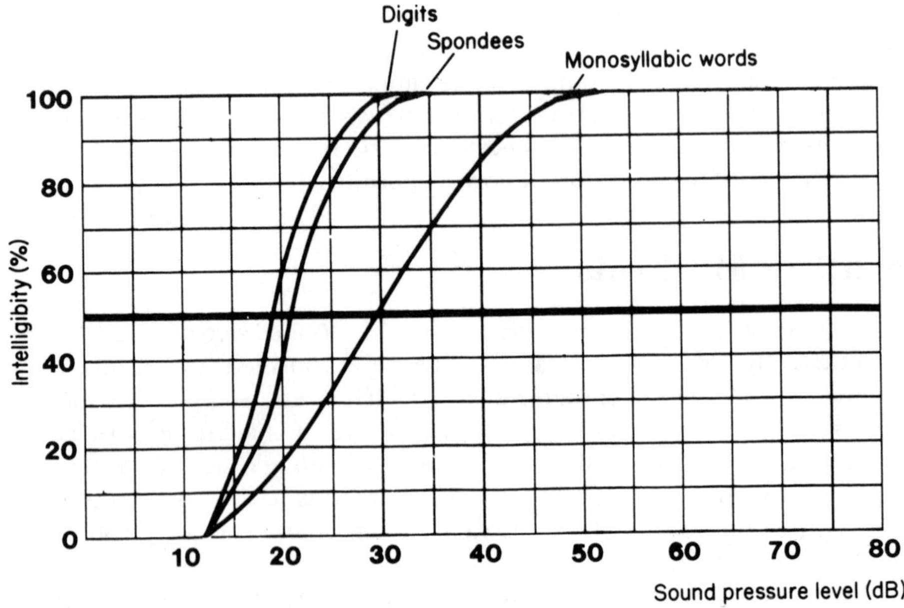

Figure 2.8 Psychometric curves for different types of speech material for normally hearing listeners.

sometimes, and they show a still steeper slope in the psychometric function (Figure 2.8). Complete sentences may be considered to be the most natural manner of presentation, but often the possibility of guessing correctly is highest for such material.

A phoneme is the smallest sound element in speech. A single phoneme or simple combinations of phonemes may be considered as the simplest form of speech stimulus. Logatomes are random combinations of phonemes, usually consonant–vowel–consonant (CVC), which sound like monosyllabic words but lack sense, i.e. are nonsense words.

Test material may be open or closed. Closed material is characterised by a limited number of alternative responses, which usually are available for the listener to read. An example of closed material is a rhyme test, when the listener has to recognise, for example, one of the following alternatives: bid, big, bill, bin, bit. In open test material, the number of possible response alternatives is unlimited.

Analysis

The analysis of speech recognition ability may be based on correctly recognised phonemes, complete words or complete sentences. A sentence may be correct literally or with regard to its meaning. When phoneme scoring is used, a detailed analysis in the form of a confusion matrix is possible. This means not only counting the correctly identified phonemes but also evaluating the confusions made among the incorrectly recognised phonemes.

The most commonly determined quantities in speech recognition testing are speech recognition threshold (SRT) and maximum speech recognition score. SRT is usually defined as the speech level at which the listener correctly recognises 50% of the presented speech material. At this level the slope of the psychometric function is steepest. When closed speech material is used, a higher probability level for correct recognition than 50% is normally used in consideration of the probability of guessing the correct answer. The maximum speech recognition score is the score obtained at the optimum speech level and vice versa – the optimum speech level is that level which yields maximum speech recognition score.

An alternative way of studying speech recognition is when the speech signal is presented against a background of noise of variable level. The test result is normally presented as the speech-to-noise ratio that corresponds to 50% correct speech recognition (Hagerman, 1984).

Articulation index (AI)

This is a measure of what proportion of the information in a normal speech signal is available in a certain listening situation. AI can have a value between 0 and 1 and is determined on the basis of speech level and noise level in 20 frequency bands, which are all assumed to contribute equally to the speech recognition (5% each). It has been shown that AI gives a relatively good estimation of speech recognition for various types of speech material (Kryter, 1962). It may also be applied to the evaluation of speech recognition performance in hearing-impaired listeners (Pavlovic, Studebaker and Sherbecoes, 1986).

Speech transmission index (STI)

This is an electroacoustic method for predicting speech recognition in a room or across some other acoustic or electronic transmission channel, where background noise, reverberation and other factors may disturb the transmission of speech. The principle of this method is to use seven octave bands of noise (125–8000 Hz centre frequencies), which are sinusoidally modulated in intensity with 100% modulation. Fourteen different modulation frequencies in steps of one-third of an octave from 0.63 to 12.5 Hz are tested, corresponding to the range for amplitude frequencies in normal speech. The calculation of STI is based on the modulation transfer function, i.e. the reduction of the intensity modulation from the originally transmitted 100% in these 7 × 14 combinations of parameters. The modulation is reduced significantly in a room with significant background noise and reverberation. A clear relation between measured STI values and speech recognition for different types of speech test material and languages has been shown (Steeneken and Houtgast, 1980).

A simplified version of this method, called RASTI (rapid speech transmission index), has been developed, where only the octave bands 500 and 2000 Hz are used, with four modulation frequencies in the 500-Hz band and five in the 2000-Hz band. This method is mainly used for the rapid estimation of speech reception properties of a room (Steeneken and Houtgast, 1985).

References

ARLINGER, S.D., JERLVALL, L.B., AHREN, T. and HOLMGREN, E.C. (1977). Discrimination of frequency ramps in subjects with cochlear hearing loss. *Acta Oto-Laryngologica* **83**, 310–316.

BONDING, P. (1979). Frequency selectivity and speech discrimination in sensorineural hearing loss. *Scandinavian Audiology* **8**, 205–215.

CACACE, A.T. and MARGOLIS, R.H. (1985). On the loudness of complex stimuli and its relationship to cochlear excitation. *Journal of the Acoustical Society of America* **78**, 1568–1573.

DENSERT, B., KINBERGER, B., ARLINGER, S. and DENSERT, O. (1986). Quantifying psychoacoustical tuning curves for clinical use. *Scandinavian Audiology* **15**, 97–103.

ELLIOTT, D.N. and FRASER, W. (1970). Fatigue and adaptation. In: Tobias, J.V. (Ed.) *Foundations of Modern Auditory Theory*, Vol. I. New York: Academic Press.

FESTEN, J.M. and PLOMP, R. (1983). Relations between auditory functions in impaired hearing. *Journal of the Acoustical Society of America* **73**, 652–662.

FLETCHER, H. (1940). Auditory patterns. *Revue of Modern Physics* **12**, 47–65.

GABRIELSSON, A. and SJÖGREN, H. (1979). Perceived sound quality of hearing aids. *Scandinavian Audiology* **8**, 159–169.

GELFAND, S.A. (1981), *Hearing – An Introduction to Psychological and Physiological Acoustics.* New York: Marcel Dekker.

HAGERMAN, B. (1984). Clinical measurements of speech reception threshold in noise. *Scandinavian Audiology* **13**, 57–63.

HOOD, J.D. (1972). Fundamentals of identification of sensorineural hearing loss. *Sound* **6**, 21–26.

IEC 645 (1979). *Audiometers.* Geneva: International Electrotechnical Commission.

ISO 131 (1979). *Acoustics – Expression of physical and subjective magnitudes of sound or noise in air.* Geneva: International Standards Organisation.

ISO 226 (1987). *Acoustics – Normal equal-loudness level contours.* Geneva: International Standards Organisation.

ISO 532 (1975). *Acoustics – Method for calculating loudness level.* Geneva: International Standards Organisation.

KRYTER, K.D. (1962). Validation of the articulation index. *Journal of the Acoustical Society of America* **34**, 1698–1702.

LEVITT, H. (1978). Adaptive testing in audiology. *Scandinavian Audiology*, Supplement 6, 241–291.

MOORE, B.C.J. (1976). Comparison of frequency DL's for pulsed tones and modulated tones. *British Journal of Audiology* **10**, 17–20.

MOORE, B.C.J. (1982). *An Introduction to the Psychology of Hearing.* London: Academic Press.

MOORE, B.C.J. and GLASBERG, B. (1986). Comparisons of frequency selectivity in simultaneous and forward masking for subjects with unilateral cochlear impairments. *Journal of the Acoustical Society of America* **80**, 93–107.

PAVLOVIC, C.V., STUDEBAKER, G.A. and SHERBECOES, R.L. (1986). An articulation index based procedure for predicting the speech recognition performance of hearing-impaired individuals. *Journal of the Acoustical Society of America* **80**, 50–57.

POULSEN, T. (1975). *Temporal Loudness Summation of Tone-Pulses, Report No. 8*, Copenhagen: The Acoustics Laboratory, Technical University of Denmark.

SCHARF, B. (1970). Critical bands. In: Tobias, J.V. (Ed.) *Foundations of Modern Auditory Theory*. New York: Academic Press.

SMALL, A. (1973). Psychoacoustics. In: Minifie, F.D., Hixon, T.J. and Williams, F. (Eds) *Normal Aspects of Speech, Hearing and Language.* New York: Prentice Hall.

STEENEKEN, H.J.M. and HOUTGAST, T. (1980). A physical method for measuring speech-transmission quality. *Journal of the Acoustical Society of America* **67**, 318–326.

STEENEKEN, H.J.M. and HOUTGAST, T. (1985). RASTI: a tool for evaluating auditoria. *Bruel & Kjaer Technical Review*, No. 3-1985, 13–30.

TANNER, W.P. and SORKIN, R.D. (1972). The theory of signal detection. In: Tobias, J.V. (Ed.) *Foundations of Modern Auditory Theory*, Vol. II. New York: Academic Press.

ZWICKER, E. (1974). Time constants (characteristic durations) of hearing. *Journal of Audiological Technique* **13**, 82–102.

ZWICKER, E. and SCHORN, K. (1978). Psychoacoustical tuning curves in audiology. *Audiology* **17**, 120–140.

Chapter 3 Statistical Aspects on Measurement Accuracy

Precision and Accuracy

A test method is characterised first by what quantity it measures. However, an equally important characteristic is the quality of the test results. Quality can be described by the two concepts of precision and accuracy. Precision concerns deviations between repeated measurements of the same quantity on the same test subject. A high precision means that repeated tests give essentially the same results. Accuracy concerns the agreement between measured values and the true value. A test may show high precision but still have poor accuracy.

Validity and Reliability

Another relevant concept pair is the validity and the reliability of a test method. Validity is concerned with the extent to which the test results are valid, i.e. reflecting the characteristic which the method aims at measuring. Validity is thus closely related to the concept of accuracy as defined above. Reliability is concerned with the extent to which identical results are obtained at repeated testing on a constant object. Reliability and precision are thus essentially synonymous concepts.

Each test method has various sources of error, which result in a certain probability of the test result deviating from the true value. A systematic error is an error which affects the test result in a certain direction. Test equipment may give rise to a systematic error due to technical shortcomings. For example, a pure-tone audiometer, whose calibration is incorrect resulting in sound levels which are too low, will cause a systematic error in the form of hearing threshold levels which are too poor being measured. Learning effects constitute another possible source of systematic errors in psychoacoustic testing.

Random errors are errors whose size and direction vary in a seemingly random manner and can be predicted only in statistical terms. Examples of factors which may cause random errors in audiometry are fluctuations in listener concentration in psychoacoustic testing and variations in sound level caused by the placement of the earphone or bone vibrator. Small changes of listener position in sound-field audiometry may have similar effects.

The results from a large number of measurements performed on a test subject under constant conditions can often be illustrated by a curve as shown in Figure 3.1. This normal distribution (gaussian curve) has a symmetrical shape around a mean value (*M*), and a more or less open bell shape, quantitatively described by the standard deviation (s.d.).

The area below the curve and between the vertical lines which cross the *x* axis at *A* and *B*, i.e. the dashed area, represents the probability of a test value falling between the values *A* and *B*. Characteristically, for the gaussian curve, values in the interval to the left of (*M*−s.d.) are about 16% of all test values, whilst between (*M*−s.d.) and *M* they are about 34%. Similarly, between *M* and (*M*+s.d.) and to the right of (*M*+s.d.), approximately 34% and 16% of the test values will fall respectively.

The quantity illustrated by Figure 3.1 can have any value, e.g. 1.98 or −39.248. Such results represent a continuous variable. In audiometry, it is usually the case that the result of a test cannot have any value; only a limited number of values are possible, e.g. integers or multiples of 5 (0, 5, 10, 15 etc.). Such values represent a discontinuous or discrete variable.

If the hearing threshold level for a pure tone of a certain frequency were to be measured a large number of times on the same listener, the result would not always be the same because of the various sources of error that influence the measurements. A possible outcome is illustrated by Figure 3.2, where *M* represents the mean value. Most of the time, the result of

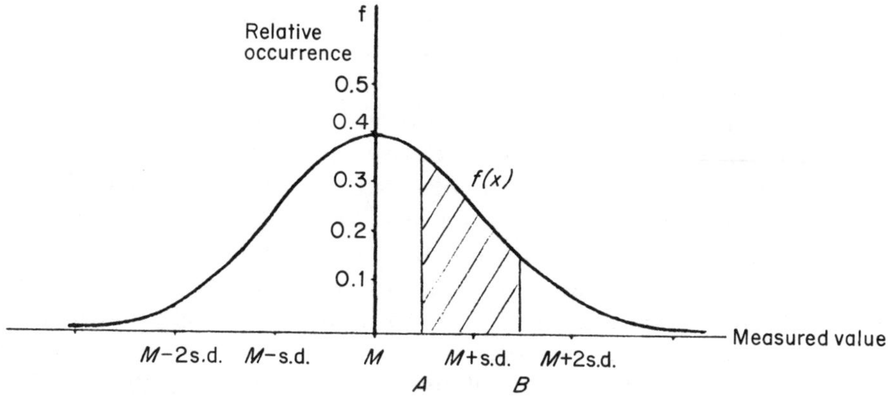

Figure 3.1 Normal distribution curve with mean value *M* and standard deviation s.d.

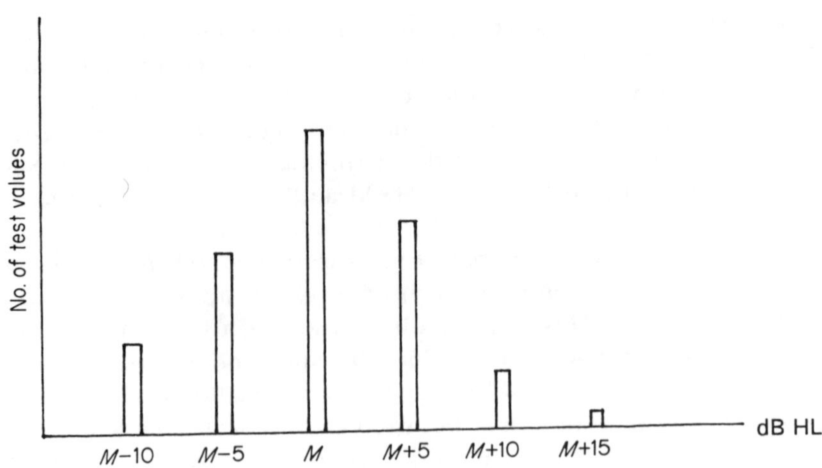

Figure 3.2 A distribution function for a discontinuous or discrete variable.

the measurement was *M*, but sometimes the result was a higher threshold level and sometimes a lower one.

Figures 3.1 and 3.2 illustrate the statistical distribution of the results from repeated measurements on one and the same test subject. The variation of this distribution is specified by the standard deviation for a single measurement. When a result of a test has been obtained and is being evaluated, a common question is whether this result is abnormal, i.e. whether it shows a significant difference when compared with an average normal value. The probability for a single test result to differ from the mean value by 1 s.d. or more is about 0.32, by 2 s.d. or more about 0.04 etc. Conversely, a test result which differs by more than 2 s.d. from the normal mean value represents a test object which, by a probability of 0.96, does not belong to the normal population.

> *Example:* Hearing thresholds have been measured on a large group of young normal-hearing listeners. At 2 kHz a mean value of 1.2 dB was obtained with a standard deviation of 6.1 dB. A patient, when tested at 2 kHz, shows a hearing threshold level of 15 dB. This value differs from the mean value of the normal population by 13.8 dB, which corresponds to $13.8/6.1 = 2.3 \times$ s.d. With a probability of almost 0.98, this hearing threshold value represents a deviation from the normal population. By a probability of almost 0.99 this test subject belongs to a population with hearing thresholds that are poorer than those of the normal population.

In the example above, the probability 0.98 represents a double-sided evaluation, i.e. only the difference between the test result and the normal mean value is compared without consideration of the sign. If the test subject had been exposed to a factor known to be able to cause hearing loss, the evaluation could have been limited to whether his hearing threshold level was significantly worse than that of the normal population or not. Then a one-sided statistical test is performed, which in the example above corresponds to the probability value of 0.99.

In clinical evaluations, a common question is whether the test result obtained on a certain patient today is the same, worse or better than corresponding results from the same test made at a previous examination. The question is, therefore, whether the difference between two test results obtained from the same test subject on different occasions is statistically significant. When evaluating such a difference, a decision has to be made about the level of significance. This is the probability or risk level that the test result will be misinterpreted, i.e. that a difference is considered present when in fact no change has occurred or, vice versa, that the difference noted is caused only by random sources of error. In order to determine the level of significance of a difference between two test results, the standard deviation for test–retest difference is of importance. This measure of variation is about 1.4 times larger than the standard deviation for a single measurement.

A common level of significance is 0.05, which corresponds to a difference between two test values of 1.96 times the standard deviation for the test–retest difference in a two-sided test. In other words, if the difference between the results obtained at two different test occasions is at least twice the standard deviation for the test–retest difference, this may be interpreted as evidence that a change has occurred. The risk that this is not the case is then less than 0.05.

> *Example*: A large number of hearing threshold determinations have been made on a listener at 1 kHz. The standard deviation for a single measurement was found to be 2.5 dB. The standard deviation for test–retest differences is then $2.5 \times 1.4 = 3.5$ dB. In order for two test results to differ significantly on the 0.05 significance level, the difference has to be 7 dB or more. If the measurements have been made using 5-dB steps, the difference will have to be the next higher multiple of 5 dB, i.e. 10 dB.

If the hearing threshold levels at a specific frequency are determined on a group of listeners of a certain age group, the results obtained will form a statistical distribution which is not perfectly symmetrical but somewhat asymmetrical or skewed. This is due to the fact that hearing thresholds for physiological reasons cannot be very much better than, say, −10 or −15 dB HL. No corresponding limit is available for poor hearing thresholds. However, when the hearing threshold levels are relatively close to normal, the asymmetry is slight and can often be neglected in statistical analysis. However, with elderly subjects, or subjects who have been exposed to noise or other harmful agents, the degree of skew is often quite evident.

In speech audiometry, asymmetrical distributions are also quite common. On assuming that repeated determinations of speech recognition scores have been made on a listener and that, on average, a score of 94% was obtained, then the possible upward variation is of course limited to 6%, since the maximum score is 100%. However, considerably larger downward variations may occur. The statistical distribution function which describes the result from speech recognition testing is known as the binomial distribution function (Hagerman, 1976; Lyregaard, 1987).

In the various audiometric test methods, where the result is expressed by a discontinuous or discrete variable, it may seem reasonable to assume that the step size of this variable is of importance for the standard deviation and the test reliability. Why then is a step size of 5 dB so common? A very large step size will of course give rise to systematic error. Using a step size of 50 dB in pure-tone audiometry would influence both precision and accuracy; then precision and reliability would be good but accuracy and validity would be extremely poor. The large step size will give rise to what is termed a 'quantisation error'.

The consequences of this source of error can be analysed mathematically (Leijon, A., personal communication). Such an analysis will show that this source of error is negligible when the slope of the psychometric function is of the order of magnitude usually found on subjects with normal hearing or inner ear lesions, and a step size of 2 or 5 dB is used in pure-tone audiometry. When frequency modulated tones are used instead of pure tones, e.g. as in sound-field audiometry, the quantisation error will be somewhat larger but still negligible from a practical point of view.

Sensitivity and Specificity

Many test methods are used for diagnostic purposes, i.e. as a basis for evaluation of what type of auditory lesion is present. As measures of merit in this respect the terms 'sensitivity' and 'specificity' are used (Turner and Nielsen, 1984). The basis for these two concepts is that in a certain group of subjects, tested with regard to the diagnosis of a certain disease, some of the subjects have this disease whilst other do not. If the test result indicates the presence of the disease, the result is called positive, whilst a negative test result indicates absence of the disease. A positive result on a subject having the disease is called true positive; a positive result on a subject who does not have the disease is called false positive. Similarly, a negative result on a patient with the disease is a false negative, whilst a negative result on a subject who does not have the particular disease is a true negative result. These concepts are illustrated in Table 3.1.

Table 3.1 Concepts of diagnosis of a disease

	Disease present	Disease absent
Positive test	True positive	False positive
Negative test	False negative	True negative

The sensitivity of a method is defined as the number of true positives in relation to the total number of subjects having the disease, i.e. sum of true positives and false negatives:

Sensitivity = True positives/No. of subjects with disease

A good method should of course have high sensitivity. The ideal is that all subjects with the disease will yield a positive result, i.e. show true positive results with no false negatives, which means a sensitivity of 100%.

Specificity is related to how reliably the method can free a subject, who does not have the disease, from the suspicion of having it:

Specificity = True negatives/No. of subjects without disease

Naturally, a good method should also have high specificity.

The results from a study on brain-stem audiometry in patients with a sensorineural hearing loss, who have a questionable diagnosis of either cochlear or retrocochlear lesion, may be taken as an example. Out of 56 patients with surgically verified cerebellopontine tumours, 55 had a pathological auditory brain-stem response (ABR) whilst one patient was within normal limits for cochlear lesions. Out of 39 patients, where history and results from all other tests including X-ray supported a diagnosis of cochlear lesion, 34 had ABR within normal limits whilst 5 had pathological ABR. The sensitivity of ABR for retrocochlear lesion according to this study is thus 55/56 = 98% whilst the specificity is 34/39 = 87%.

Depending on how the limits are chosen between positive and negative results of the test, its sensitivity and specificity can be altered. An increase in sensitivity is obtained at the expense of reduced specificity and vice versa. The choice of limit is usually based on an evaluation of the severity of the disease and to what extent successful treatment is available. Considering, for example, cerebellopontine angle tumours, there is general agreement that the disease is serious and that it can be treated successfully. Therefore, good diagnostic tests for this disease must have a very high sensitivity, i.e. the test method must be able to detect as many as possible of the patients having the disease. The disadvantage of a relatively lower specificity is an increase in the number of patients without tumour who are referred for computer-aided X-ray testing. This provides an additional cost and a risk of unnecessary worry for these patients, but this is usually considered acceptable in the light of the reduced risk of missing a patient having a tumour.

In the diagnosis of otosalpingitis by means of tympanometry, the disease is less serious than in the tumour case and there is no generally accepted successful method of treatment. In such cases the choice of limit between positive and negative test results usually leads to a lower sensitivity in order to avoid a specificity that is too low.

References

HAGERMAN, B. (1976). Reliability in the determination of speech discrimination. *Scandinavian Audiology* **5**, 219–228.

LYREGAARD, P. (1987). Towards a theory of speech audiometry tests. In: Martin, M. (Ed.) *Speech Audiometry*. London: Taylor & Francis.

TURNER, R.G. and NIELSEN, D.W. (1984). Application of clinical decision analysis to audiological tests. *Ear and Hearing* **5**, 125–133.

Chapter 4
Common Sources of Error in Audiometry

Test methods which are absolutely exact and free of errors do not exist. Experience also shows that the very simplest method in the audiometric test battery is influenced by sources of error. If a pure-tone audiogram is repeated after 5 minutes, the probability that the new one will be identical to the first one is very small. For more complex methods, which may concern comparison of different test sounds, the probability may be even smaller that a repeat test yields the same result as the first test. Physiological, psychological, psychoacoustic as well as electroacoustic factors may contribute to the total error.

A general overview of the various possible sources of error in audiometry may be structured as follows.

Physiological Factors

In the auditory pathways of the central nervous system, spontaneous activity is present even when in a completely silent environment. This activity may be regarded as physiological noise. If a sound signal is very weak and inaudible, it is completely masked by this physiological noise and the spontaneous activity in the nervous pathways is not influenced at all by the sound. However, if the sound is loud and clearly audible it gives rise to high activity in the nerves which is considerably greater than the spontaneous activity. At levels close to the auditory threshold, a sound will barely influence the nervous activity and the firing rates will barely start to increase above the spontaneous activity level. However, phase synchronisation appears at this level, i.e. the nerve impulses tend to appear in a relatively constant phase for a periodic sound wave.

As for the detection of a sound against a background of acoustic noise, there is random uncertainty in the detection of a sound close to the auditory threshold caused by this physiological noise. The listener does not clearly perceive the auditory character of the sound, but reacts mainly on a diffuse feeling of some change in the acoustic environment. This uncertainty, which can be considered as masking by the physiological noise, is one possible source of error in audiometry with test signals close to the auditory threshold.

Abnormal physiological noise in the form of tones or ringing or hissing sounds (tinnitus) may, of course, give rise to additional difficulties in detecting a test sound. Fluctuating tinnitus especially causes an additional source of error in audiometry.

Another type of physiological noise is generated by the circulatory system, mainly in blood vessels close to the ear under test, by the respiratory system and by contracted muscles (Berger and Kerivan, 1983). This is mainly a source of error when weak sounds are presented by means of earphones, in which situation the test ear is occluded. Noise generated by the circulatory system often appears as periodic pulse-synchronous sounds, whilst respiratory noise and that from muscle contractions usually have the character of a low-pitched noise. The masking effect of this type of physiological noise is most evident in the low frequency range, where the occlusion effect is largest.

Another physiological phenomenon, which may influence the test result, is adaptation in the auditory pathways. Adaptation means a gradual reduction of the activity in the sense organ when exposed to a constant stimulus of long duration. This has the effect that mainly the beginning and the end of a tone pulse are detected when listening at levels close to threshold. These transient parts are very important whilst the almost constant part between has much less significance for detection. This explains why the listener often responds to the test tone only after its end when it is presented very close to threshold.

Other phenomena of a similar nature are habituation and fatigue. Habituation means that the reaction to a certain stimulus decreases when it is presented repeatedly. Fatigue constitutes a reduced reaction in the sense organ to a sound after stimulation, at levels that are more intense than normal.

The duration of a tone pulse also influences its audibility and loudness. This phenomenon is called temporal integration and is level dependent. Close to normal auditory thresholds, the tone pulse duration must be at least 0.5 s for maximum audibility. If the tone-pulse duration is shorter, it is perceived as less loud. At higher sound levels this integration time is shorter and is reduced to about 50 ms at high sound levels (Poulsen, 1975).

Psychological Factors

In psychoacoustic tests, the actively participating listener is a necessary requirement. The listener is expected to detect, discriminate or recognise and produce some kind of response, such as pressing a signal switch or answering by words. Thus, the result of the test may be influenced by the listener's ability and willingness to cooperate.

The *ability* may be influenced by factors such as fatigue, worry, anxiety, insecurity or an uncomfortable test room. Distracting events in the test surroundings, e.g. people running back and forth outside the test room window, may also disturb the listener's ability to concentrate on the test. Therefore, such factors must be eliminated or at least minimised as far as possible.

The *willingness* or the motivation to have the highest concentration and cooperation possible may be influenced by the actual reason for the hearing test. Depending on whether it is the result of the patient's own expressed desire to be helped with a hearing problem, or whether the patient was more or less forced to the clinic and considers the test rather needless, the test result will be influenced. Insurance evaluations, where the test result may have an effect on a monetary compensation to be awarded is another possible factor. In such cases, the effect is usually one of aggravation, i.e. the result is somewhat worse than the actual hearing loss, or simulation, i.e. the result indicates a hearing loss although the patient's hearing in reality is within normal limits.

The listener's interpretation of the test instructions may also affect the result. Therefore, the formulation of instructions is of importance as well as checking that the listener has understood them correctly before the actual test is started.

However, when a very precise and standardised formulation is used for the instruction of the patient, the actual interpretation may vary from one individual to another. In a detection task such as pure-tone audiometry, the meaning of words like 'faint tone' or 'weakest audible tone' may vary, depending on the degree of certainty the individual listener requires before he or she feels ready to respond.

Also, in impedance audiometry and electrophysiological test methods, psychological factors may influence the result. Brain-stem response audiometry is a method which is very sensitive to the degree of relaxation of the patient under test. A tense patient will produce disturbing electric activity from the muscles in the head and neck region. Movements and muscular activity may also disturb the testing procedure in impedance audiometry.

Methodology

The way in which a test is performed can naturally influence the outcome of the test. Methodology involves several factors: how the listener is instructed, how the test signals are presented, how the listener's responses are interpreted by the tester, how the output from an impedance audiometer or the electric responses recorded in the electrophysiological methods are evaluated etc.

The instruction to the listener is of particular importance in psychoacoustic test methods. A formulation where the listeners are encouraged to guess may give a result that differs from one obtained when they are told to respond only when they feel certain about having detected a sound. Another factor may be the number of alternative responses the listener may make use of. In a lateralisation experiment, for example, two alternatives (right or left) or three alternatives (right, middle or left) may be used; the influence on the test result is evident.

Test results should be as independent as possible of the person performing the test and of when and where it takes place. Therefore it is desirable to use a standardised method including a uniform instruction of the listener.

Learning Effects

In psychoacoustic test methods, learning effects are always present to some degree. The more difficult the listener's task, the more time will be required for the learning procedure and the more important it is to allow the listener sufficient training before the actual testing is started.

In simple detection tasks, the learning period is usually quite short. In pure-tone audiometry, usually only the first test frequency requires a few extra presentations of test signals until the training may be considered sufficient from a practical point of view. Looking at group mean values from serial testing, however, slight improvements of the hearing thresholds in the order of a decibel over a surprisingly long period may be found (Robinson and Shipton, 1982).

In speech audiometry, there is always the risk of the listener learning the test words being used. This aspect of the learning effect can be considered as undesirable. Therefore, it is important not to use identical speech test material at repeated testing within short periods. However, it is difficult to make two word lists of exactly equal difficulty, because the listener's vocabulary has some effect on the outcome of the test. If the listener has a pronounced dialect and is used to listening to others with the same dialect, a speech test performed with the usual dialect-free test lists may be more difficult than for another listener. This problem will be even more pronounced when a speech test is performed on a listener in a language other than his or her native one, since this increases the demand of hearing all the acoustic details of the test words in order to recognise them.

Central Masking

In monaural audiometry, the contralateral ear sometimes has to be masked to prevent the test signal from being heard in that ear. Noise is normally used as a masker, presented on a level sufficient to make cross-hearing impossible. However, the fact that this masking noise is delivered to the non-test ear has a certain influence on the perception of the test signal in the test ear. This is not caused by the masking noise being audible in the test ear (a situation called over-masking which is to be avoided) but arises in the central auditory pathways, and this is the reason why the phenomenon is called central masking. In pure-tone audiometry, it increases the hearing threshold level obtained in the test ear by approximately 0.1 dB per dB masking noise level above the masked ear's hearing threshold for the noise (i.e. dB SL), on average (Robinson and Shipton, 1982).

Ambient Sounds

If the ambient sound level in the test room is too high, the test signal may be masked by it. Acceptable ambient sound levels therefore depend on the type of test signal (tone, speech or other) and the test sound level to be used. How the test signals are presented is also of importance. Earphones provide a certain attenuation of the ambient sounds. This frequency-dependent attenuation varies with the mechanical construction of the earphone and its contact with the listener's ear or skull. For the most commonly used audiometric earphone, Telephonics TDH-39 with cushion MX-41/AR, of supra-aural type, sound attenuation data have been presented by Michael and Bienvenue (1981) and Arlinger (1986). The sound attenuation is usually quite modest for frequencies up to 500–1000 Hz. Due to this and to the frequency dependence of the human hearing thresholds, the requirements on the ambient sound levels for pure-tone audiometry are most severe in the frequency range around 500 Hz.

In bone-conduction audiometry, one ear, the test ear, is usually unoccluded. In sound-field audiometry, when the signal is presented from a loudspeaker in the test room, both ears are normally open. In such tests, the ambient sound levels have to be lower than when earphones are used for the same type of test sound and levels. The difference is most evident in the frequency range above 500 Hz.

If the ambient sound level in a test room can be varied experimentally while the hearing thresholds of a listener are being measured, the following will occur: when the ambient noise is inaudible, the hearing threshold measured is the true one; if the ambient noise level is increased gradually, the hearing threshold level recorded will start to increase. This is caused by masking and occurs when the noise level in the third octave band, the centre of which corresponds to the test tone frequency, has reached the level of a few decibels below the test tone level as measured in the listener's ear. If the ambient noise level continues to increase, the hearing threshold value recorded will also increase; however, this does not occur at the same rate but more slowly at first. Not until the third octave noise level is in the range 10–20 dB SL will the hearing threshold value recorded increase at the same rate as the increase of the ambient noise level (Berry, 1973; Shipton and Robinson, 1975).

This is the background for the requirements on ambient sound levels given in the *Manual of Practical Audiometry*, Volume 1. The tables refer to pure-tone audiometry with the lowest true hearing threshold levels to be recorded equal to 0 dB HL with a maximum masking of 2 dB. This value (2 dB) is the highest threshold shift that may occur due to masking from ambient noise in an ear, the true hearing threshold level of which is 0 dB HL if the specified requirements are fulfilled. If a maximum masking of 5 dB can be tolerated, the ambient noise level may be 8 dB higher than those specified in the tables (ISO 8253, 1989).

When measuring the ambient noise levels in a test room to be used for pure-tone audiometry, it is desirable to measure in one-third octave levels. The reason for this is that the masking of a tone by a broad-band noise is mainly caused by that part of the noise which is contained in a rather limited frequency band around the test tone frequency – the critical band. The one-third octave band is a good technical approximation of the critical band. Sometimes, only whole octave band filters may be available for the measurements. From the octave levels measured, an approximate evaluation of the usefulness of the test room for pure-tone audiometry can be made, but it will be less reliable than when one-third octave levels are known.

Audiometric Equipment

The technical equipment being used for audiometry is, of course, also a factor that contributes to the reliability of the testing. Calibration of the equipment has to be performed at regular intervals. In addition, the tester must continually check the various functions of the equipment. The choice of suitable interval between successive electroacoustic calibrations depends on the type of equipment, how often it is being used, whether it is stationary or mobile etc. Even when daily subjective listening control of the various functions does not indicate any problem, the interval should not exceed one year.

In the calibration procedure, the essential functions of the audiometric equipment is measured by means of electroacoustic test equipment with sufficient accuracy and, when needed, corrections are made. The special test equipment required may be available at larger audiology centres, and at distributors and manufacturers of audiometric equipment. In addition to the test equipment being available, a thorough knowledge of audiometric equipment is also required, including its clinical use, and knowledge about relevant national and international standards. The IEC standard 645 (1991) at present concerns only pure-tone audiometers. However, corresponding standards covering equipment for speech audiometry and impedance audiometry will soon be published. Reference equivalent threshold sound pressure and vibratory force levels are specified in the ISO standards 389 (1985) and 7566 (1987) for air and bone conduction, respectively. Calibration values for narrow-band masking noise in pure-tone audiometers are given in ISO standard 8798 (1987).

For impedance audiometers and for equipment used in electrophysiological tests, the design of the equipment often has some influence on the results obtained. Displays and recorders may vary in sensitivity, resulting in varying accuracy in the evaluation of test results and making comparisons of results obtained on different types of equipment more difficult. This can, for example, influence stapedius reflex thresholds and reflex decay test results (Jerger, Mandlin and Lewis, 1977) or latencies of different components in an electric response obtained in electric response audiometry (ERA). In ERA equipment, bandwidth and type of filtering in the electrophysiological amplifier is of considerable importance, and also the transduction properties of the earphone for short-duration clicks (Arlinger, 1981; Laukli, 1983). For ERA equipment, no standardisation is available.

Placement of Transducers

The placement of an earphone or a bone vibrator on the ear or skull of the listener, or the placement of the listener relative to the loudspeaker, are other possible sources of error. The difficulty in obtaining exactly the same placement at one test as was used in a previous test is obvious.

Supra-aural earphones, which are normally used in audiometry, mainly provide two possible types of error. The earphone is expected to fit closely to the external ear. If this tight fit is not obtained, sound energy will leak out and result in lower sound level in the ear canal for a certain electric signal level fed to the earphone. This mainly affects the lowest frequency range, and often gives rise to falsely poor (by up to 15 dB) hearing thresholds in pure-tone audiometry at frequencies up to 500 Hz.

The earphone is to be placed with its sound outlet facing the ear canal entrance. Variations by a few millimetres up and down or forward and backward can give rise to measurable variation in sound levels reaching the ear drum at the highest frequencies – 6 kHz and over. This is due to the fact that the sound wavelength is sufficiently small for such variations in position to influence the wave pattern in the ear canal (Erlandsson et al., 1980).

In sound-field audiometry, large variations in test sound level may arise in the test room if this is not anechoic – a very special type of room where all surfaces have very high sound absorption. This problem is especially pronounced when the test signal is a pure tone, because of standing wave patterns in the room, caused by interaction between the directly transmitted sound and various reflected sound components. One way of reducing this problem to an acceptable level in regular audiometric test rooms, which have significant acoustic damping but are not anechoic, is to use frequency-modulated (FM) tones or narrow-band noise (Walker, Dillon and Byrne, 1984; Arlinger and Jerlvall, 1987).

References

ARLINGER, S. (1981). Technical aspects on ABR – stimulation, recording and signal processing. *Scandinavian Audiology* Suppl. 13, 41–53.

ARLINGER, S. (1986). Sound attenuation of TDH-39 earphones in a diffuse field of narrow-band noise. *Journal of the Acoustical Society of America* **79**, 189–191.

ARLINGER, S. and JERLVALL, L. (1987). Reliability in warble tone sound field audiometry. *Scandinavian Audiology* **16**, 21–27.

BERGER, E.H. and KERIVAN, J.E. (1983). Influence of physiological noise and the occlusion effect on the measurement of real-ear attenuation at threshold. *Journal of the Acoustical Society of America* **74**, 81–94.

BERRY, B.F. (1973). *Ambient Noise Limits for Audiometry.* Teddington: NPL Acoustics Report AC60, National Physical Laboratory.

ERLANDSSON, B., HÄKANSSON, H., IVARSSON, A. and NILSSON, P. (1980). The reliability of Békésy sweep audiometry recording and effects of the earphone position. *Acta Oto-Laryngologica Supplementum* **366**, 99–112.

IEC 645 (1991). *Audiometers Part 1: Pure Tone Audiometers.* Geneva: International Electrotechnical Commission.

ISO 389 (1985). *Standard Reference Zero for the Calibration of Pure Tone Air Conduction Audiometers.* Geneva: International Standards Organisation.

ISO 7566 (1987). *Standard Reference Zero for the Calibration of Pure Tone Bone Conduction Audiometers.* Geneva: International Standards Organisation.

ISO 8253 (1989). *Acoustics – Audiometric Test Methods, Part 1: Basic Pure Tone Air and Bone Conduction Threshold Audiometry.* Geneva: International Standards Organisation.

ISO 8798 (1987). *Acoustics – Reference Levels for Narrow-Band Masking Noise.* Geneva: International Standards Organisation.

JERGER, J., MAULDIN, L. and LEWIS, N. (1977). Temporal summation of the acoustic reflex. *Audiology* **16**, 177–200.

LAUKLI, E. (1983). Stimulus waveforms used in brainstem response audiometry. *Scandinavian Audiology* **12**, 83–89.

MICHAEL, P.L. and BIENVENUE, G.R. (1981). Noise attenuation characteristics for supra-aural audiometric headsets using the models MX-41/AR and 51 earphone cushions. *Journal of the Acoustical Society of America* **70**, 1235–1238.

POULSEN, T. (1975). *Temporal Loudness Summation of Tone-Pulses*, Report No. 8. Copenhagen: The Acoustics Laboratory, Technical University of Denmark.

ROBINSON, D.W. and SHIPTON, M.S. (1982). A standard determination of paired air- and bone-conduction thresholds under different masking noise conditions. *Audiology* **21**, 61–82.

SHIPTON, M.S. and ROBINSON, D.W. (1975). *Ambient Noise Limits for Industrial Audiometry.* Teddington: NPL Acoustics Report AC69, National Physical Laboratory.

WALKER, G., DILLON, H. and BYRNE, D. (1984). Sound field audiometry: Recommended stimuli and procedures. *Ear and Hearing* **5**, 13–21.

Chapter 5 Psychoacoustic Methods with Pure-tone Stimuli

Psychoacoustic test methods using pure-tone stimulation play a very important role in audiometry for the determination of hearing thresholds as well as for tests of auditory characteristics at suprathreshold stimulus levels. In the *Manual of Practical Audiometry*, Volume 1, this section contains 24 different methods. Because the background for several of these methods is more or less the same, this chapter has been structured in a different fashion from that in Volume 1. In the six sections that follow, the majority of methods are discussed, but a few less commonly used methods are not explicitly represented.

In the first section on pure-tone air-conduction audiometry, screening audiometry and insert masking are also discussed. The section on bone-conduction audiometry also includes the placement of the bone vibrator on the subject's forehead, the Weber test, the occlusion test and the Gellé test. The third section concerns Békésy audiometry with fixed frequency as well as with frequency sweep.

The section on loudness balancing concerns both the binaural and monaural tests. The threshold tone decay test is presented in the fifth section whilst the last section concerns sound localisation in a free sound field and by means of phase audiometry.

Pure-tone Air-conduction Audiometry

Indication

Pure-tone air-conduction audiometry concerns the determination of hearing thresholds for pure tones, presented monaurally by means of an earphone. The test is a basic part of a routine evaluation of hearing. It may be performed to provide information for diagnosis as well as for the selection and fitting of hearing aids.

Physiological and psychoacoustic background

In pure-tone audiometry, the auditory ability to detect pure tones at certain standardised frequencies is determined. In normal clinical applications, the frequency range 125–8000 Hz is covered, corresponding to the frequency range of the main components of the spectrum of human speech.

An increasing interest has been shown for extended high frequency audiometry (the range from 8 to 20 kHz), but several problems remain to be solved before this will become a standardised test range. Such problems include the shape of the earphone and its coupling to the ear, the lack of a standardised artificial ear or acoustic coupler for frequencies above 10 kHz, and the significant age dependence of hearing thresholds in this range (Fausti et al., 1979; Osterhammel and Osterhammel, 1979).

In addition to the test frequency, the human auditory sensitivity depends on how the tones are presented: monaurally or binaurally, by earphones or in a sound field. Normal pure-tone audiometry makes use of monaural earphone presentation. For this situation, internationally standardised reference values, corresponding to the average normal hearing thresholds, are specified in ISO 389 (1985), to be used for the calibration of pure-tone audiometers.

The important outcome of a pure-tone audiometric test is not the absolute hearing thresholds in decibel sound pressure level (dB SPL) but

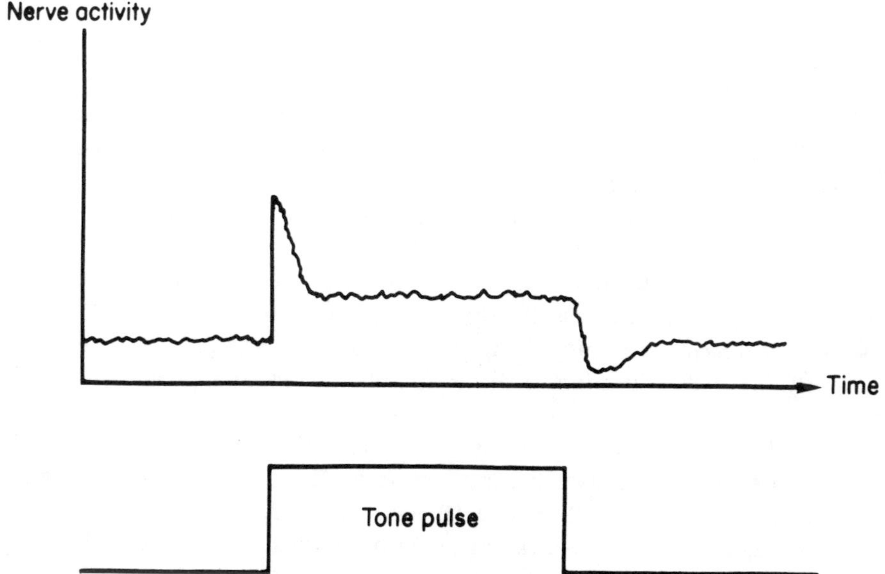

Figure 5.1 Neuronal activity at constant and at a change in excitation.

any deviation from normality. Therefore, the hearing level (HL) scale of decibels is used, where 0 dB for each frequency is defined as corresponding to the average threshold of hearing for a large group of young (18–30 years), otologically normal persons of both sexes (Robinson, Shipton and Hinchcliffe, 1981; ISO 389, 1985).

Pure-tone audiometry is a detection test, i.e. the listener's task is to detect barely audible tone pulses. In the range around the hearing threshold, the listener is usually uncertain of whether he or she hears a tone or not. Therefore, the instruction of the patient is very important. A clear difference in results is easily obtainable if the listener is encouraged to be certain before responding, as compared to when he is encouraged to respond as soon as he thinks he heard a tone.

Physiologically, changes in a signal from the environment excite the auditory nerve paths more than a constant signal (Figure 5.1). The marked change in nerve activity, when a change occurs in the acoustic environment, will soon diminish, however. This phenomenon is called adaptation. A common perception of this physiological fact is that, at levels close to the auditory threshold, a diffuse feeling of change is perceived at the moments when the onset and the offset of the tone pulse occur, whilst nothing can really be heard in between.

Therefore, it may seem desirable to present tone pulses with very sharp onset and offset, i.e. with infinitely short rise and fall times. However, such abrupt changes give rise to broadening of the spectrum (the frequency contents) of the tone pulse. The faster the rate of change of level at onset and offset, the broader the frequency spectrum of the pulse. The listener can hear this effect as clicks being added to the beginning and the end of the tone. This is a possible cause of error, because a listener could well detect such clicks without being able to hear the actual tone due to the clicks containing energy over a wide frequency range. For this reason, rise and fall times of the tone pulses are chosen in the range 20–50 ms as a compromise, considering the wish to have fast changes to excite the neurons as effectively as possible, but not fast enough to cause a significant spectral broadening.

Temporal integration has the effect that the perception of a sound is affected by the duration of the signal (Pedersen and Salomon, 1977). For normally hearing people, temporal integration results in a reduced detectability if the duration of the tone pulse is below approximately 0.5 s. Shorter tone pulses have to be increased in level in order to remain audible. For durations below 0.2 s, the hearing threshold level of normally hearing listeners decreases by approximately 10 dB when the tone pulse duration is reduced by a factor of 10. The effect of temporal integration is usually less pronounced for listeners with cochlear hearing loss. To avoid any influence from temporal integration on the results of pure-tone audiometry, pulse durations longer than 0.5 s are used.

However, if the interval between the beginning and the end of the tone pulse is made too long, the relation between them becomes less clear and the listener feels less certain. Therefore, tone pulse durations in the range 1–2 s are used in pure-tone audiometry. For the same reason, intervals between consecutive tone pulses should not be shorter than this value of 1–2 s. In addition, the intervals should be varied in a random pattern to avoid the risk of the listener detecting a steady rhythm in the presentation pattern of the tones and responding because of that rather than because of hearing a tone. Another important factor to reduce the risk of the listener guessing when a tone is presented is to prevent him or her from seeing when the controls of the audiometer are changed and the interrupter activated.

The actual determination of a hearing threshold can be made in several ways. Signals must be presented at levels both above and below the threshold level. This can be achieved with ascending signal levels, starting from inaudible and being increased to audible levels, or with descending signal levels, starting from audible and being reduced to inaudible levels, or a combination of both – bracketing (Carhart and Jerger, 1959). The average difference between hearing thresholds determined with ascending and with bracketing technique is small (Arlinger, 1979), but on a single listener significant differences may occur. Therefore, a standardised method is of importance. The normal, standardised method is an ascending one (ISO 6189, 1983; ISO 8253, 1989).

Theoretically, the hearing threshold at a certain frequency should represent that signal level at which 50% of the presented test tones are detected. However, such an exact definition of the hearing threshold requires a large number of test tones to be presented, which in turn leads to a time-consuming test, increasing listener fatigue. In practical, clinical, pure-tone audiometry, the definition of hearing threshold level – the threshold criterion – is that level at which the listener first responds three times in repeated series of ascending stimulus level. The ascending series should be repeated at most five times (ISO 6189, 1983; ISO 8253, 1989). This criterion corresponds to a detection level in the range 60–100%. The difference between this definition and the theoretically most logical, 50% correct detection is, however, limited to at most a few decibels and is of no clinical importance. It is important to use a well-defined and standardised technique to reduce variation in the test results. The reduction of such variations is desirable to allow a reliable comparison of audiograms for a listener, obtained at different times and/or clinics. Also, when comparing results obtained on different individuals or evaluating the statistical outcome from groups of listeners, the standardised technique improves reliability.

The normal step size in the variation of the test sound level is 5 dB. This may seem a rather large step, and a smaller step size might be expected to result in better precision in the test. However, this is not the case (Jerlvall and Arlinger, 1986) and the 5-dB step size appears to be close to optimum. This is related to the fact that the ability to detect a difference or change in sound level close to the auditory threshold is of the order of 5 dB. A smaller step size does not increase the precision but increases testing time, because a larger number of ascending series of stimuli are needed before the threshold criterion is fulfilled, i.e. three responses are obtained on the same level. However, a smaller step size will result in a somewhat better (higher) threshold value, a fact of limited clinical interest.

Screening

In some applications, fast sorting of a group of people may be required, e.g. into the two categories normal/abnormal hearing, in order to concentrate more detailed evaluations only on those who have abnormal results. For such purposes, screening audiometry is the natural choice. The outcome of a screening test is to determine if a listener's hearing threshold is above or below the screening level at one or more test frequencies. A common screening level is 20 dB HL, which is the limit for a statistically significant deviation from 0 dB hearing threshold level.

The choice of screening level should be made according to the aim of the particular test, what population is being tested and with regard to the practical circumstances for the test (ambient sound levels in the test room, time available etc.). The most common use of screening audiometry is for testing school children and in occupational hearing conservation programmes. In the latter case, it is important to choose as low a screening level as possible, because the main aim of the testing is to detect hearing losses and deterioration in hearing as early as possible. Often screening audiometry is combined with a full determination of hearing thresholds at those frequencies where the test subject fails the screening test.

Interaural attenuation

The capacity of the skull to separate the two ears acoustically is limited. This leads to the phenomenon called cross-hearing, which means that a sound, presented by means of a transducer placed on one side of the listener's head, will also reach the inner ear of the other side. The degree of cross-hearing in air conduction can be tested on subjects with unilateral total deafness and normal hearing on the other ear. When test tones are presented by means of an earphone on the deaf ear they will be audible when their level is raised to, on average, 60 dB HL but sometimes it can be as low as 40 dB HL. This is due to the earphone on the deaf ear generating vibrations, which are transmitted to the skull and reach the inner ear on the normal side by means of bone conduction.

The transcranial attenuation tends to be lower for low frequencies than for high (Zwislocki, 1953; Lidén, Nilsson and Andersson, 1959). This is explained by the effective transcranial attenuation not only being determined by the actual transfer of mechanical energy from the earphone to the skull and inner ear directly, but also being influenced by the occlusion effect.

Occlusion effect

The occlusion effect is the fact that a bone-conducted signal will reach the inner ear at a higher level if the auditory canal is occluded, e.g. by an earphone, provided that the middle ear is normal. This increase in level can be as high as 20–30 dB at the lowest audiometric test frequencies, whereas it is negligible above 2 kHz. There are probably two reasons for the occlusion effect. One is that bone-conducted sound radiates from the wall of the ear canal into the air. With the ear unoccluded, this sound leaks out into the outside, but with the ear occluded, this leakage is prevented. The other reason is that the occluding earphone is set into vibration by the skull vibrations, thereby generating an additional contribution to the total pressure in the auditory canal.

Masking

As a rule, pure-tone audiometry is performed as a monaural test, i.e. the hearing thresholds are determined for each ear separately. If there is a risk that the test signal is transmitted to the non-test side by means of cross-hearing at or above the hearing threshold of the non-test ear, this has to be masked by masking sound. In the past, broad-band noise was used; however, today narrow-band noise, generated by band-pass filtering white noise with a centre frequency coinciding with the tone frequency to be masked, is used since this is the most efficient type of masker for pure tones. A bandwidth corresponding to the critical bandwidth in hearing is a suitable minimum bandwidth. Noise with frequencies within this band contributes to the masking of the tone in the centre of the band, whilst noise outside this band adds little to the masking but causes fatigue and makes the noise unnecessarily loud. At frequencies from about 1 kHz, critical bandwidth is very close to one-third octave.

Noise with a very narrow bandwidth takes on a tonal character. Since it is essential that the character of the masker is distinctly different from that of the test tone, to avoid the listener mixing them up, a somewhat wider band than the critical band is normally used.

The level of the masking noise which is necessary to mask a cross-heard tone reliably can be calculated. It is then important to assume that the smallest transcranial attenuation which can occur is 40 dB, to be on the safe side. Since the real transcranial attenuation is often higher than 40 dB, sufficient masking level is often obtained at a lower level.

If the masking level is increased to a sufficiently high level, the masking noise may become audible in the test ear via cross-hearing, thereby interfering with the listener's ability to detect the test tone. This is called over-masking. The level that may cause over-masking can be calculated by assuming a transcranial attenuation of 40 dB. Since the real transcranial attenuation is often higher than 40 dB, higher masking levels than this limit can often be used until over-masking really occurs. Thus, the formula just estimates the highest safe level of the masking noise.

The method used to adjust the level of the contralateral masking noise, which is described in ISO 8253 (1989) and in Volume 1 of the *Manual of Practical Audiometry*, is based on finding the masking plateau. The likely course is illustrated in Figure 5.2 when testing a patient having a

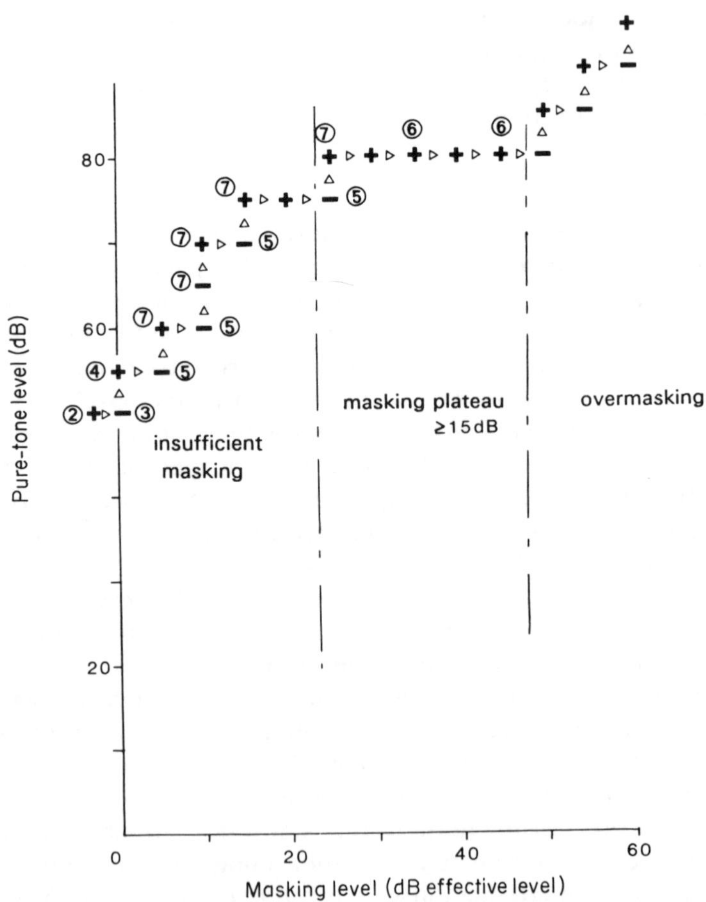

Figure 5.2 Illustration of the procedure for determination of the masked threshold of a patient with unmasked thresholds obtained at 50 and 0 dB HL, respectively.

true hearing threshold at 80 dB on the test ear and 0 dB on the non-test ear. When testing the poorer ear without masking, the first response is obtained at 50 dB. When a contralateral masker is presented at 0 dB effective masking level, this tone will become inaudible, because it was detected by the better ear now being masked by the noise. Every increase of the test tone level will make the tone audible again, whereupon every increase in masking level will mask it. This goes on until the masking plateau is reached.

The beginning of the masking plateau is determined by the test tone level reaching the actual hearing threshold of the test ear. The test tone will now be detected in the test ear rather than by cross-hearing to the non-test ear, which is being masked at a level sufficient to make the tone inaudible in that ear. The end of the plateau is determined by the highest masking level which can be used without giving rise to over-masking.

According to the international standard for pure-tone audiometers (IEC 645, Part 1, 1991), the narrow-band masking noise should be calibrated in effective masking level. The effective masking level of a certain noise is defined as the pure-tone level, expressed in dB HL, to which the hearing threshold for the test tone is raised in the presence of the masking noise. If a normally hearing listener listens to a tone in noise and the detection threshold for the tone is 55 dB HL, the effective masking level of that noise is 55 dB. International standard ISO 8798 (1987) has specified how narrow-band noise should be calibrated in dB SPL in order to provide a scale of effective masking level.

The values for transcranial attenuation presented above concern the conventional audiometer earphone Telephonics TDH-39 or TDH-49 with cushion MX-41/AR. If another type of earphone is used, having different weight, contact pressure against the ear etc., other values of transcranial attenuation may be valid. In pure-tone audiometry on some patients, in particular those with severe bilateral conductive losses, the masking dilemma is often a source of problem. This dilemma means that over-masking occurs at a level lower than the lowest sufficient masking level, thus making it impossible to establish a masking plateau.

One way of reducing this problem is to present the masking noise by means of a transducer which offers higher transcranial attenuation than the conventional one (Hosford-Dunn et al., 1986). The most common solution is insert masking, which means using an insert earphone for the presentation of the masking noise. The noise levels produced by an insert earphone in different ears may vary considerably because of differences in acoustic coupling between the earphone and ear and in the acoustic impedance of the ear. Therefore, it is not of value to try to calibrate the audiometer for a particular earphone. Instead, a good approach is to determine the hearing threshold for the masking noise when it is presented by the particular insert earphone. Recently, however, a special insert earphone has been produced which has approximately equivalent sensitivity and frequency dependence as the Telephonics TDH-39 and is relatively insensitive to variations in acoustic loading offered by different ears. This earphone will thus make a reliable calibration in effective masking level possible (Killion, Wilber and Gudmundsen, 1985).

When contralateral masking has to be used, to make sure that the subject hears the test tone in the test ear, this may give rise to central masking. Central masking means that a sound, presented to one ear, influences the perception of another, usually simultaneous, sound presented to the other ear. In other words the presence of a masking noise in one ear interacts with the ability to detect the test tone in the other ear. The hearing threshold is elevated by an average of 1–2 dB per 10 dB of masking level above the hearing threshold for the noise, i.e. per 10 dB SL (Robinson and Shipton, 1982). Considering the masking levels commonly used in clinical applications, 5 or 10 dB of the measured hearing threshold level may be due to central masking.

Equipment

Air-conduction pure-tone audiometry can be performed with pure-tone audiometers which fulfil the requirements of IEC 645 Part 1 (1991), types 1–4. When masking is required, the choice will be limited to types 1 or 2. A type 3 audiometer may have masking noise other than the standardised narrow-band noise and a type 4 audiometer has no masking noise at all.

The calibration of the tone levels, i.e. electroacoustic measurements and, if necessary, adjustment to correct values, is performed by placing the earphone under test on a special acoustic test load – an acoustic coupler as specified in IEC 303 (1970). This so-called 6 cm^3 coupler is to be used for two specific audiometer earphones, Telephonics TDH-39 with cushion MX-41/AR and Beyer DT 48, for which calibration data are specified in ISO 389 (1985) in terms of reference equivalent threshold sound pressure levels.

The purpose of using this coupler is to present to the earphone an acoustic load which is approximately equivalent to that of an average human ear. Thereby, the sound levels recorded by the test microphone in the coupler will correspond fairly well with those obtained with the earphone on a human ear. This approximation is reasonably good at frequencies up to 2–3 kHz, but at higher frequencies the coupler is too simple a model of the human ear. A better device is available and is specified in an IEC standard, IEC 318 (1970). This is called an artificial ear and is made to represent the acoustic impedance of the average human ear up to 10 kHz. In ISO 389, Addendum 1 (1983) are specified reference equivalent threshold sound pressure levels for supra-aural earphones other than the two covered by ISO 389 (1985) which are intended to be calibrated on the acoustic coupler. These are excluded to avoid a slight ambiguity which would appear if either of the two sets of reference levels were used for the TDH-39 and Beyer DT48 earphones.

When testing the earphone it is placed on the coupler or artificial ear and pressed down with a specified force of 4.5 ± 0.5 N. For the calibration to be valid, the earphone headband must provide the same force. It is thus important to check that the headband is not deformed or adjusted from its original form and tension.

Sources of error and test accuracy

Pure-tone audiometry puts very high requirements on the ambient sound levels on the test site when testing patients with near normal hearing, as the method involves measuring the lowest audible test tone level. The ambient sound levels must be sufficiently low in order to assure that no masking of the test tones occurs. The earphones provide some attenuation of the ambient sounds (Michael and Bienvenue, 1981; Arlinger, 1986) and the higher this attenuation, the higher ambient sound levels may be permitted.

The masking from ambient noise of a test tone is mainly determined by that part of the frequency spectrum of the ambient sound which is within the critical band centred around the test tone. But also ambient sounds at considerably lower frequencies may mask the tone if the noise level is sufficiently high due to the upward spread of masking. This is the reason for specifying different requirements on ambient sound levels, depending on the lowest test tone frequency (ISO 8253, 1989).

As a rule, a special sound-attenuating test booth is required to obtain ambient sound levels that permit measurements of hearing thresholds down to 0 dB HL. Sometimes, special sound-attenuating earphone enclosures are used as a substitute. However, this is often a questionable solution for two reasons: one is that the attenuation obtained in addition to the earphone's own attenuation is sometimes relatively small, particularly in the low frequency region where the need for attenuation is highest. The other is the risk that the earphone will not generate correct sound levels. This is caused by the fact that the audiometer earphone is of the supra-aural type, i.e. made to make tight contact with the pinna. The extra enclosure reduces the force that presses the earphone against the pinna, thus increasing the risk for sound leakage into the enclosure cavity, causing a reduction in tone level (Roeser and Glorig, 1975).

The placement of the earphone on the pinna is supposed to result in a tight coupling with the sound opening of the earphone being placed exactly opposite to the entrance of the auditory canal. If a tight coupling is not achieved, sound leaks out, mainly in the low frequency range, resulting in test tone levels that are too low and thus hearing threshold levels which are too poor are obtained. The placement of the earphone in relation to the ear canal entrance mainly affects the highest test frequencies (Erlandsson et al., 1980).

Of all different factors which may influence the test and cause errors, the listener's ability to concentrate on the listening task seems to be the most difficult one to control with the techniques normally used. To make this source of error as small as possible, it is important to eliminate all likely reasons for distraction in the test situation. It is also essential to adapt the duration of the test sessions in order to let the listener relax as often as desired.

The test accuracy in pure-tone audiometry has been evaluated by means of test–retest experiments on listeners, whose hearing with all probability has not changed between the two test occasions. Standardised methodology has been followed and the middle-ear function has been checked by means of tympanometry at each test occasion. The standard deviations for single threshold measurements determined at these experiments have been in the range 2–5 dB and standard deviations for test–retest difference in the range 3–7 dB (Jerlvall, Dryselius and Arlinger, 1983). Thus, with the 5-dB step size and the requirement of a difference of at least two standard deviations in order to consider a measured change as statistically significant, it has to be 10–15 dB. As a simple general rule of thumb, the 15 dB figure is easy to remember.

By analysing the mean value of several test frequencies, test–retest accuracy can be improved (Erlandsson et al., 1980). However, the measurement errors at neighbouring frequencies co-vary somewhat, and the use of such mean values for improved accuracy usually requires a computer for rational handling.

Clinical interpretation

Considering test accuracy and the biological variability of the normally hearing group of age range 18–30 years, the hearing of which forms the basis for the reference levels corresponding to 0 dB HL, the limit between normal and abnormal hearing threshold levels is usually drawn at 20 dB HL. Values better than 20 dB thus do not differ significantly from zero and represent normal auditory sensitivity. However, significant changes may still occur within this normal range, and this can be of importance to discover. A test subject who at one test has threshold levels around −5 dB which at a later test have dropped to 15 dB, definitely shows a significant deterioration, although the values are still within the normal range.

The shape of the pure-tone audiogram gives certain diagnostic information, too. A conductive loss due to otosclerosis often has a low frequency dominated hearing loss (Figure 5.3). Also otosalpingitis may give rise to a

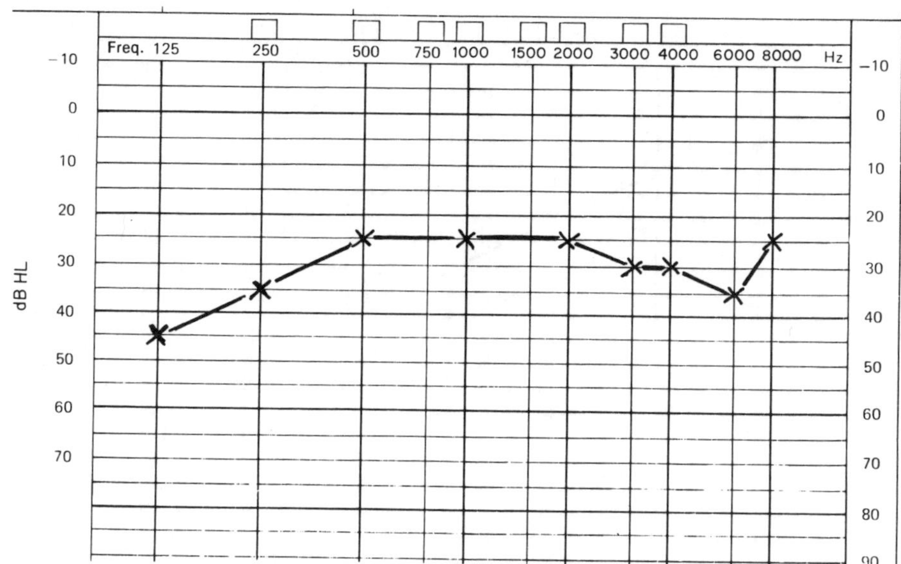

Figure 5.3 Example of pure-tone air-conduction audiogram in otosclerosis.

low frequency loss, often combined with a loss in the high frequency range. Sensorineural hearing impairments are usually greatest at the high frequency range, e.g. in presbyacusis or noise-induced hearing loss (Figures 5.4 and 5.5). However, other shapes also occur, such as in cases with the early stage of Menière's disease, where a low frequency dominated loss is common.

The topical diagnosis, i.e. the decision of the localisation of the lesion, is usually based on both air- and bone-conduction audiograms. In addition, the results from other test methods are considered together with history and otoscopy. Sometimes a vestibular test battery is also used to reach a diagnostic conclusion. Thus, in general, the pure-tone audiogram is only a part of the total puzzle to be solved. However, in some cases the pure-tone audiogram is of great significance, and a general rule is naturally to strive for the very best validity and reliability of each part of the test battery.

With regard to functional hearing capacity, the pure-tone audiogram is a measure of limited validity. Two patients with quite similar audiograms may differ considerably in the functional consequences of the hearing loss and meet quite different problems in various everyday listening conditions. Such differences may be illuminated by means of other test methods which describe functional characteristics of the ear other than auditory sensitivity. However, the possibilities for making practical use of the results of such tests are still very limited. Therefore, the pure-tone audiogram is still the single most important basis for, for example, hearing aid fitting (see Chapter 13).

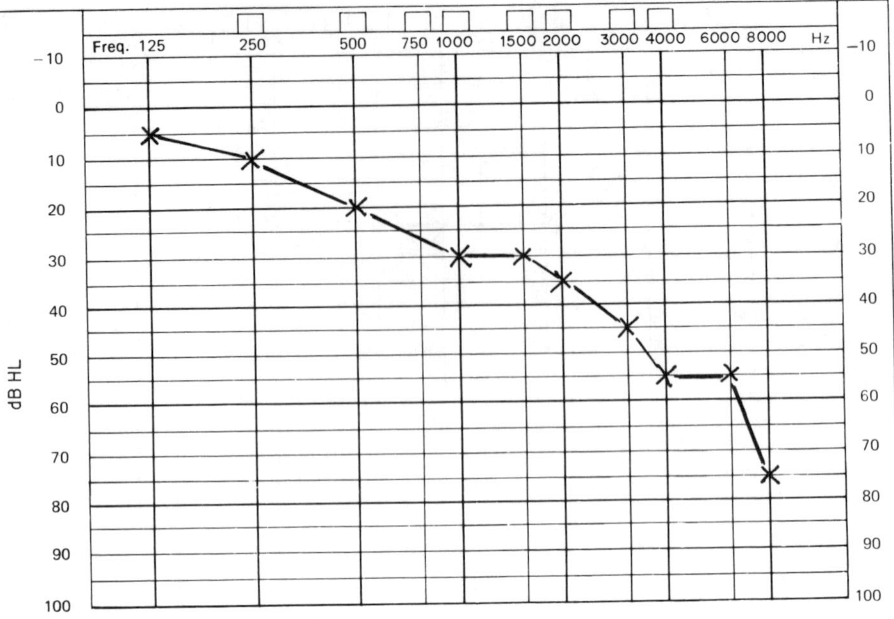

Figure 5.4 Example of pure-tone air-conduction audiogram in presbyacusis.

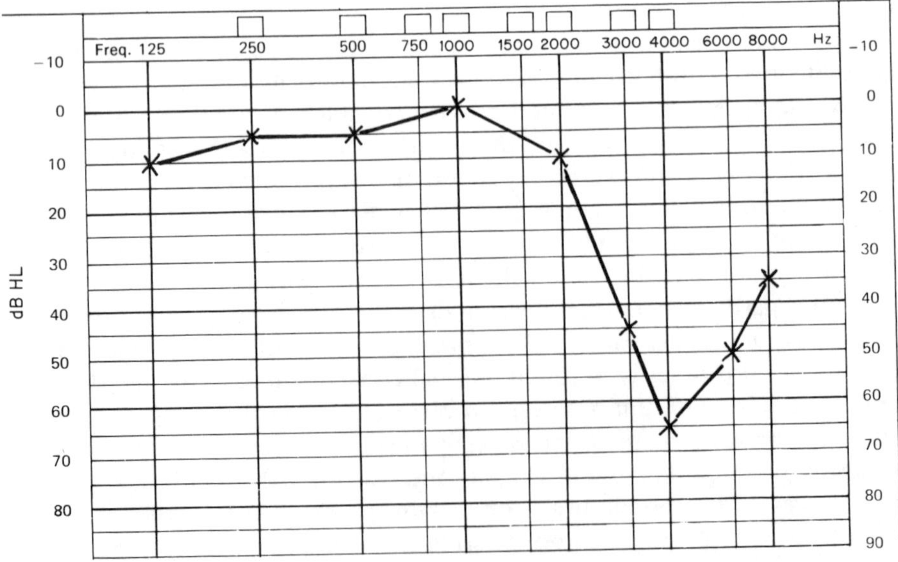

Figure 5.5 Example of pure-tone air-conduction audiogram in noise-induced hearing loss.

The pure-tone audiogram is often used to express the degree of hearing loss. Often the multi-figure information of the audiogram is condensed into a single average measure. The classic average value is based on the hearing threshold levels at 500, 1000 and 2000 Hz. These frequencies are assumed to represent the most important frequency range with regard to speech recognition. This average hearing threshold has also been shown to have good statistical correlation with the speech recognition threshold determined in a silent listening situation.

However, when speech has to be recognised in a noisy background, higher frequencies are of increasing importance. Therefore, evaluations of degree of handicap and similar applications need to take account of hearing thresholds at frequencies higher than 2000 Hz. The American Medical Association has suggested a mean value for the four test frequencies: 500, 1000, 2000 and 3000 Hz (Ward, 1983). In England, a three frequency average based on 1000, 2000 and 4000 Hz has been recommended (BAOL/BSA, 1983). Insurance evaluation cases, with, for example, noise-induced hearing loss, increasingly takes into account the higher frequencies, sometimes up to 6000 Hz.

Still another method to condense the complex information of a pure-tone audiogram is offered by the use of a classification system (Klockhoff et al., 1973). Such systems have mainly been used on results from audiometry on noise-exposed populations. The system according to Klockhoff et al. is based on dividing the audiogram form into five parts. The frequency range is split into two parts: a lower from 500 to 2000 Hz and a higher from 3000 to 6000 Hz. The lower frequency range is divided into two level ranges and the higher frequency range into three level ranges. Each ear is classified by a value from one to five depending on how the audiogram curve runs through these five parts. The classification value 1 refers to an essentially normal curve, 2 refers to a slight high frequency loss, 3 to a moderate and 4 to a severe high frequency loss, and 5 indicates other types of loss.

Pure-tone Bone-conduction Audiometry

Indication

Pure-tone bone-conduction audiometry concerns the determination of hearing thresholds for pure tones, presented by means of a bone vibrator placed on the subject's skull, usually behind one ear or on the forehead. The measurement is usually a complement to air-conduction audiometry mainly to evaluate the middle-ear function. The occlusion test, Gellé test and Weber test are special methods which also make use of bone-conducted stimuli.

Physiological and psychoacoustic background

A complete pure-tone audiogram contains both air- and bone-conduction hearing thresholds for both ears of a subject. In bone-conduction testing, a bone vibrator, usually a small electromagnetic transducer, is placed on the skull. The placement in the normal clinical procedure is behind the ear, on the relatively plane surface behind the entrance of the auditory canal (planum mastoideus). The placement of the bone vibrator is less well defined than the placement of a supra-aural earphone on the outer ear. A consequence of this is a greater difficulty in finding the same placement in a retest.

Normally, the placement of the vibrator is adjusted until the listener perceives the bone-conducted signal as loudly as possible, taking care that the vibrator or its headband does not touch the outer ear. The signal level to be used in this adjustment should be relatively high in order to make use of the greater ability to note changes in loudness at higher sound levels than close to hearing threshold.

The signal from the bone vibrator reaches the inner ear via at least three possible routes (Tonndorf, 1976): first, the vibrations may reach the cochlea directly through the skull, giving rise to small changes in cochlear shape, which in turn causes a fluid flow in the scala media and thereby hair cell stimulation. This is the inner ear component. Secondly, the ossicles in the middle ear will be set in motion relative to the surrounding skull bone. This is a consequence of their mass and the elasticity of their mounting within the middle-ear cavity. The effect will be a vibration of the stapedial footplate relative to the oval window, which will add a fluid flow component in the inner ear; this is the middle-ear component. Its magnitude depends on the mechanical properties of the ossicular chain, including the coupling to the inner ear via the oval window and to the outer ear via the ear drum. Thirdly, the skull vibrations will give rise to a sound radiation into the external auditory canal through vibration of its soft walls, in particular in the outer cartilaginous part. This outer ear component can reach the inner ear in the normal way through the middle ear.

These three main components add up to a certain degree of stimulation of the inner ear. The three parts are added as vectors, which means that the sum is determined by both magnitudes and relative phase of the three components. When adding two vectors of equal magnitude, but opposite phase, the sum will be zero, whilst if they have equal phase the sum will be twice the magnitude of each single component. The relative importance of the three components is frequency dependent, since magnitude as well as phase angle varies with frequency.

As a very first approximation, the function of the inner ear determines the bone-conduction hearing thresholds. However, when considering the complex nature of the bone-conduction pathways to the inner ear, it is easy to realise that the function of the middle ear also has an influence since this affects the middle- and outer-ear components. This is the reason why bone-conduction hearing thresholds often are improved after middle-ear surgery. This improvement thus reflects the influence of the middle ear on bone conduction and of course has nothing to do with any change in inner-ear function due to surgery.

If the outer ear is blocked, e.g. by the placement of an earphone on or in it, a considerable increase in the outer ear component is obtained, resulting in a higher than normal bone-conducted signal level reaching the inner ear if the middle ear has normal sound transmission properties. The increase may be as high as 20–30 dB at 250 Hz. This phenomenon is called the occlusion effect and is considered to depend on two factors (Goldstein and Hayes, 1965; Dirks and Swindeman, 1967; Edgerton and Klodd, 1977). One is that the outer-ear component increases in magnitude because of sound, radiated into the ear canal, being prevented from leaking out into the free air, but limited to a relatively small closed cavity by the occlusion. The other factor is a relative motion between the occluding earphone and the skull, dependent on the earphone mass and the elasticity in the contact between earphone and ear. This, in turn, gives rise to an additional sound pressure component in the external ear canal, added to the original outer ear component. For these reasons, it is necessary to have the test ear unoccluded in bone-conduction audiometry.

The occlusion effect is made use of in the occlusion test. If the middle ear has normal mobility and intact ossicular chain, the increase in the outer-ear component caused by the occlusion of the outer ear will reach the inner ear and result in an improvement of the bone-conduction threshold measured in the lower frequency range as compared to the unoccluded state.

In the Gellé test, the influence of relative over- and under-pressure in the external auditory canal on bone-conduction thresholds is examined. By loading the ear drum with a static pressure, the middle-ear component is changed, resulting in a reduced inner-ear stimulation in the low and mid-frequency range. Also the outer ear component is affected by the reduced sound transmission from the ear canal to the middle ear. Thus, if the middle-ear function is normal, a static over- or under-pressure in the ear canal will make the bone-conduction hearing thresholds worse. An alternative evaluation is to look for a change in sound lateralisation from the test ear to the non-test ear when the over- or under-pressure is applied.

The Weber test is also based on the complex signal transmission in bone conduction and mainly on the effect of the middle-ear state on the middle-ear component (Tonndorf, 1976). A fluid-filled middle ear is considered to damp the ossicular vibrations. Also, swelling of the mucous lining of the middle-ear space may give rise to an increased mechanical loading of the ossicles. This will lead to an increase in the net stimulation that reaches the inner ear in the low frequency range. When ossicular fixation is present, i.e. as in otosclerosis, the dominating effect is assumed to be a change in phase angle of the middle-ear component, resulting in an increased bone-conduction level reaching the inner ear in the low frequency range. In cases of ossicular disruption, both mass, elasticity and damping of the middle-ear component are changed. Again, the most common finding is an increase in the bone-conducted signal level reaching the inner ear. However, no clear scientific explanation has been given for this.

The Weber test is mainly used for lateralisation experiments. If symmetrical inner-ear conditions are present, a unilateral conductive component will mean that bone-conducted test signals, mainly in the lower frequency range, will be lateralised to the ear with the conductive lesion.

Carhart's notch is a phenomenon that refers to otosclerotic ears showing an extra bone-conduction hearing loss of on average 15 dB centred on 2000 Hz (Carhart, 1950). This may be explained by the middle- and outer-ear components being effectively eliminated by the disease and the inner-ear component being changed by the fixation of the stapedial footplate in the oval window. This will have some influence on bone-conduction hearing thresholds at low frequencies, in keeping with the discussion on the Weber test above and this quite specific influence at 2000 Hz.

The bone vibrator may also be placed on the listener's forehead. An advantage with this placement is that the listener does not know in advance in which ear he will hear the test tone. Further, the forehead is sometimes a better and more accessible surface for a stable placement of the vibrator. However, the vibration transmission from the forehead to the inner ear is less efficient than from behind the ear. The bone-conduction hearing threshold levels are usually 10–15 dB worse with this placement, as indicated when using an audiometer calibrated for mastoid placement of the vibrator (Haughton and Pardoe, 1981; Frank, 1982).

Most bone vibrators which are currently available commercially have a limited capacity to produce undistorted signals. A considerable problem exists with non-linear distortion mainly at low frequencies. In addition, the non-linear mechanical properties of the skull seem to be a possible additional source of distortion (Arlinger, Kylen and Hellqvist, 1978). For these reasons, bone-conduction signal levels in pure-tone audiometers are usually limited to the frequency range from 250 Hz to 4000 or 6000 Hz with levels up to a maximum of 60–70 dB HL, but at 250 Hz they are typically 40 dB HL. Considering the non-linear distortion in the most commonly used vibrator type (Radioear B-71) and human skull, care should be applied in the interpretation of bone-conduction threshold levels worse than 20 dB HL at 250 Hz and 30 dB HL at 500 Hz. At higher levels, there is a significant risk that the listener will hear harmonic distortion products rather than the fundamental, i.e. components with higher frequency than the one selected on the audiometer.

There is a certain risk that sound may be radiated into the surrounding air from the outer surfaces of the vibrator at audible levels (Shipton, John and Robinson, 1980). This weakness constitutes a risk for obtaining too good a test result if the listener hears the air-conducted sound from the vibrator at lower levels than the bone-conducted sound. The problem seems to concern mainly the higher frequency range above 3 kHz. It may be eliminated by the use of a porous ear plug in the external ear canal of the test ear. However, the plug must not be placed in the ear canal when frequencies lower than 3000 Hz are tested because of the occlusion effect.

The methodology in bone-conduction hearing threshold determination is exactly the same as in air-conduction testing. However, to be sure about which ear the listener perceives the test tone to be in, the non-test ear has to be masked by narrow-band noise. This requirement is based on the fact that the interaural attenuation in bone conduction is essentially zero (Nolan and Lyon, 1981).

When bone-conduction hearing thresholds are determined without the use of contralateral masking, the results obtained represent the sensitivity of the best ear; whether this is left or right is, however, not always known reliably. Sometimes information is available to this end, e.g. from the patient's medical records, and then of course the test results are valid. However, the threshold values obtained without masking are on average 2–3 dB better. This is due to the values used for the calibration of bone-conduction audiometers (ISO 7566, 1987) being determined with the use of contralateral masking (Richter and Brinkmann, 1981; Robinson and Shipton, 1982), which gives rise to an average of 2–3 dB of central masking. Since it is usually not known which ear is best, this usually being part of the reason for performing the audiometry, the general rule is that bone-conduction hearing thresholds must be determined with the use of contralateral masking for evaluating a specific ear.

Equipment

Bone-conduction measurements should be performed by means of pure-tone audiometers which fulfil the requirements of IEC 645 (1991) type 1 or 2. The international standard for the calibration of bone-conduction pure-tone levels is ISO 7566 (1987). When calibration is to be performed, the vibrator is placed on a mechanical coupler, sometimes called an artificial mastoid, which offers the vibrator approximately the same mechanical working conditions as when placed on a human skull behind the outer ear. This coupler is standardised in the document IEC 373 (1988). An accelerometer, built into the coupler, generates an electric signal which is a measure of the vibration signal magnitude from the vibrator.

Sources of error and test accuracy

Most sources of errors are common for air- and bone-conduction measurements. However, there are also some differences, which cause the uncertainties of the two signal presentation forms to co-vary only to a limited extent. In ears with normal middle-ear function air- and bone-conduction audiograms coincide on average, i.e. the average air–bone gap is zero. This means that on some of those ears, bone-conduction hearing thresholds are somewhat worse than air-conduction thresholds, whilst on others they are somewhat better. The reason for this is partly that separate sources of error influence the results of air- and bone-conduction testing. Therefore, it is wrong, in principle, to say that a bone-conduction threshold cannot be worse than an air-conduction threshold for the same frequency and ear.

In bone-conduction testing, the test ear should be open to avoid the occlusion effect. When determining bone-conduction thresholds without the use of contralateral masking, the contralateral ear also has to be open. The requirement for an open test ear leads to a higher sensitivity to ambient noise than in air-conduction testing. In the latter case, earphones are always placed on both ears and provide a certain attenuation of ambient sounds. This is the reason for the more stringent requirements on permissible ambient noise levels for bone-conduction testing than for air-conduction testing.

The placement of the vibrator on the listener's skull is a source of error specific to bone-conduction testing. Also, variations in the mechanical characteristics of the skin and the underlying soft tissues contribute to the test uncertainty. Contact between the vibrator or its headband and the outer ear must be avoided, otherwise the pinna may amplify the vibrations giving rise to a significant air-borne component. The risk of an air-borne component, radiated from the outer shell of the vibrator as mentioned previously, is also a possible source of error.

Studies of test–retest reliability in bone-conduction hearing thresholds have shown a somewhat poorer reliability than in air-conduction testings. Standard deviations for single measurements of 3–7 dB and for test–retest difference of 4–10 dB have been found (L. Jerlvall and S.D. Arlinger, unpublished results). Thus, a change or difference in bone-conduction hearing thresholds should be 10–20 dB in order to be statistically significant.

In the same study, test–retest variations of the air–bone gap were also evaluated, because these are often of considerable clinical importance. The standard deviation for single measurements was about 3 dB and for test–

retest difference about 4 dB for a group of normally hearing listeners. However, a group of hearing-impaired subjects showed considerably greater uncertainty with standard deviations for a single air–bone gap determination in the range 5–8 dB and for test–retest difference in the range 7–11 dB. This means that an air–bone gap is significantly larger than zero if it is 15 dB or more and a change in air–bone gap is significant if it exceeds about 20 dB.

Clinical interpretation

The complete pure-tone audiogram provides important information about the type of hearing loss. When air- and bone-conduction curves coincide, i.e. when the air–bone gap is at most 10 dB, this is an indication of the lesion being sensorineural, i.e. localised to the inner ear or higher. If, however, the air–bone gap is significant, i.e. 15 dB or more, this indicates a disturbed middle-ear function – a conductive loss. If both air- and bone-conduction hearing thresholds are outside the normal range, i.e. over 20 dB HL, with air-conduction thresholds significantly poorer than bone-conduction thresholds, a combined hearing loss is present, i.e. the function of both the middle ear and the inner ear and/or higher auditory pathways is abnormal. Figures 5.6–5.9 illustrate some typical air- and bone-conduction audiograms in different types of hearing impairment.

Again it is important to stress that the bone-conduction hearing thresholds, not only reflect the cochlear function, but are also influenced by the state of the middle ear. This is confirmed by the very common finding that bone-conduction hearing thresholds improve after reconstructive middle-ear surgery.

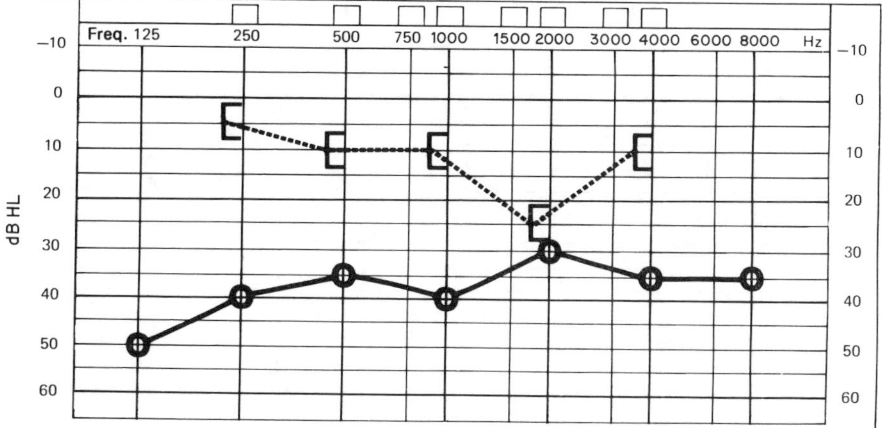

Figure 5.6 Example of air- and bone-conduction pure-tone audiogram in an ear with otosclerosis.

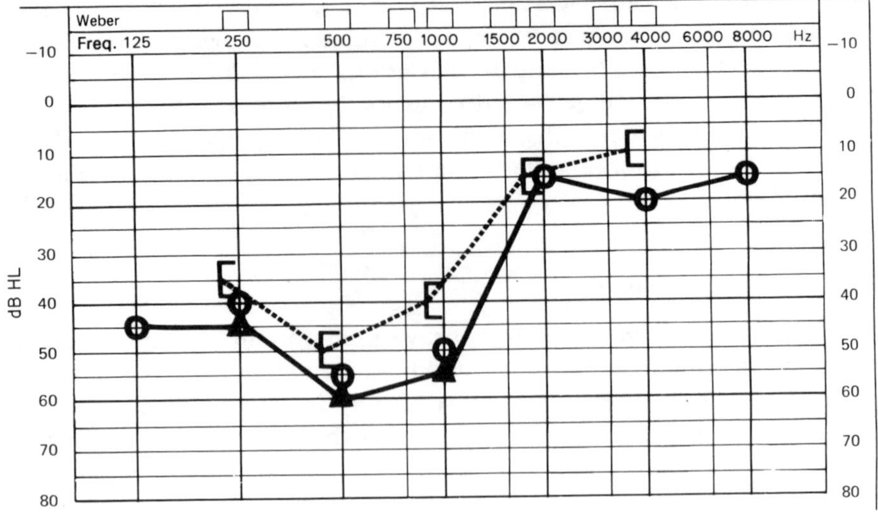

Figure 5.7 Example of air- and bone-conduction pure-tone audiogram for an ear with Menière's disease.

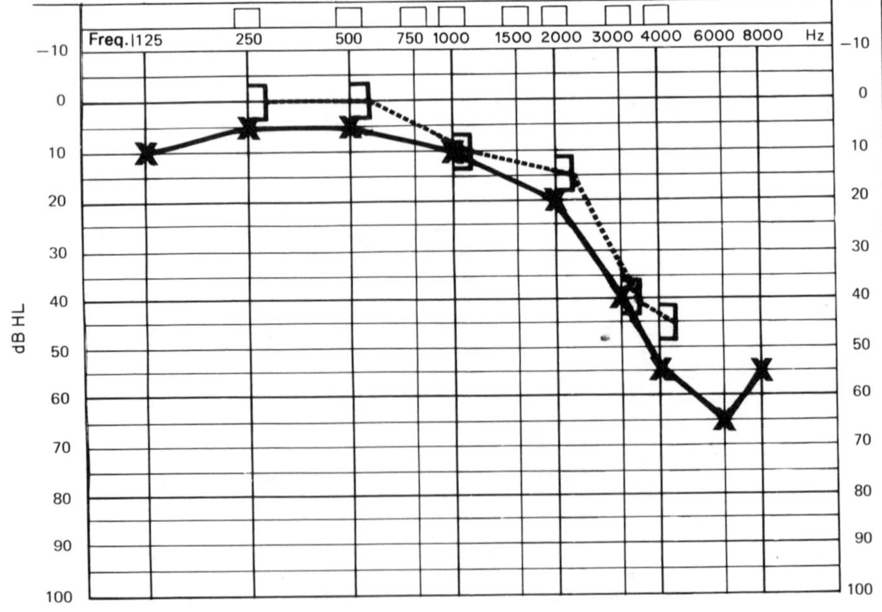

Figure 5.8 Example of air- and bone-conduction pure-tone audiogram for an ear with noise-induced hearing loss.

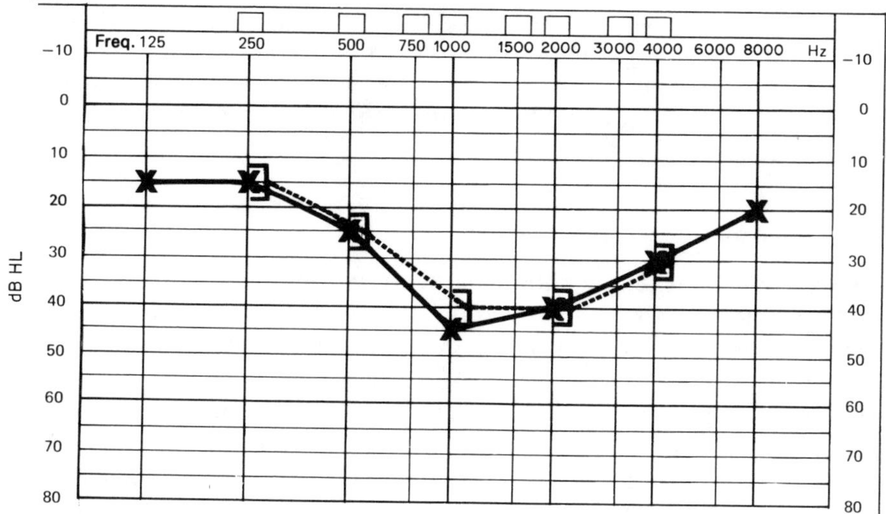

Figure 5.9 Example of air- and bone-conduction pure-tone audiogram for an ear with hereditary sensorineural hearing loss.

A positive occlusion test, i.e. improved hearing thresholds in the lower frequency range (up to and including 1 kHz) when the outer ear is occluded, indicates normal middle-ear function. Thus, if no change in bone-conduction thresholds is seen due to occlusion, this supports the diagnosis of a conductive lesion.

Similarly, a positive Gellé test, i.e. bone-conduction thresholds affected by variations in static air pressure in the ear canal, indicates normal middle-ear conditions whilst a negative Gellé test indicates a conductive disorder.

For both the occlusion test and the Gellé test, it is important to make sure that contralateral masking has been used in the tests, otherwise a negative result may be due to the test tone having been heard in the wrong ear.

If the Weber test results in the low-frequency bone-conducted signals being lateralised to the ear with significantly poorer air-conduction thresholds, this indicates a conductive lesion in that ear. The interpretation of the Weber test at frequencies over 1 kHz is, however, unclear.

Békésy Audiometry

Indication

The Békésy method of self-recording audiometry may be used as an alternative to manual pure-tone audiometry for the determination of hearing thresholds, e.g. in a hearing conservation programme. The test is usually performed at a number of fixed frequencies.

The test is also sometimes used as part of the evaluation of sensorineural or non-organic hearing loss. In such cases, the test is often performed with a sweep frequency.

Psychoacoustics

Békésy (1947) developed the first self-recording audiometer. The test method, where it is used, is based on the automatic reduction of the test tone level as long as the listener indicates that the tone is audible by pressing a switch. As soon as he or she releases the switch, the tone level will increase again. It is always easier to follow an audible tone which is decreasing in level than to detect a previously inaudible tone. The level where the patient indicates that the tone becomes inaudible is therefore always lower than the level at which it returns to audibility. This phenomenon can be termed 'hysteresis'. The test tone level will therefore vary up and down around the hearing threshold between the limits of audibility and inaudibility. A graphic recording will show a zig-zag curve. The hearing threshold level is estimated by calculating the mean value of a number of such turning-points, corresponding to when the listener released or depressed the switch. Since the test procedure is not identical with the procedure used in conventional pure-tone audiometry, the results are not directly comparable. However, the difference is usually small (Erlandsson et al., 1979).

It should be noted that the Békésy procedure is only one of several possible methods for automatic recording of hearing thresholds. The Békésy procedure was relatively simple to accomplish with the technology available in the late 1940s. However, with today's computerised equipment other test procedures can also be automatically controlled.

The distance between the turning-points in the recording (the excursion width) is influenced by the listener's uncertainty close to threshold and his or her ability to detect and react quickly to the changes in test tone level. The excursion width is thus related to the listener's ability to detect small changes in sound level, and thus indirectly related to his or her difference limen for intensity. A reduced excursion width when testing with a continuous test tone is quite a common finding in listeners with cochlear hearing loss and abnormal loudness function (Brunt, 1985).

For a differential diagnosis of cochlear vs retrocochlear lesion, the Békésy audiogram is recorded with the use of pulsed tone first, followed by continuous tone. The recording made by the pulsed tone normally yields results which are quite close to the conventionally determined hearing thresholds. If the patient suffers from abnormal adaptation at the hearing threshold, the Békésy threshold will deteriorate successively during testing when a continuous tone is used. This application of Békésy audiometry can thus be considered a kind of threshold tone decay test. When influence on the test result from adaptation is to be avoided, pulsed test tone should be used.

Equipment

Békésy audiometers may have facilities for testing with fixed frequencies or sweep frequencies and with pulsed or continuous tone. When used for hearing threshold determination only, pulsed tones at fixed frequencies are the preferred combination. For differential diagnostic applications, all facilities are usually required. For correct interpretation of the test results, the rate of change of test tone level is an important characteristic and generally 2.5 dB/s has been used (Brunt, 1985). The step size used for tone level changes is also of importance. Békésy himself originally used a step size of 2 dB, but commercially available equipment generally makes use of much smaller steps and modern equipment is capable of producing a continuous variation in level.

To be able to discover threshold decay when testing at fixed frequencies, the recording should continue for 2–3 minutes at each frequency. When testing with a sweep frequency, rate of frequency change may influence the test result. The usual rate of sweep is one octave per minute.

Sources of error and test accuracy

For this test the correct instruction of the listener is as important as for any other psychoacoustic test. Since the technical construction of the equipment determines the test rate, the method sometimes requires more concentration and endurance by the test subject than manual test methods.

With hearing losses that increase steeply with increasing frequency, the standard rate of change of test tone level and frequency may be insufficient to follow the threshold curve. One way to reduce this problem is to test with the frequency sweep in both positive and negative directions.

Tinnitus may sometimes cause difficulties for the listener to detect the test tone, in particular at higher frequencies when using a continuous tone. When this occurs an abnormally large excursion width may result. The listener may also mistakenly confuse the tinnitus with the test tone and press the subject's switch continuously. The test tone becomes inaudible but the listener hears and responds to the tinnitus, causing the test to show erroneously low threshold values.

When large differences in hearing thresholds exist between the two ears, masking should be used when testing the poorer ear. However, considerable difficulties exist in obtaining correct masking, in particular when testing with sweep frequencies. Not all commercially available Békésy audiometers are equipped with facilities for contralateral masking.

The standard deviation of a single threshold determination using Békésy audiometry has been found to be in the range 2.4–3.4 dB in the frequency range 0.5–6 kHz when using sweep frequencies (Erlandsson et al., 1979). Thus, a change in hearing threshold at a certain frequency for a particular test subject should be 7–10 dB in order to be considered statistically significant at the 5% level.

As is the case for conventional pure-tone audiometry, the Békésy method is sensitive to variations in the individual response criterion of the listener, i.e. how certain of hearing the test tone he or she needs to be before responding. In this respect other automatic test procedures may yield more reliable results.

When using the test method for differential diagnosis, an important part of the evaluation is based on differences in the responses to pulsed and continuous test tones. In pathological cases, this difference is large enough to make the practical test accuracy of a single threshold determination of less importance. However, when using Békésy audiometry for the determination of hearing thresholds or for following changes in thresholds during the course of a disease or treatment, the test accuracy is of course of central importance.

Clinical interpretation

Three characteristics are important in the evaluation of the results of Békésy audiometry:

- The relation between hearing thresholds determined by means of Békésy audiometry and by means of conventional pure-tone audiometry.
- The excursion width of the threshold recording.
- The separation between thresholds for continuous and pulsed test tones.

When used for hearing threshold determination the results are interpreted in the same way as with other methods for threshold determination. The results obtained with pulsed test tones are strongly correlated with those obtained by means of conventional pure-tone audiometry (Erlandsson et al., 1979).

The normal excursion width is 5–15 dB for both continuous and pulsed test tones. When using pulsed tones, the width is usually in the same range in subjects with hearing impairment. However, for continuous test tones, a reduced excursion width is often found in subjects with cochlear hearing loss although normal width also occurs fairly often (Brunt, 1985).

The threshold curve recorded when using a continuous test tone may differ somewhat from that of a pulsed tone (up to 20 dB, continuous usually being worse than pulsed). In cases with retrocochlear hearing loss, the difference may be considerably larger (more than 20 dB). Often the threshold curves coincide at low frequencies and begin to separate in the mid-frequency range. No significance has been found in the frequency at which the separation begins (Brunt, 1985). A reverse tracing, i.e. starting the frequency sweep at the highest test frequency and sweeping downwards, may give additional information. Often the reverse tracing with continuous tone shows increasing separation from the pulsed tone recording at low frequencies, and the normal and the reverse sweeps mirror each other in this respect (Kärjä and Palva, 1970; Palva, Kärjä and Palva, 1970, 1978; Jerger and Jerger, 1974; Palva et al., 1978).

When Békésy audiometry is used for differential diagnosis, the result is often classified in one of five types as shown in Figure 5.10 (Jerger, 1960; Brunt, 1985).

Békésy audiograms of type I occur in normal hearing and in conductive hearing loss, but may occur also in cochlear hearing loss. Type II is common in cochlear hearing loss. Type III or IV indicates retrocochlear hearing loss. Type V is usually found in cases with non-organic hearing loss, e.g. with simulated or aggravated hearing loss.

The sensitivity in diagnosing retrocochlear hearing loss by using this classification system may be estimated as 50–60%. In a study of 363 cases with verified acoustic neuromas, 57% showed pathological Békésy audiograms of type III or IV (Johnson, 1977). For large tumours, the sensitivity was 72% whilst for medium and small tumours it was 47% and 39%, respectively. In several studies, cited by Brunt (1985), with a total of 198 cases of cochlear impairments, such as Menière's disease, acoustic trauma or presbyacusis, all patients had Békésy audiograms of type I or II. Thus, the specificity of this method of classifying Békésy audiograms can be estimated to be close to 100%.

Since the sensitivity in diagnosing retrocochlear lesions is relatively low and the time needed to carry out the testing relatively long, the method has to a large extent been replaced by other faster methods with higher sensitivity, e.g. stapedius reflex thresholds, reflex decay and brain-stem response audiometry.

Loudness Balance Tests

Indication

The methods may be used as part of the diagnostic evaluation of sensorineural hearing loss. The alternating binaural loudness balance (ABLB) test evaluates differences in the loudness function between the two ears at the test frequency. The alternating monaural loudness balance

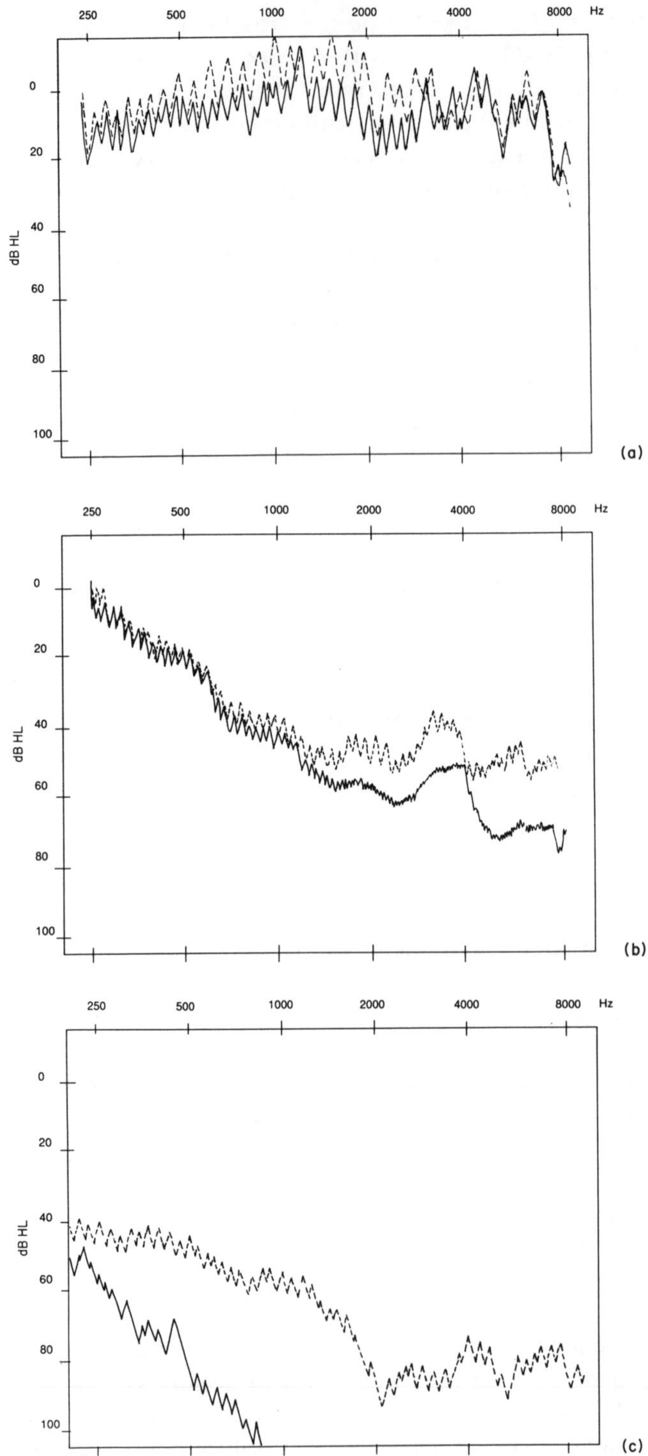
250
500
1000
2000
4000
8000
Hz
0
20
40
60
80
100
dB HL
(a)
250
500
1000
2000
4000
8000
Hz
0
20
40
60
80
100
dB HL
(b)
250
500
1000
2000
4000
8000
Hz
0
20
40
60
80
100
dB HL
(c)

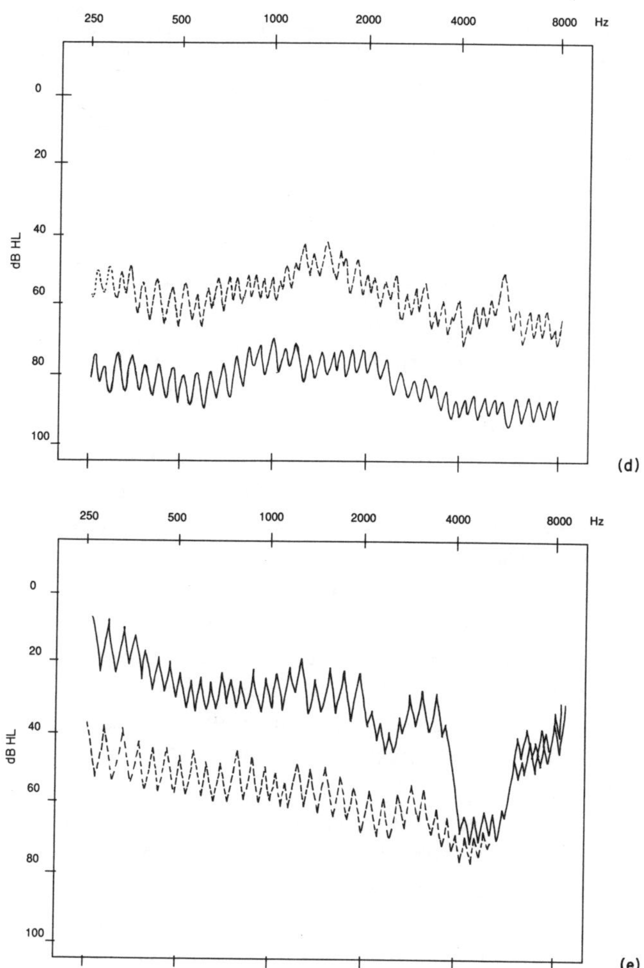

Figure 5.10 Examples of the five different types of Békésy audiograms: (a) type I, (b) type II, (c) type III, (d) type IV, (e) type V. Dashed lines represent pulsed test tone and fully drawn lines continuous test tone.

(AMLB) test evaluates loudness differences between different test frequencies on the same ear. In order to indicate the presence of recruitment of loudness, the loudness function has to be normal on one ear or at one frequency, respectively.

Psychoacoustics and physiology

Loudness balancing is based on two test sounds being presented one after the other, i.e. a two-interval test. One is defined as the reference sound and the other as the test sound. In the binaural test, the reference and the test sounds are presented to different ears. In the monaural test, the reference and the test sound are tones of different frequencies. The listener's task is to decide which of the two sounds is loudest (two-alternative forced choice). Equal loudness for the two sounds is present when the subject chooses the two sounds an equal number of times. A three-alternative variant may also be used where the third response alternative is 'equally loud'. Normal results from loudness balance experiments are internationally standardised (ISO 226, 1987) in the form of isophon curves (see Figure 2.1 in Chapter 2).

Listeners with hearing loss caused only by a middle-ear disorder usually have a normal loudness function. Also, in cases with retrocochlear lesions, it is often within normal limits. However, listeners with a cochlear hearing impairment usually have an abnormally rapid growth of loudness when the sound level is increased above their hearing threshold. Fowler (1937) termed this phenomenon 'recruitment of loudness'. The phenomenon is of considerable practical importance for the hearing-impaired person, especially when a hearing aid is to be fitted and used.

The reduced dynamic range of the impaired inner ear appears in different ways. The loudness discomfort level (LDL) is usually near normal, sometimes even lower than normal, whilst the most comfortable level (MCL) typically shows a moderate elevation in comparison to the hearing threshold shift. Thus, the differences between threshold and MCL and LDL are considerably smaller than normal. A similar reduction in difference holds for the stapedius reflex threshold relative to the hearing threshold. Complex sounds with variations in sound level, such as human speech and music, are also perceived as having abnormally wide ranges in loudness. For wide-band sounds, loudness appears to be influenced in a complex way not only by the sound level but also by the bandwidth in relation to the auditory frequency resolution, which is often abnormal in sensorineural hearing loss.

The physiological mechanism behind the subjective perception of loudness is not clearly understood. A review of the neurophysiological background is given by Phillips (1987). The firing rate, the number of action potentials or impulses per second, in an activated neuron increases with sound level within certain limits. In addition, the number of active neurons increases with increasing sound level, both because different neurons with the same characteristic frequency have different activation thresholds and because other neurons with characteristic frequencies surrounding the test frequency become activated. In addition, the synchronisation of impulse activity in different nerve fibres improves as sound level increases.

It is not clear which of these mechanisms contribute to the abnormal loudness function in cochlear hearing loss. Certain experimental results can be explained by models based on reduced frequency resolution and abnormal growth of nerve activity within each frequency band (Florentine and Zwicker, 1979). A classic hypothesis is based on the fact that the limited frequency resolution of the individual sensory cells has to give rise to an abnormal loudness growth (see Figure 2.4 in Chapter 2). The hearing threshold is reached at that level where the most sensitive hair cell becomes activated. If the sound level is increased somewhat further, many surrounding hair cells will rapidly become activated if their frequency selectivity is poor. If this explanation were correct, the loudness growth for a pure tone should be influenced by masking noise bands on either side of the tone. Results from such experiments indicate, however, that reduced frequency selectivity cannot be the main cause of recruitment of loudness (Moore et al., 1985).

According to another hypothesis, abnormal micromechanical characteristics of the cochlea could give rise to abnormal frequency selectivity as well as loudness growth (Tonndorf, 1980). Both phenomena might be due to a mechanical interaction between the stereocilia of the hair cells and the tectorial membrane. This leads to the cells being unresponsive at low vibration amplitudes of the basilar membrane, but responding with relatively normal activity once the vibration amplitude is large enough to bridge the gap between stereocilia and tectorial membrane.

The evaluation of the results of loudness balance tests assumes that one of the two test sounds which are compared is perceived with relatively normal loudness function. This condition is fulfilled in the ABLB test with two test tones of equal frequency if one ear is within normal limits at this test frequency. In the AMLB test, one of the test tones has to be at a frequency where the hearing threshold and the loudness function are within normal limits.

Equipment

Clinical audiometers often provide facilities for automatic stimulus presentation for the ABLB test. The monaural loudness balance test requires an audiometer with two independent tone oscillators or an additional external oscillator.

Sources of error and test accuracy

The test accuracy of a single loudness balancing of a pair of test tones is determined by the listener's ability to detect small differences in loudness. In addition, the accuracy is influenced by the step size with which the test tone level is varied. If the true balance is exactly in between the two levels tested, the test error will be largest, i.e. equal to half the step size. If the step size is significantly larger than the smallest change in sound level that can be detected by the listener, the accuracy would be unnecessarily poor.

For this reason, Hood (1969, 1977) recommends the use of a step size of 1 or 2 dB when the test tone level to the poorer ear is varied in the ABLB test.

In the clinical application of the test, the easier method is to use a step size of 5 dB. This corresponds to a somewhat large change in loudness when recruitment is present. A change of 5 dB in the normal ear, however, corresponds well to the just detectable change in sound level at low levels. For this reason, some listeners may find it easier to evaluate the difference in loudness if the level is changed in steps of 5 dB in the poorer ear. However, in that case test accuracy would be less than optimal.

Another problem may be that the listener makes a systematic misjudgement, e.g. by overestimating the loudness in the ear where the tone level is varied. The order of presentation and the time interval between the tone presentations could also influence the results. When the requirements on test accuracy are very high, the procedure should be randomised to counterbalance the effects of these sources of error as far as possible.

The corresponding conditions are valid also in monaural loudness balance testing (AMLB). Best accuracy is achieved when the sound level is varied at that test frequency where the hearing is relatively normal if the level is changed in steps of 5 dB.

Clinical interpretation

For clinical evaluation, the test results may be classified into the two main categories of recruitment or absence of recruitment. Recruitment is present if loudness balance is reached at approximately the same sound level in the two ears in spite of one ear having significantly elevated hearing thresholds. Brunt (1985) suggests a more detailed classification with five degrees, which are illustrated in Figure 5.11. The corresponding criteria may be applied to the results of the AMLB test.

Test results of the over-recruitment type (Figure 5.11e) may be seen as an extreme case within the category of complete recruitment (Figure 5.11a), indicating a cochlear hearing loss. Similarly, results of the decruitment type may be considered as a variant of no recruitment (Figure 5.11b), indicating retrocochlear hearing loss in cases of sensorineural lesions.

When loudness balance testing is used for the purpose of diagnosing retrocochlear lesions, its sensitivity has been estimated to be around 50%. Johnson (1977) found results of the no recruitment type in 50% of a total of 171 cases with verified acoustic tumours, the sensitivity being poorer for small tumours. Among patients with large tumours, 72% of the patients showed no recruitment while only 37% of the cases with medium and 24% of those with small tumours yielded this result. Other studies show sensitivity figures in the range 33–90% (Brunt, 1985).

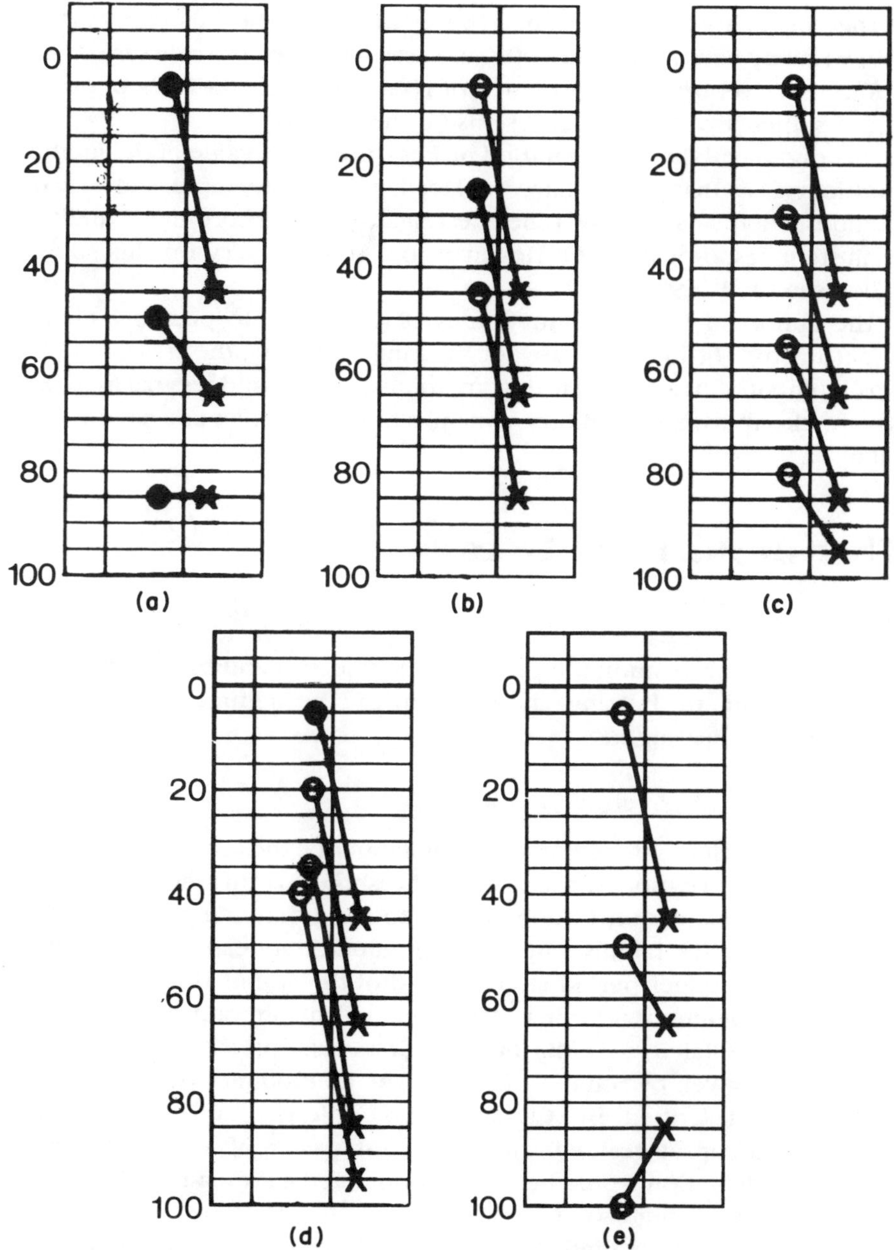

Figure 5.11 Illustration of classification of the results from the ABLB test: (a) complete recruitment – loudness balance is obtained at the same hearing level ± 10 dB whilst the difference close to threshold exceeded 30 dB. (b) No recruitment – loudness balance is obtained at the same sensation level ± 10 dB. (c) Partial recruitment – in between the results in (a) and (b). (d) Under-recruitment – equal loudness is achieved at a clearly higher sensation level in the poorer ear. (e) Over-recruitment – loudness balance is obtained at clearly lower hearing level in the poorer ear.

The specificity of the test may be estimated to be 70–100%. Hood (1969) found recruitment in 100% of cases with Menière's disease. Other studies have reported the presence of recruitment in 73–85% of groups of test subjects with cochlear lesions (Brunt, 1985).

The low sensitivity of the method makes the clinical value of the method questioned by many who have replaced it by more rapid and reliable methods, such as stapedius reflex testing, and the recording of auditory brain-stem responses (ABR). However, opinions do vary on this subject (Thomsen et al., 1981).

The abnormal loudness function is of considerable practical clinical value in the fitting and use of hearing aids. In the research and development of hearing aid fitting, methods such as loudness balance tests which take the whole auditory dynamic range into account have a clear value.

Threshold Tone Decay

Indication

The test is used to study the presence of abnormal auditory adaptation at the threshold of hearing. It is used in the clinical evaluation of sensorineural hearing loss.

Physiology and psychoacoustics

Sound stimulation of long duration may influence the auditory function by a gradual deterioration of the hearing threshold – a threshold decay. This is a form of adaptation (Hood, 1956) to be differentiated from fatigue. Adaptation ceases rapidly once the stimulus disappears whereas fatigue remains for a longer period after the end of the stimulation.

The phenomenon was first described in the literature more than a century ago (Raleigh, 1882) but the first description of a clinical test method was given by Schubert (1944). The method most commonly used today was described by Carhart (1957). Jerger and Jerger (1975) presented a suprathreshold adaptation test, assuming that symptoms of abnormal adaptation would be most pronounced after loading the auditory sense organ with high sound levels.

The mechanisms behind threshold decay are not clearly known. What is known is that the more the auditory nerve is damaged, the more rapid the threshold decay and the wider the frequency range engaged. Comparisons have been made with similar phenomena which affect peripheral nerves that are partly disabled through the action of anaesthesia. When stimulated, the first nerve impulses are transmitted in a normal way but, on continuous stimulation, the firing rate is reduced because of the abnormally prolonged recovery of the individual neurons after each action potential (Davis, 1962).

In some cases only a moderate change in auditory threshold is found, but the listener reports a change in character of the test tone. This might be due to the spread of excitation on the basilar membrane to areas with relatively intact nerve supplies with stable and normal firing characteristics (Green, 1985). Deficiencies in the supply of neurochemical transmitters may also be a possible mechanism (Ylikoski and Lehtosalo, 1985).

Equipment

A pure-tone audiometer of type 1 or 2 as specified in IEC 645 (1991) is used. The importance of continuous stimulation without any interruption of the test tone is stressed in several reports (e.g. Sörensen, 1962). Thus, no interruption should be allowed when the test tone level is changed. On some modern digital audiometers, however, the test tone is automatically switched off for a few hundred milliseconds when a change in attenuator setting is made. This may affect the test result.

Some audiometers have a special programme for the tone decay test which then provides continuous stimulation. This programme setting may lock the level of a contralateral masking noise. If this is the case, it is important to set the masking noise level high enough to provide sufficient masking for a tone decay of up to 40 dB. On some audiometers, the easiest solution might be to connect a special attenuator, with impedance matched to the earphones and with 5-dB step size and 40-dB range, to one of the earphone outputs.

Sources of error and test accuracy

As pointed out above, any interruption of the test tone is a possible source of error. If it occurs by accident, the test should be repeated from the beginning after letting the patient rest for a few minutes. Since the test usually is part of a larger test battery, due regard has to be given to the patient's need for rest after a preceding test before starting a decay test.

When masking is used and its level has to be increased, it is important to increase the masking level before the test tone level is increased to make sure that the patient does not respond to the change in noise level.

Tinnitus may be a source of confusion for many patients, in particular when tonal in character and within the frequency range being tested.

The threshold tone decay test has a relatively high sensitivity to detect retrocochlear lesions – 90% according to Reimer (1987). However, the specificity is lower and false positive results may thus occur to a considerable extent. Test–retest reproducibility has been measured in an unpublished study. The standard deviation for test–retest difference was found to be about 9 dB on a group of subjects with cochlear hearing loss and about 4 dB on subjects with normal hearing.

Clinical interpretation

A threshold tone decay of up to 5 dB is considered negligible, between 10 and 25 dB moderate, and 30 dB or more pathological. The test is most sensitive at high frequencies. If no decay is found at 2 kHz, lower test frequencies may often be omitted. The combination of pathological decay at 2 kHz, but no decay at 500 Hz and 1 kHz, is not uncommon and is difficult to interpret. The lower the test frequency at which pathological decay is found, the stronger the indication of a retrocochlear lesion. For this reason, and because high test tone levels are often needed, test frequencies of 4 kHz and higher are not used.

Threshold tone decay of 30 dB or more is considered as an indicator of retrocochlear hearing loss. The most common diagnosis is acoustic neuroma (Johnson, 1968), but also other causes occur, e.g. nerve degeneration, inflammatory processes, trauma etc. (Johnson, 1966).

It is quite common for the listener to perceive a change in tone quality during the continuous stimulation. The tone may be perceived as atonal, metallic or otherwise distorted. Some authors consider such changes to be most common in retrocochlear disease (Green, 1985). Therefore, such changes should be noted at the time of testing.

Sound Localisation

Indications

Directional hearing can be studied by means of sound localisation in a free sound field and phase audiometry. These tests may be used in the evaluation of sensorineural hearing loss and suspected brain-stem lesions, i.e. they have both audiological and neurological applications.

A drawback with the sound localisation test in a free sound field is the need for an anechoic room. The test requires several measurements and requires a long test time. Phase audiometry is much more rapid but gives the patient a difficult task.

Physiology and psychoacoustics (Figure 5.12)

In humans, directional hearing in the horizontal plane is of most importance. The basic acoustic factors that enable directional hearing are the following:

- Interaural intensity difference.
- Interaural time or phase difference.

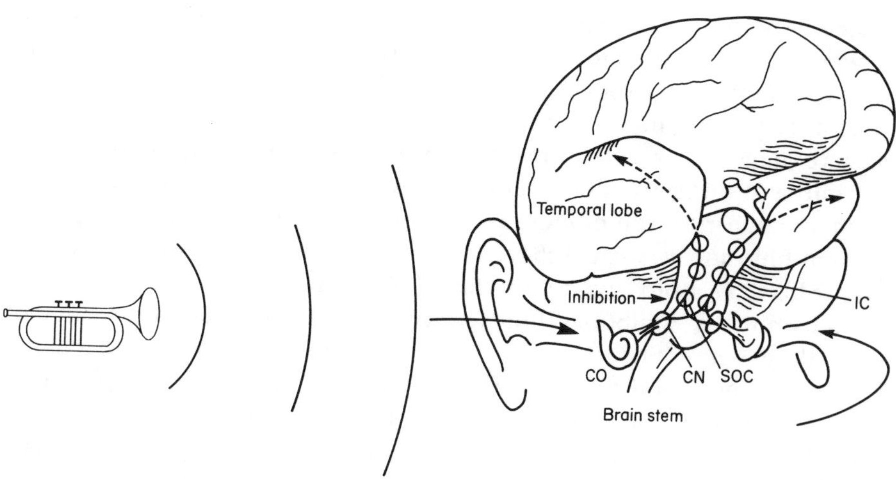

Figure 5.12 Schematic illustration of the auditory pathways and the physiological background for directional hearing. The sound excites the cochlea, auditory nerve and brain-stem pathways. The impulse flow travels via the cochlear nuclei (CN) and superior olive (SOC) across the lateral lemniscus and inferior colliculus (IC) to the primary auditory projection areas in the cortex. The sound is assumed to reach the right ear first and is somewhat delayed to the left ear. A fusion of the left and right information occurs in the superior olive in the brain stem.

In addition, the listener may make use of the following characteristics (Searle et al., 1976):

- Monaural spectral variations due to head shadow.
- Interaural spectral differences caused by the frequency-dependent acoustic characteristics of the pinna.
- Monaural spectral variations due to the frequency-dependent characteristics of the pinna.
- Spectral variations due to sound reflected by the shoulders.

The interaural intensity difference is based on the sound reaching the ear that is turned towards the source at a somewhat higher level than the other ear, which is in the acoustic shadow of the head. This intensity difference occurs for sounds whose wavelength is smaller than the width of the human head. Therefore, it is of significance only at frequencies above about 1 kHz.

The interaural time difference is due to the difference in travelling distance for the sound from its source to the two ears. The maximum time difference is about 0.7 ms, occurring when the sound comes directly to one side. This time difference is utilised mainly for low frequency sounds. At higher frequencies, above about 1.4 kHz, the time difference may exceed one period. When seen as a phase difference for a periodic sound, it would then be ambiguous and unreliable as a basis for the perception of the direction of a sound source.

In a free sound field the ability to localise a sound source is better for low-frequency sounds than for high-frequency sounds (Nordlund, 1964).

Time and intensity differences activate the superior olive in the brain stem. Excitatory and inhibitory signals interact to coordinate the information on time and intensity differences. Nerve cells in the superior olive are controlled by both excitatory fibres from the contralateral cochlear nucleus and by inhibitory fibres from the ipsilateral cochlear nucleus. Ascending nerve fibres transmit the information higher up to centres where the interaural time and intensity differences become represented by the activity in specific nerve cells. Such cells which are sensitive to a specific interaural time difference have been found in animal experiments (Moller, 1983). The activity in such cells form the basis for the perception of direction to a sound source (Hall, 1965). Intensity and time differences may partly be used independently.

The superior olive complex is the first station in the brain stem that receives binaural information. A brain-stem lesion at the level of the superior olive or somewhat higher in the pons may disturb the directional hearing ability. Since it depends on an intact and exactly timed information from the inner ears, it is also sensitive to disorders in the first (auditory nerve) or second order neurons. However, a purely peripheral lesion in the cochlea does not disturb the analysis of interaural time differences to any large extent. Directional hearing, however, may be influenced by a peripheral hearing loss which is large enough to affect the possibilities for making use of interaural intensity differences (Rosenhall, 1985).

For cortical lesions the situation is more complex. In such cases the binaural fusion taking place in the brain stem is not disturbed. Some cortical lesions, mainly in the temporal lobe, may still influence the patient's spatial orientation, which may affect directional hearing.

When testing directional hearing in a free sound field, test sounds are presented from different directions in the horizontal plane. The patient's task is to identify the perceived direction on an angular scale in the room.

In phase audiometry, the smallest detectable interaural time difference is determined. The patient listens dichotically by means of earphones. The signal to one earphone is delayed and the patient's task is to lateralise the sound. After each stimulus he or she has to say whether the sound was heard displaced to the left or to the right.

In trials with only two alternative responses, the probability for guessing the correct one is 50%. Therefore, the interaural time difference threshold is usually defined as that which the listener hears correctly at 75% of the trials. Phase audiometry may also be performed as a screening procedure, using a predetermined interaural time difference selected for a value that provides correct lateralisation for normally hearing listeners in essentially 100% of all trials.

Equipment

A test of directional hearing in a free sound field has to be carried out in an anechoic room. Low frequency sounds are used such as 500-Hz tone pulses, low-pass filtered noise with a cut-off frequency of about 1 kHz or band-pass filtered noise around 500 Hz. The test sound is presented from a loudspeaker that can be moved to different positions and is invisible behind a screen. In front of the screen, an angular scale is clearly visible. The true position of the loudspeaker can be read electronically from outside the anechoic room. Another method is to use several loudspeakers with fixed positions. Since slight differences in electroacoustic characteristics between such loudspeakers usually occur, this may aid the listener in identifying the active loudspeaker and thus affect the test reliability.

The same type of stimulus sound should be used for phase audiometry as for directional audiometry in a free sound field. The sound is presented dichotically via earphones and with adjustable interaural time difference. Time differences in the range from 0 to 500 μs (microseconds) should be available. The sound levels to the two earphones must be individually adjustable. Currently, there is a lack of standardised equipment for phase audiometry.

Phase audiometry can be performed in an ordinary audiometric test room. The stimulus level is set to the listener's most comfortable level, i.e. about 60 dB HL or higher. Thus, the requirements of ambient sound levels in the test room are very moderate.

For pure tones in the low frequency range a time difference can always be expressed as a phase difference with the relation:

$$\text{Phase difference (in angular degrees)} = \text{Time difference (in } \mu\text{s)} \times \text{frequency (kHz)} \times 0.36$$

For a 500-Hz tone one angular degree corresponds to 5.56 μs.

Sources of error and test accuracy

Being psychoacoustic test methods, both methods used assume good cooperation by the patient. The localisation test in a free sound field is an identification test and the instructions are straightforward and easy to understand. The test requires relatively good hearing thresholds in the low frequency range. Two types of test results may be obtained: one is the spread, expressed as the standard deviation of the errors in the patient's responses; the other is the mean of the errors in the responses. Clinically, the former, i.e. the standard deviation, is of the greatest importance.

Test reliability data in sound localisation tests have not been reported.

Assuming that the standard deviation determined for the errors in the directional responses is based on 20 trials, the reliability (standard deviation) of a single measurement can be estimated, on theoretical grounds, to be approximately 16% of the measured standard deviation. Two test results from the same subject should differ by at least 28% of the larger of the two values for the difference to be statistically significant ($P<0.05$).

Phase audiometry is a detection test which puts great demands on the listener's cooperation. Small interaural time differences are difficult to detect because the listening situation and the test sounds do not represent a very normal listening task. The aim of the test is to determine the smallest detectable interaural time difference.

The test reliability is influenced to a large degree by the type of test procedure used. The statistical variation in the test results may vary between methods, and systematic differences may also occur. Therefore, results and normal data obtained with different procedures cannot always be compared.

In a clinical variant of phase audiometry (Nilsson and Lidén, 1976), an automatic descending procedure can be used. Starting with a large time difference, this is reduced in steps of first 10 μs and later 5 μs, as long as the listener's lateralisation remains correct. The threshold is defined as that time difference at which the listener gives an erroneous response three times when the delay is presented to the same ear. The test accuracy of the method has not been reported. However, individual results from repeated measurements on 10 normally hearing subjects have been reported (Nilsson and Lidén, 1976). From these results the accuracy can be analysed but a learning effect seems to exist. The threshold value measured improved on average 13 μs during the course of six measurements. This improvement was significant ($P<0.05$). The intra-individual standard deviation (for the last three measurements) was 13 μs. Two test results obtained on the same subject, therefore, should differ by at least 36 μs in order for the difference to be statistically significant ($P<0.05$).

Clinical interpretation

For sound localisation in a free sound field, normative data based on 51 listeners of various age with normal hearing or noise-induced hearing loss have been reported (Nordlund, 1964). Later, data from another 100 normally hearing subjects in the age range 15–35 years were published (Nilsson et al., 1973). The standard deviation of the target pattern was on average 2.3 angular degrees. An upper limit for normal results of 12 angular degrees was proposed in both reports. This limit corresponds to the mean plus three standard deviations. In some cases, the patient may always lateralise the test sound to one side. Such a result must of course be considered pathological, although the variation may be small.

The average normal interaural time difference threshold has been found to be 17 μs for 500-Hz pure tones, 14 μs for a noise band in the range 425–600 Hz, and 11 μs for a series of clicks (Klump and Eady, 1956). These measurements were made on nine normally hearing subjects. The threshold was defined as the 75% level of the psychometric function on two alternative trials.

For the clinical variant of phase audiometry studied by Nilsson and Lidén (1976), normal data for 500-Hz pure tones have been presented, based on 60 young subjects. The average interaural time difference threshold for this particular procedure was 48 μs with a standard deviation within the group of about 20 μs. An upper limit for normality was set to 105 μs (mean plus three standard deviations). Häller (1977) found an average normal threshold of 20 μs as measured on 10 normally hearing subjects. The large difference in mean value between the two studies is probably due to the different test procedures and threshold criteria used.

Using the procedure and upper limit of normality suggested by Nilsson and Lidén (1976), the sensitivity of phase audiometry for diagnosing acoustic tumours has been determined as 78% (Lidén and Rosenhall, 1985). To allow a meaningful interpretation, no significant hearing loss should be present on any ear at 500 Hz. The specificity of the test is 91% if the hearing thresholds at 500 Hz do not exceed 35 dB and 83% if not exceeding 40 dB. At the worst 500-Hz thresholds, the interpretation of the result from phase audiometry becomes very unreliable (Rosenhall, 1985). This is probably true for both conductive and sensorineural hearing losses. Hearing impairment at frequencies above 500 Hz is of no importance for the test result. Therefore, patients with a large high-frequency hearing loss may be successfully tested.

References

ARLINGER, S.D. (1979). Comparison of ascending and bracketing methods in pure tone audiometry. *Scandinavian Audiology* **8**, 247–251.

ARLINGER, S.D. (1986). Sound attenuation of TDH-39 earphones in a diffuse field of narrow-band noise. *Journal of the Acoustical Society of America* **79**, 189–191.

ARLINGER, S.D., KYLEN, P. and HELLQVIST, H. (1978). Skull distortion of bone conducted signals. *Acta Oto-Laryngologica* **85**, 318–323.

BAOL/BSA (1983). BAOL/BSA method for assessment of hearing disability. *British Journal of Audiology* **17**, 203–212.

BÉKÉSY, G. VON (1947). A new audiometer. *Acta Oto-Laryngologica* **35**, 411–422.

BRUNT, M.A. (1985). Békésy audiometry and loudness balance testing. In: Katz, J. (Ed.) *Handbook of Audiology*, 3rd edn, pp. 273–291. Baltimore: Williams & Wilkins.

CARHART, R. (1950). Clinical application of bone conduction audiometry. *Archives of Otolaryngology* **51**, 798–808.

CARHART, R. (1957). Clinical determination of abnormal auditory adaptation. *Archives of Otolaryngology* **65**, 32–39.

CARHART, R. and JERGER, J. (1959). Preferred method for clinical determination of pure-tone thresholds. *Journal of Speech and Hearing Disorders* **24**, 330–345.

DAVIS, H. (1962). A functional classification of auditory defects. *Annals of Otology, Rhinology and Laryngology* **7**, 693–704.

DIRKS, D. and SWINDEMAN, J.G. (1967). The variability of occluded and unoccluded bone-conduction thresholds. *Journal of Speech and Hearing Research* **10**, 232–249.

EDGERTON, B.J. and KLODD, D.A. (1977). Occlusion effect in bone conduction pure tone and speech audiometry. *Journal of the American Auditory Society* **2**, 151–158.

ERLANDSSON, B., HÅKANSSON, H., IVARSSON, A. and NILSSON, P. (1979). Comparison of the hearing threshold measured by manual pure-tone and by self-recording (Békésy) audiometry. *Audiology* **18**, 414–429.

ERLANDSSON, B., HÅKANSSON, H., IVARSSON, A. and NILSSON, P. (1980). The reliability of Békésy sweep audiometry recording and effects of the earphone position. *Acta Oto-Laryngologica Supplementum* **366**, 99–112.

FAUSTI, S.A., FREY, R.H., ERICKSON, D.A., RAPPAPORT, B.Z., CLEARY, E.J. and BRUMMETT, R.E. (1979). A system for evaluating auditory function from 8000 to 20000 Hz. *Journal of the Acoustical Society of America* **66**, 1713–1718.

FLORENTINE, M. and ZWICKER, E. (1979). A model of loudness summation applied to noise-induced hearing loss. *Hearing Research* **1**, 121–132.

FOWLER, E.P. (1937). The diagnosis of diseases of the neural mechanism of hearing by the aid of sounds well above threshold. *Transactions of the American Otological Society* **27**, 207–219.

FRANK, T. (1982). Forehead versus mastoid threshold differences with a circular tipped vibrator. *Ear and Hearing* **3**, 91–92.

GOLDSTEIN, D.P. and HAYES, C.S. (1965). The occlusion effect in bone conduction hearing. *Journal of Speech and Hearing Research* **8**, 137–148.

GREEN, D.S. (1985). Tone decay. In: Katz, J. (Ed.) *Handbook of Clinical Audiology*, 3rd edn, pp. 304–318. Baltimore: Williams & Wilkins.

HALL, J.L. (1965). Binaural interaction in the accessory superior-olivary nucleus of the cat. *Journal of the Acoustical Society of America* **37**, 814–823.

HÄLLER, U. (1977). Construction of an automatic phase audiometer (in Swedish). *Technical Report*, Department of Biomedical Engineering, University of Linköping.

HAUGHTON, P.M. and PARDOE, K. (1981). Normal pure tone thresholds for hearing by bone conduction. *British Journal of Audiology* **15**, 113–121.

HOOD, J.R. (1956). Fatigue and adaptation of hearing. *British Medical Bulletin* **112**, 125–130.

HOOD, J.D. (1969). Basic audiologic requirements in neuro-otology. *Journal of Laryngology and Otology* **83**, 695–711.

HOOD, J.D. (1977). Loudness balance procedures for the measurement of recruitment. *Audiology* **16**, 215–228.

HOSFORD-DUNN, H., KUKLINSKI, A.L., RAGGIO, M. and HAGGERTY, S. (1986). Solving audiometric masking dilemmas with an insert masker. *Archives of Otolaryngology Head and Neck Surgery* **112**, 92–95.

IEC 303 (1970). *IEC Provisional Coupler for the Calibration of Earphones Used in Audiometry.* Geneva: International Electrotechnical Commission.

IEC 318 (1970). *An IEC Artificial Ear, of the Wide Band Type, for the Calibration of Earphones Used in Audiometry.* Geneva: International Electrotechnical Commission.

IEC 373 (1988). *Mechanical Coupler for Measurements of Bone Vibrators.* Geneva: International Electrotechnical Commission.

IEC 645 (1991). *Audiometers. Part 1: Pure tone audiometers.* Geneva: International Electrotechnical Commission.

ISO 226 (1987). *Acoustics – Normal equal-loudness level contours.* Geneva: International Standards Organisation.

ISO 389, ADDENDUM 1 (1983). *Acoustics – Standard Reference Zero for the Calibration of Pure Tone Air Conduction Audiometers.* Geneva: International Standards Organisation.

ISO 389 (1985). *Acoustics – Standard Reference Zero for the Calibration of Pure Tone Air Conduction Audiometers.* Geneva: International Standards Organisation.

ISO 6189 (1983). *Acoustics – Pure Tone Air Conduction Threshold Audiometry for Hearing Conservation Purposes.* Geneva: International Standards Organisation.

ISO 7566 (1987). *Acoustics – Standard Reference Zero for the Calibration of Pure-tone Bone Conduction Audiometers.* Geneva: International Standards Organisation.

ISO 8253 (1989). *Acoustics – Audiometric Test Methods, Part 1: Basic Pure Tone Air and Bone Conduction Threshold Audiometry.* Geneva: International Standards Organisation.

ISO 8798 (1987). *Acoustics – Reference Levels for Narrow-Band Masking.* Geneva: International Standards Organisation.

JERGER, J. (1960). Békésy audiometry in analysis of auditory disorders. *Journal of Speech and Hearing Research* **3**, 275–287.

JERGER, J. and JERGER, S. (1974). Audiological comparison of cochlear and eighth nerve disorders. *Annals of Otology, Rhinology and Laryngology* **83**, 275–285.

JERGER, J. and JERGER, S. (1975). A simplified tone decay test. *Archives of Otolaryngology* **101**, 403–407.

JERLVALL, L. and ARLINGER, S. (1986). A comparison of 2 and 5 dB step size in pure tone audiometry. *Scandinavian Audiology* **15**, 51–56.

JERLVALL, L., DRYSELIUS, H. and ARLINGER, S. (1983). Comparison of manual and computer-controlled audiometry using identical procedures. *Scandinavian Audiology* **12**, 209–213.

JOHNSON, E.W. (1966). Confirmed retrocochlear lesions. *Archives of Otolaryngology* **84**, 247–254.

JOHNSON, E.W. (1968). Auditory findings in 200 cases of acoustic neuromas. *Archives of Otolaryngology* **88**, 598–603.

JOHNSON, E.W. (1977). Auditory test results in 500 cases of acoustic neuromas. *Archives of Otolaryngology* **103**, 152–158.

KÄRJÄ, J. and PALVA, A. (1970). Reverse frequency-sweep Békésy audiometry. *Acta Oto-Laryngologica Supplementum* **263**, 225–228.

KILLION, M.C., WILBER, L.A. and GUDMUNDSEN, G.I. (1985). Insert earphones for more interaural attenuation. *Hearing Instruments* **36**(2), 34–36.

KLOCKHOFF, I., DRETTNER, B., HAGELIN, K.W. and LINDHOLM, L. (1973). A method for computerized classification of pure tone screening audiometry results in noise exposed groups. *Acta Oto-Laryngologica* **75**, 339–340.

KLUMP, R.G. and EADY, D.R. (1956). Some measurements of interaural time difference thresholds. *Journal of the Acoustical Society of America* **28**, 859–860.

LIDÉN, G. and ROSENHALL, U. (1985). New dimensions in the assessment of auditory function. Special tests I. In: Myers, E. (Ed.) *New Dimensions in Otolaryngology – Head and Neck Surgery*, Volume I, pp. 174–177. Amsterdam: Elsevier.

LIDÉN, G., NILSSON, G. and ANDERSSON, H. (1959). Narrow-band masking with white noise. *Acta Oto-Laryngologica* **50**, 116–124.

MICHAEL, P.L. and BIENVENUE, G.R. (1981). Noise attenuation characteristics for supra-aural audiometric headsets using the models MX-41/AR and 51 earphone cushions. *Journal of the Acoustical Society of America* **70**, 1235–1238.

MOLLER, A. (1983). *Auditory Physiology.* New York: Academic Press.

MOORE, B.C.J., GLASBERG, B.R., HESS, R.F. and BIRCHALL, J.P. (1985). Effects of flanking noise bands on the rate of growth of loudness of tones in normal and recruiting ears. *Journal of the Acoustical Society of America* 77, 1505–1513.

NILSSON, R. and LIDÉN, G. (1976). Sound localization with phase audiometry. *Acta Oto-Laryngologica* **81**, 291–299.

NILSSON, R., LIDÉN, G., ROSÉN, M. and ZÖLLER, M. (1973). Directional hearing, three different methods. *Scandinavian Audiology* **2**, 125–131.

NOLAN, M. and LYON, D.J. (1981). Transcranial attenuation in bone conduction audiometry. *Journal of Laryngology and Otology* **95**, 597–608.

NORDLUND, B. (1964). Directional audiometry. *Acta Oto-Laryngologica* **57**, 1–18.

PALVA, T., KÄRJÄ, J. and PALVA, A. (1970). Forward vs. reversed Békésy tracings. *Archives of Otolaryngology* **9**, 449–452.

PALVA, T., JAUHIAINEN, T., SJÖBLOM, J. and YLIKOSKI, J. (1978). Diagnosis and surgery of acoustic tumours. *Acta Oto-Laryngologica* **86**, 233–240.

PEDERSEN, C.B. and SALOMON, G. (1977). Temporal integration of acoustic energy. *Acta Oto-Laryngologica* **83**, 417–423.

PHILLIPS, D.P. (1987). Stimulus intensity and loudness recruitment: neural correlates. *Journal of the Acoustical Society of America* **82**, 1–12.

OSTERHAMMEL, D. and OSTERHAMMEL, P. (1979). High-frequency audiometry. Age and sex variations. *Scandinavian Audiology* **8**, 73–81.

RAYLEIGH, L. (1882). Acoustical observations. IV. *Philosophical Magazine* **13**, Series 5, 340–347.

REIMER, Å. (1987). Quantitative interpretation of audiological test battery. I. *Scandinavian Audiology* **16**, 101–108.

RICHTER, U. and BRINKMANN, K. (1981). Threshold of hearing by bone conduction. *Scandinavian Audiology* **10**, 235–237.

ROBINSON, D.W. and SHIPTON, M.S. (1982). A standard determination of paired air- and bone-conduction thresholds under different masking conditions. *Audiology* **21**, 61–82.

ROBINSON, D.W., SHIPTON, M.S. and HINCHCLIFFE, R. (1981). Audiometric zero for air conduction. *Audiology* **20**, 409–431.

ROESER, R.J. and GLORIG, A. (1975). Pure tone audiometry in noise with Auraldomes. *Audiology* **14**, 144–151.

ROSENHALL, U. (1985). The influence of hearing loss on directional hearing. *Scandinavian Audiology* **14**, 187–189.

SCHUBERT, K. (1944). Hörermudung und Hördauer. *Hals-, Nasen- und Ohrenheilkunde* **51**, 41–46.

SEARLE, C.L., BRAIDA, L.D., DAVIS, M.F. and COLBURN, H.S. (1976). Model for auditory localization. *Journal of the Acoustical Society of America* **60**, 1164–1175.

SHIPTON, M.S., JOHN, A.J. and ROBINSON, D.W. (1980). Air-radiated sound from bone vibration transducers and its implications for bone conduction audiometry. *British Journal of Audiology* **14**, 86–99.

SÖRENSEN, H. (1962). Clinical application of continuous threshold recording. *Acta Oto-Laryngologica* **54**, 403–422.

THOMSEN, J., NYBOE, J., BORUM, P., TOS, M. and BARFOED, C. (1981). Acoustic neuromas. *Archives of Otolaryngology* **107**, 601–607.

TONNDORF, J. (1976). Bone conduction. In: Keidel, W.D. and Neff, W.D. (Eds.) *Handbook of Sensory Physiology*, Vol. V/3. Berlin: Springer-Verlag.

TONNDORF, J. (1980). Acute cochlear disorders: the combination of hearing loss, recruitment, poor speech discrimination and tinnitus. *Annals of Otology, Rhinology and Laryngology* **89**, 353–358.

WARD, W.D. (1983). The American Medical Association/American Academy of Otolaryngology formula for determination of hearing handicap. *Audiology* **22**, 313–324.

YLIKOSKI, J. and LEHTOSALO, J. (1985). Neurochemical basis of auditory fatigue – a new hypothesis. *Acta Oto-Laryngologica* **99**, 353–363.

ZWISLOCKI, J. (1953). Acoustic attenuation between the ears. *Journal of the Acoustical Society of America* **25**, 752–759.

Chapter 6 Psychoacoustic Methods using Speech Stimuli

Out of 12 different speech audiometric methods which are presented in Volume 1, only those of most practical clinical importance will be discussed here. Under the heading 'Routine speech audiometry' speech recognition threshold, maximum speech recognition score and uncomfortable loudness level for speech are discussed. In addition, distorted speech audiometry is included because of its special applications in the diagnosis of central auditory lesions.

Routine Speech Audiometry

Indication

Speech recognition threshold, maximum speech recognition score and uncomfortable loudness level for speech are routine tests in audiological evaluations as well as in hearing aid fitting and evaluation before and after middle-ear surgery.

Physiology and psychoacoustics

The ability to recognise speech is one of the most important functions of the auditory system. The auditory sense organ has its best sensitivity to sounds in the frequency range that corresponds to human speech. The measurement of speech recognition threshold and of maximum speech recognition score are therefore meaningful tests to quantify social communication ability.

The most important frequency range in the speech spectrum is about 0.5–4 kHz. Voiced speech sounds are generated in the larynx by the vibrations of the vocal folds. The periodicity of the vibrations of the vocal folds, the fundamental frequency, is in the range 100–150 Hz for a male voice and 200–300 Hz for a female. Acoustic resonances in the pharyngeal and nasal cavities and the mouth filter the sound that is generated in the larynx. Certain bands of harmonics are amplified by these resonance phenomena. Such bands are called formants and they give rise to spectral patterns that are characteristic for different voiced speech sounds, in particular vowels (Wright, 1987). In general, consonants have more of their energy in the higher frequency range whereas vowels dominate the low and mid-frequency range. Since hearing impairments are usually more pronounced in the high frequency range, consonant recognition is typically affected more by a hearing loss than vowel recognition (Figure 6.1).

Speech recognition threshold (SRT)

The purpose of the test is to determine the speech level at which 50% of the presented speech material is correctly recognised by the test subject. Usually, isolated bisyllabic test words are used.

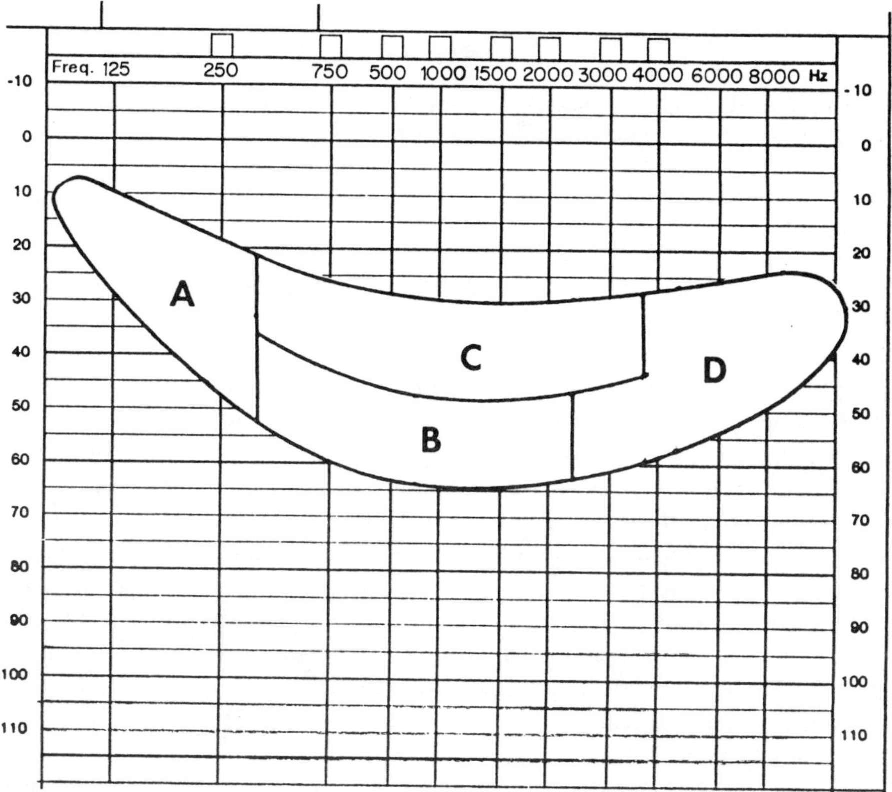

Figure 6.1 Illustration in audiogram format of the speech spectrum. Area A represents the fundamental frequency range, B is the main area for vowels, C for voiced consonants and D for voiceless consonants.

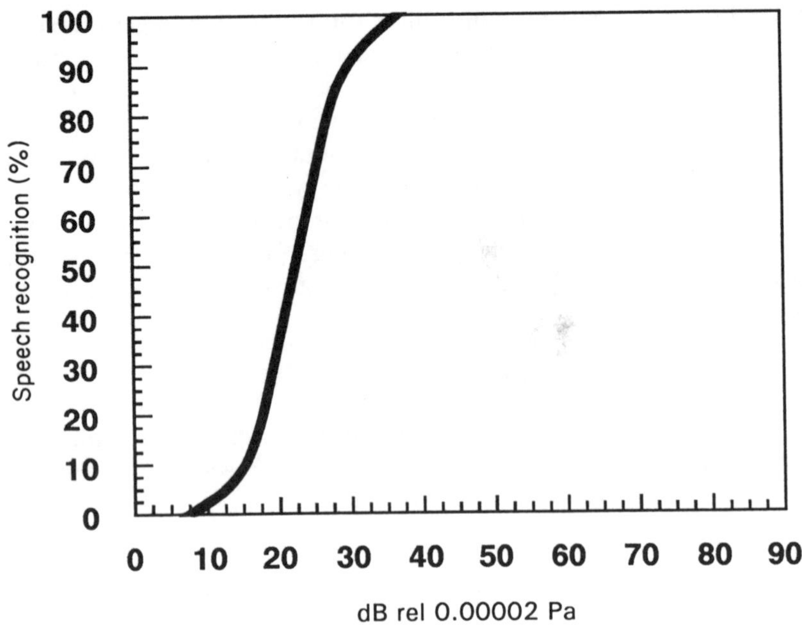

Figure 6.2 The average normal psychometric function for speech, i.e. percentage correctly recognised test words as a function of speech level, for spondees.

The construction of test lists is usually based on North American studies (e.g. Hudgins et al., 1947), assuming well-known common test words, which have a phonetic distribution that reasonably represents that of normal speech and which are approximately equally difficult to recognise. With homogeneous test word material, the psychometric function has a steep slope (Figure 6.2). Spondees, bisyllabic words with equal stress on the two syllables, have been shown to fulfil this criterion. Due to the steep slope of the psychometric function the accuracy of the SRT value obtained is better than for test words with less steep slope, e.g. monosyllabic words.

Schill (1985) found a 10% increase in speech recognition for each decibel of increase in level around SRT. When presented monaurally via an earphone, the average normal speech recognition threshold corresponds to a mean speech level in the range 20–25 dB SPL with some variation due to language and to the exact method by which the speech level is measured.

The speech recognition threshold is usually 8–10 dB above the speech detection threshold, i.e. the lowest level at which the listener can just detect the presence of the speech signal. This measure has been used for the estimation of hearing thresholds in children (Schill, 1985).

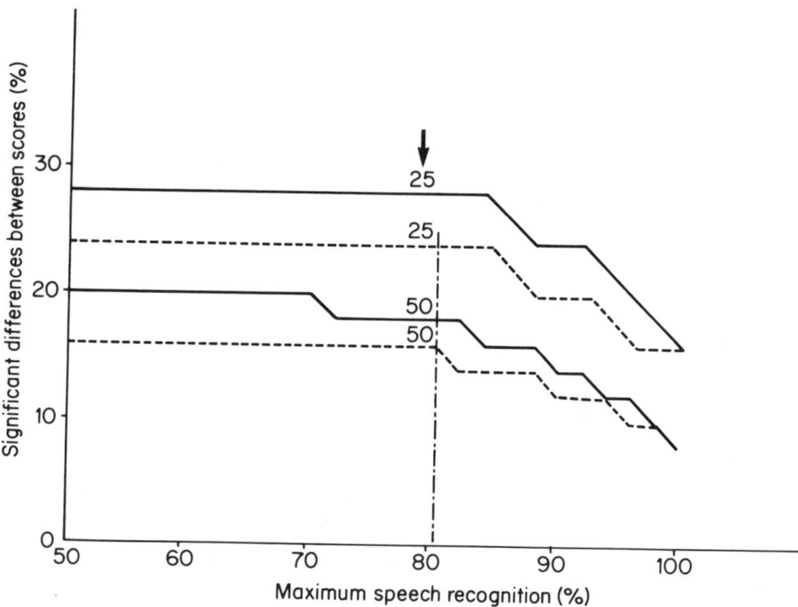

Figure 6.3 Smallest statistically significant difference in test scores between two measurements for $P<0.05$ and $P<0.1$, respectively, when using 25 and 50 word test lists as a function of the highest of the two scores compared; (—)5%; (----)10%.

Maximum speech recognition score

In this test, maximum speech recognition is determined by means of monosyllabic test words, presented as phonetically balanced (PB) lists. In general, the maximum speech recognition score is found at about 30 dB above the speech recognition threshold. Historically, North American telephone companies first studied speech recognition tests very early and in 1910 Campbell had already developed a test method. Fletcher and Steinberg published their method in 1930, using test lists of 50 words which since then have been the common form of test lists in use in the USA and many other countries. Sometimes a carrier phrase is used before the actual test word, e.g. 'Now you will hear . . .' to make it easier for the speaker to keep the speech level constant and natural and for the listener to be prepared to respond when the test word is uttered.

When using phonetically balanced test lists it is essential to use the complete list of 50 words. If only half of the list, 25 words, is used, test accuracy suffers (Hagerman, 1979) (Figure 6.3). The reliability of the results obtained depends on the listener's maximum speech recognition score. For example, the standard deviation is about 4% for a score in the

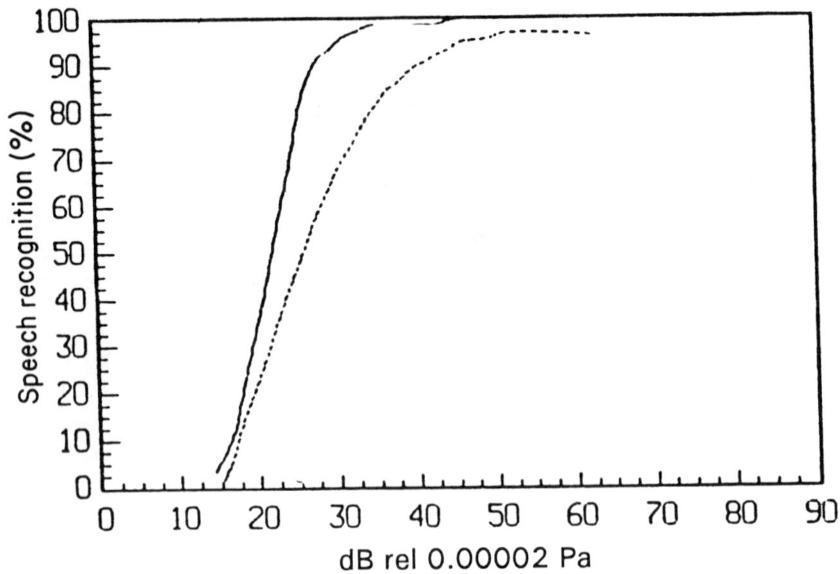

Figure 6.4 Average normal speech recognition score for monosyllabic test words (---) rises more slowly with increasing speech level than that for spondees (—).

range 90–98%, whereas it is about 10% for the range below 58% (Hagerman, 1976).

Monosyllabic words contain less redundancy than bisyllabic words, i.e. the listener has to identify relatively more phonemes in order to recognise the word. Due to this fact, the slope of the psychometric function for monosyllabic words is less than that for spondees (Figure 6.4).

A listener with a high frequency hearing loss usually has more problems recognising monosyllabic than bisyllabic test words. This is due to the consonants, with their main energy in the higher frequency range, having relatively more importance for the intelligibility of the monosyllabic words.

In some listeners with hearing loss, speech recognition shows a maximum for a certain speech level with lower scores obtained at higher levels. This phenomenon is called roll-over (Penred, 1985). It is usually more pronounced for older listeners and in certain pathological cases, such as those with retrocochlear lesions.

Uncomfortable loudness level for speech

At this test the lowest speech level which is perceived as uncomfortably loud is determined. One application of importance is in the procedure of fitting a hearing aid. The uncomfortable loudness level for speech and for pure tones often shows a far from perfect correlation. Explanations for this finding may be one of the following:

- The listener accepts a different level for a sound that carries information than for one that does not.
- The speech signal contains many components at a high level but of short duration.
- The correlation between the hearing level for speech and the hearing level for pure tones assumes that listeners have a hearing loss of relatively constant magnitude over the whole frequency range.

The instruction of the test subject is of course of considerable importance for the outcome of the test.

A general argument against these routine speech audiometric tests is that they do not reflect ordinary speech listening situations because the speech signal is presented in silence over an earphone. Therefore, an increasing interest has recently been shown in speech tests in background noise presented in a sound field, especially as part of a hearing aid fitting procedure.

It is important to note that peak levels in a speech test material are considerably higher than the average speech level and the attenuator setting being used. Typically, the dynamic range of speech is ±10–15 dB around the level of the calibration signal on the recording, which usually corresponds approximately to the average speech level. The equipment is usually calibrated in such a way that the calibration signal produces a sound level of around 20 dB SPL (Figure 6.5), varying somewhat between different speech materials. The actual sound pressure level from individual speech sounds may thus reach 35 dB above the value of the attenuator setting being used.

Equipment

Speech audiometry should be performed using equipment that fulfils the requirements of IEC 645 Part 2 (1991). The frequency response curve of the audiometer should be flat within ± 3 dB in the range 250–4000 Hz. Between 125 and 250 Hz a tolerance of +0/−10 dB is accepted and from 4 to 6.3 kHz the tolerance is ± 5 dB. The response curve should be measured on an acoustic coupler or artificial ear as applicable, depending on the type of earphone used.

The electric input of the audiometer, to which a tape or compact disc (CD) recorder is to be connected for playback, should have a relatively high input impedance (10–50 kΩ) and a sensitivity in the range 0.1–1 V. A signal level indicator on the audiometer having temporal characteristics corresponding to the VU-meter (volume unit meter) according to IEC 268-10 (1976), is used to monitor the calibration and speech input signals. The

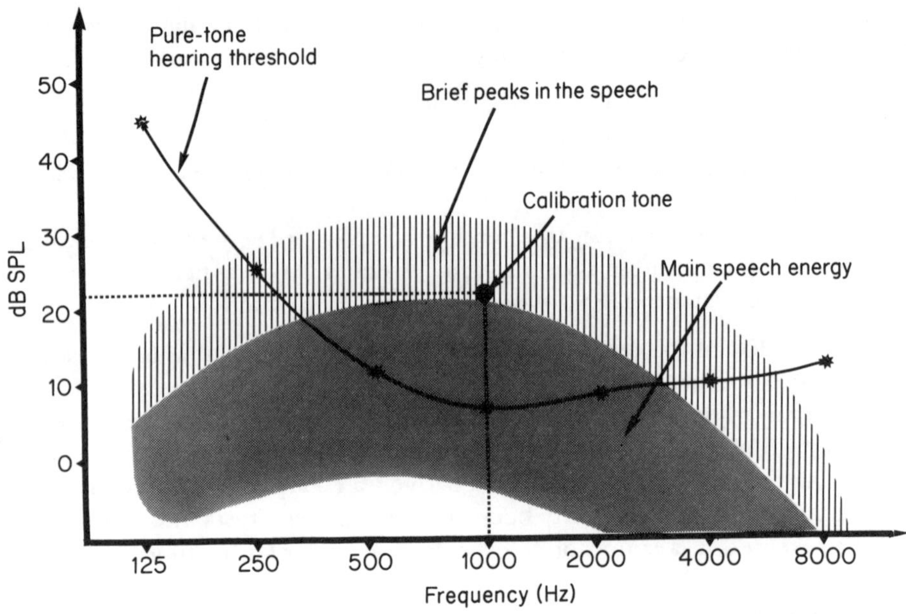

Figure 6.5 Illustration of the relation between average normal thresholds of hearing for pure tones (0 dB HL) and speech at a level which corresponds to barely recognisable speech, i.e. 0 dB HL for speech. A typical calibration signal of a speech recording is also shown (1 kHz tone at 22 dB SPL for 0 dB attenuator setting).

VU-meter should have a specified reference point, usually corresponding to a scale reading of 0 dB. The VU-meter is a relatively slow indicator and, therefore, its response to the speech signal does not show the peak levels present but reflects the average speech signal level. The sensitivity of the equipment is adjusted to make the calibration signal, usually recorded at the beginning of the test material at a level close to the average speech signal level, produce a VU-meter reading of 0 dB, i.e. at the reference point. The IEC 645 Part 2 (1991) standard specifies that the audiometer should be capable of handling signal levels of at least 9 dB above the level corresponding to 0 dB on the signal level indicator with acceptable low non-linear distortion.

According to IEC 645 Part 2, the reference calibration level of a speech audiometer should be 20 dB SPL, as measured in an acoustic coupler or artificial ear as appropriate. This means that the sound level produced by the calibration signal in the audiometer earphone and the audiometer input sensitivity is appropriately adjusted to give a signal level indicator reading at the reference point. The setting of the audiometer attenuator should be 0 dB, i.e. the hearing level scale for speech should have this reference calibration level of 20 dB SPL as its zero value. Theoretically, 0 dB HL for a speech test material should correspond to that speech level at which the average normally hearing listener recognises just 50% of the material presented. Thus, the producer of the speech test material has to determine this speech level by testing a sufficient number of young otologically normal subjects and then record the calibration signal at a level relative to the average speech level which makes an attenuator setting of 0 dB HL correspond to this normal average speech recognition threshold. The difference between the calibration signal level and the average speech level depends on the type of test items (digits, mono- or bisyllabic words, sentences) and language. Typically, the difference in level is of the order of a few decibels.

In practice, the calibration of the audiometer is undertaken with the attenuator at a point in the middle of its range, e.g. 60 dB. The sound level produced by the earphone in an acoustic coupler or artificial ear, when activated by the calibration signal and with the signal level indicator at its reference point, should be 80 dB SPL.

The masking noise must be weighted random noise with a flat spectrum up to 1 kHz and sloping by 12 dB per octave from 1 to 6 kHz. Its sound pressure level, as measured in the appropriate acoustic coupler or artificial ear, should be 20 dB +5/−3 dB above the value of the masking attenuator setting.

Sources of error and test accuracy

A patient's skill and knowledge in the language used in the test is a factor of significant importance. This may influence the usually good correlation between speech recognition threshold and the average pure-tone hearing thresholds. Test subjects who are used to a strong dialect may also experience difficulties in recognising the standardised speech test material. Some training effect is usually seen and it is therefore important not to use too few and too small sets of test items.

Hagerman (1979) studied the test accuracy of speech recognition threshold determination using Swedish bisyllabic test words. For normally hearing subjects he obtained a standard deviation of about 2 dB. For subjects with sensorineural hearing loss the standard deviation was found to be in the range 3–6 dB.

If a poor correlation is obtained between the pure-tone audiogram and the optimum speech recognition score, the test should be extended to levels above, as well as below, the most comfortable loudness level. This is because the most comfortable loudness level for speech does not always coincide with the level that produces maximum speech recognition. A rule of thumb is to test at several speech levels if the first score obtained is less than 70%.

When testing the uncomfortable loudness level for speech, it is essential that the listener has understood the instructions correctly. They must be formulated in an unambiguous way and always be presented in the same manner.

The rules for when to use contralateral masking in speech audiometry are based on the conservative assumption of a skull attenuation of 40 dB. Thus, if the difference between the speech test level and the average pure-tone hearing thresholds (0.5, 1 and 2 kHz) for air or bone conduction of the contralateral ear is 40 dB or more, masking should be used. However, if the pure-tone audiogram has a very steep slope, masking may be required at smaller differences or the pure-tone average should be based on 0.5 and 1 kHz only.

As a rule, a sound-insulated test room is required for reliable speech audiometry. However, the requirements on ambient sound levels in the test room are not as high as for pure-tone audiometry because higher sound levels are being used in speech audiometry. The need for the supra-aural earphone to fit the test ear tightly is also of less importance in speech audiometry. This is because leakage mainly influences the low frequency range which is of less importance with regard to speech recognition.

Clinical interpretation

The three parts of routine speech audiometry – speech recognition threshold, maximum speech recognition score and uncomfortable loudness level for speech – are of importance for evaluation of the following:

- The localisation of the lesion.
- The social hearing function.
- The validity of the pure-tone audiogram.
- The prospects for reconstructive middle-ear surgery.
- The prospects for hearing aid fitting.

Speech recognition threshold

One important value of the speech recognition threshold is to verify the validity of the pure-tone audiogram. Normally, the speech recognition threshold agrees with the average pure-tone hearing thresholds of 0.5, 1 and 2 kHz within ± 10 dB (Hagerman, 1979). However, for listeners whose pure-tone audiogram slopes more than 20 dB per octave, the difference between speech threshold and pure-tone average threshold may exceed 10 dB; also language difficulties and reduced mental capacity may give rise to a larger than normal difference.

A speech recognition threshold which is significantly better than the pure-tone average may indicate a non-organic hearing loss. Another indication for this type of problem is the listener who consistently responds by repeating only half of the bisyllabic test words with no evident change when the speech level is increased.

Maximum speech recognition score

A patient with hearing thresholds within the normal range or with a conductive hearing impairment should be expected to have a score in the range 92–100%. A cochlear hearing loss at 3 kHz and over has very little influence on the maximum speech recognition score when tested in quiet. Thus, a hearing threshold within the normal range at 2 kHz and below should mean a speech score in the range 92–100%. When the pure-tone thresholds are normal up to 1 kHz, speech scores around 70% can be expected. Normal thresholds up to 500 Hz, and a significant loss at higher frequencies, are typically associated with speech scores around 50% (Lidén, 1954) (Figure 6.6). Different kinds of cochlear lesions may have different effects on speech recognition. Patients with Menière's disease, for example, often have poorer speech recognition than expected from the pure-tone audiogram. Patients with congenital mid-frequency hearing loss, with trough-shaped or 'cookie-bite' audiograms, however, often have better speech recognition scores than expected.

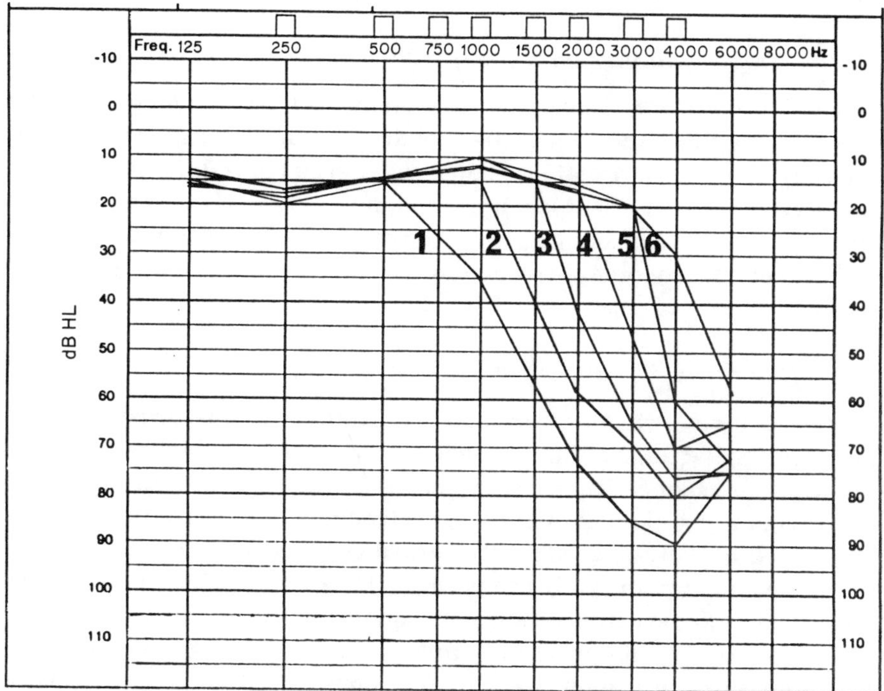

Figure 6.6 Maximum speech recognition scores in quiet are typically 50% for audiogram curve 1, 70% for curve 2, 83% for curve 3, 93% for curve 4, 96% for curve 5 and 98% for curve 6 (from Lidén, 1954).

In retrocochlear lesions, a relatively poor correlation is often found between the pure-tone audiogram and speech recognition. Extreme cases may have pure-tone hearing thresholds within normal limits but significantly reduced speech recognition. Thomsen (1982) showed significantly poorer maximum speech recognition scores in a group of patients with cerebellopontine angle tumours compared to patients with cochlear lesions.

Central lesions may also give rise to speech recognition scores that are markedly poorer than expected from the pure-tone audiogram. This is, for instance, often the case in elderly listeners with presbyacusis.

The reliability of the test scores is poorest for listeners with relatively poor scores (Hagerman, 1976). Thus, larger differences between test and retest are needed to indicate a significant difference for a listener with relatively poor speech recognition than for one with scores close to normal (see Figure 6.3). For example, if the better test score was 80%, the worse one has to be 64% or less, i.e. the difference is 16% or more, in order to be statistically significant ($P<0.1$, test list of 50 words). If the better score had been 90%, a difference of 12% would be equally significant. For test lists of half the size, i.e. 25 test items each, the corresponding differences have to be 24% and 20%, respectively.

Uncomfortable loudness level for speech

For people with normal hearing, the uncomfortable loudness level for speech is found in the range 80–100 dB HL. An abnormal (increased) speech recognition threshold together with normal or reduced uncomfortable loudness level for speech is commonly found in subjects with cochlear hearing impairment. In a typical patient with retrocochlear impairment the uncomfortable loudness level for speech is higher than normal.

Evaluation of speech audiometry for middle-ear surgery

In preoperative evaluations, speech recognition is considered to be an important characteristic. In cases with otosclerosis, the bone-conduction pure-tone thresholds may be abnormal, seeming to indicate a significant sensorineural component. A good speech recognition score may then be interpreted to indicate a relatively normal cochlear function. Conversely, poor speech recognition results may indicate a true sensorineural component and may constitute a contraindication for middle-ear surgery.

Postoperatively, the speech recognition threshold is a good indicator of the patient's practical ability to hear. According to Pfaltz, Pfaltz and Schmid (1975) the two categories 'socially acceptable hearing' and 'socially unacceptable hearing' are defined by the borderline speech recognition threshold better or worse than 35 dB HL. The maximum speech recognition score should also be included in the postoperative evaluation. Sometimes, in spite of closure of the air–bone gap and improved speech recognition threshold, the maximum speech recognition score may become worse because of a sensorineural component due to the surgical process.

Speech recognition scores may improve over time after middle-ear surgery. This may be considered as a slow training effect in an ear that received little acoustic stimulation before the surgery.

Evaluation of speech audiometry in hearing aid fitting

The speech recognition ability of the hearing-impaired person is no clear indicator for the possibility of successful hearing aid fitting. Naturally, an ear which shows good speech recognition should be expected to show good results also with a properly fitted hearing aid. But an ear with relatively poor speech recognition does not indicate that a hearing aid fitting will fail.

Often binaural hearing aids can be shown to be of advantage. However, if the patient for one reason or another prefers monaural fitting, the ear with best speech recognition score is often preferred to fit. An abnormally low uncomfortable loudness level indicates possible fitting problems because of the reduced dynamic range.

The use of speech audiometry in connection with hearing aid fitting is discussed further in Chapter 13.

Distorted Speech Audiometry

Indication

Distorted speech audiometry is used to diagnose auditory lesions in the first order neuron (cochlear nerve), in the brain stem and in the primary auditory centre in the temporal lobes of the cortex.

Physiology and psychoacoustics

Routine pure-tone and speech audiometry typically shows normal test results in subjects with central auditory lesions. The reason for this is the large redundancy, both with regard to the number of neurons involved in the auditory pathways from the brain stem and up, i.e. inner redundancy, and with regard to the information content of a normal speech signal in quiet, outer redundancy.

The inner redundancy has been studied by estimating the number of sensory cells and nerve cells on various levels (Bredberg, 1968, 1981). In a normal inner ear the number of hair cells is of the order of 20 000. A quarter of them are inner hair cells and three-quarters are outer hair cells.

The number of cells in the spiral ganglion and the number of axons in the cochlear nerve is around 30 000 (Rasmussen, 1940). In the cochlear nuclei the number of nerve cells in humans has been estimated to be around 100 000 (Hall, 1964). In the lateral lemniscus, approximately 200 000 nerve cells exist on each side. In the inferior colliculus in the order of 350 000 nerve fibres are part of the auditory pathways, and at the medial geniculate body the number has grown to more than half a million. Each primary auditory area in the cortex is estimated to have around 1.5 million cells. The auditory pathways cross the midline in the pons. This means that each ear is mainly projected on the contralateral temporal lobe. However, a small part of the neurons also leads to the ipsilateral temporal lobe. In addition, there are several cross-communications between the right and left sides on several levels in the central auditory system.

From this background, it is evident that the number of sensory cells in the inner ear is relatively small. A rather limited lesion in the cochlea may therefore lead to a relatively large functional loss. This is one important reason why the cochlear lesion is the most common cause of hearing loss. Within the central pathways, the number of neurons is much larger. Therefore central auditory lesions may occur often without evidence of functional effects that can be shown by conventional audiometric tests such as pure-tone audiometry. In cases of considerable cell loss, the neural signals can still be transmitted, reaching the temporal lobes and give rise to an auditory perception.

Outer redundancy means that the speech signal itself contains an excess of information in relation to its linguistic meaning. This is the reason why a normally hearing listener can recognise speech in noisy surroundings and when the speech signal has been subjected to severe distortion. The listener in his or her linguistic interpretation makes use of all his previous knowledge about the language, the speaker and the subject being discussed. Thereby he or she has considerable advanced knowledge about which sequences of sounds are possible or likely to occur. These limitations are the basis for redundancy both from a formal physical aspect and with regard to the message being conveyed (Fry, 1970; Stevens and House, 1972; Lundborg et al., 1975). Several levels of redundancy exist.

Acoustic – articulatory level

The acoustic pattern of speech in time and frequency cannot vary arbitrarily since it is determined by acoustic filtering processes in the speech organ with its given anatomical limitations.

Phonetic level

The various speech sounds occur only in some permissible combinations, and some sequences are more common than others.

Lexical level

Only some of the possible sound sequences are used as meaningful words in the language being used.

Syntactic level

Utterances are built according to the rules of the language concerning how words and sentences can be combined.

Semantic level

Only a limited number of the semantically correct sentences have a reasonable meaning.

Pragmatic level

In every given speech situation, social rules regulate which utterances are possible and how they are to be interpreted.

In information theory, the amount of information and redundancy are exactly defined quantities, usually quantified in the unit bits. Hedelin, Huber and Leijon (1988) have measured the statistical distribution function of all speech sounds – allophones – and combination of speech sounds in the Swedish language. By this procedure, the phonetic redundancy could be estimated. Their results show that if all speech sounds were equally common and could occur in arbitrary combinations, an average of 5.7 bits of information could be transmitted by each allophone. However, in reality only 3.3 bits/allophone are transmitted because many combinations of speech sounds seldom or never occur. The other types of redundancy in human speech are of course much more difficult to measure and quantify.

Speech test material can be distorted in several ways, thus reducing its redundancy on one or several of these levels. In order to be able to test central auditory function with speech tests, the redundancy has to be reduced. Commonly used means of achieving this are to introduce amplitude or frequency distortion, or to distort the temporal pattern. The interpretation of the distorted speech signal then presents the central auditory system with a more difficult test. Using a moderate degree of distortion, the listener will still score high because of the inner redundancy and the remaining outer redundancy. However, in a listener with a central disorder, the inner redundancy will be reduced to such an extent that a significant loss in recognition of the distorted speech signal will occur.

Several types of speech tests for the diagnosis of central disorders have been presented (Mueller, 1985; Musiek, 1985; Musiek and Baran, 1987). The tests are either dichotic, i.e. both ears are stimulated simultaneously but with different speech signals, or monotic, where one ear is tested at a time with low redundancy speech.

In Swedish, several types of distorted speech test lists have been produced (Korsan-Bengtsen, 1973). One test is dichotic (competing speech) and three are monotic. One application of the dichotic test is to present monosyllabic test words at 35 or 40 dB SL to one ear and competing sentences to the other ear at 50 dB SL. In another variant, different sentences are presented to the two ears at 50 dB SL. The listener is asked to repeat the message delivered to one ear at a time or to repeat both sentences which were presented simultaneously. This latter version is more difficult than the first.

In time-compressed speech, the speech rate has been increased in the recording without any concomitant pitch change. Normal speech rate is in the range 110–140 words per minute. Korsan-Bengtsen used two higher rates – 220 and 300 words per minute. In chopped or interrupted speech, the speech signal is periodically interrupted with an on–off ratio of one, i.e. the speech segments let through and the silent intervals in between are of equal length. Interruption rates of 10, 7 and 4 per second were used. When the silent intervals are relatively short, the inner redundancy can bridge and automatically connect the information-carrying elements. With increasing intervals, the difficulty to recognise the speech signal increases.

In the English language the staggered spondaic word test (SSW) has been used for central diagnosis (Katz, 1962; Lukas and Genchur-Lukas, 1985). This is a dichotic test: pairs of spondees are used in combinations where the second syllable of the first word is very similar to the first syllable in the second word. The two words are presented with a time difference corresponding to the duration of one syllable, i.e. the two similar syllables, the second in the first word and the first in the second word, are presented simultaneously. Alternate pairs are presented to left and to right ear first and the listener is asked to repeat both bisyllabic test words.

Dichotic tests using full sentences have also been used to diagnose central auditory lesions as well as monotic tests where the syntactic or semantic redundancy has been reduced (Willeford, 1985).

In addition to the purpose of diagnosing central auditory lesions, dichotic tests may also be used to evaluate neurological disorders, such as aphasia, and for the determination of which cerebral hemisphere is dominant for speech perception.

Equipment

Distorted speech audiometry requires the same equipment and test room facilities as routine speech audiometry. The speech test lists should be recorded on tape or compact disc. Dichotic presentation requires a two-channel audiometer.

Sources of error and test accuracy

Distorted speech audiometry presumes normal or near-normal peripheral auditory function, i.e. the pure-tone hearing threshold levels should be essentially normal. A slight loss in the high frequency range may be accepted. The maximum speech recognition score, as determined by means of standard phonetically balanced test lists in quiet, should be within normal limits. Distorted speech tests are difficult to interpret and should be avoided if the maximum speech recognition score is less than 70–80%. A relatively moderate peripheral hearing loss may also cause abnormal results in distorted speech audiometry, and the test will then lose most of its diagnostic potential. The test should be performed in the patient's native language. Naturally, the patient must be alert and capable of reliable cooperation.

No reports have been published on test reliability. As is the case with conventional speech audiometry, reliability is influenced by the total number of statistically independent test words in the list used and by the listener's speech recognition score (Hagerman, 1976). The variability is largest, i.e. reliability is poorest, when the test score is around 50% (see Figure 6.3). If the test list contains 50 independent test words of approximately equal difficulty and the result in one test is 90%, a change or difference has to be more than 14% in order to be statistically significant ($P<0.05$).

The test lists available in Swedish each contain 25 common sentences with four key words each, i.e. 100 test words in all. Since the words within each sentence have a relation with regard to syntax and meaning, they cannot be considered totally independent. However, the variation in difficulty between the different words is probably larger in distorted speech test lists than in common speech test lists which would reduce the test variability. As an approximate estimate, the same test reliability which is valid for conventional test lists of 50 phonetically balanced monosyllabic test words may be used also for interrupted speech.

Clinical interpretation

Normal test results for the monotic test lists according to Korsan-Bengtsen (1973) have to be split according to listener's age since young normally hearing subjects perform somewhat better than elderly subjects with normal hearing thresholds. Table 6.1 presents normal data for young and elderly. The borderline values are based on the mean value minus three standard deviations.

An alternative evaluation is by comparison of the test results for left and right ears. A difference in score of 15%, e.g. 90% in one ear and 75% in the other ear, can be considered as significant and as indicating abnormality in the pathways connected with the poorer ear, i.e. mainly on

Table 6.1 Percentage of normal test scores for distorted speech audiometry shown by young (mean 26 years) and elderly (mean 55 years) listeners

	Young		Elderly	
	Mean	Borderline	Mean	Borderline
Chopped speech (7/s)	98	91	93	78
Increased speech rate	98	92	93	70
LP-filtered speech	95	83	88	58

Data according to Korsan-Bengtsen (1973).

the contralateral side. If the better ear has a poorer score than 90%, the risk of false positive results increases, but the difference of 15% or more is still relatively acceptable as a rule of thumb to indicate abnormality.

The test result can indicate central auditory lesions, but without the power for detailed topical diagnosis within the central pathways (Ödkvist et al., 1987). In order to differentiate between cortical, brain-stem and retrocochlear lesions other test methods are needed.

References

BREDBERG, G. (1968). Cellular pattern and nerve supply of the human organ of Corti. *Acta Oto-Laryngologica Supplementum* 236.

BREDBERG, G. (1981). Innervation of the auditory system. *Scandinavian Audiology* Suppl. 13, 1–10.

CAMPBELL, G.A. (1910). Telephonic intelligibility. *Philosophical Magazine Journal of Science* **19**, 152–159.

FLETCHER, H. and STEINBERG, J.C. (1930). Articulation testing methods. *Journal of Acoustical Society of America* **1**, 1–97.

FRY, D.B. (1970). Speech reception and perception. In: Lyons, J. (Ed.) *New Horizons in Linguistics.* London: Penguin Books.

HAGERMAN, B. (1976). Reliability in the determination of speech discrimination. *Scandinavian Audiology* **5**, 219–228.

HAGERMAN, B. (1979). Reliability in the determination of speech reception threshold (SRT). *Scandinavian Audiology* **8**, 195–202.

HALL, J.G. (1964). The cochlea and the cochlear nuclei in neonatal asphyxia. *Acta Oto-Laryngologica Supplement* 194.

HEDELIN, P., HUBER, D. and LEIJON, A. (1988). *Probability Distribution of Allophones, Diphones and Triphones in Phonetic Transcription of Swedish Newspaper Text.* Technical Report No. 8, Department of Information Theory, Gothenburg, Chalmers Technical University.

HUDGINS, C.V., HAWKINS, J.E., KARLIN, J.E. and STEVENS, S.S. (1947). The development of recorded auditory tests for measuring hearing loss for speech. *The Laryngoscope* **57**, 57–89.

IEC 268-10 (1976). *Sound system equipment. Part 10: programme level meters.* Geneva: International Electrotechnical Commission.

IEC 645-2 (1991). *Audiometers. Part 2: equipment for speech audiometry.* Geneva: International Electrotechnical Commission.

KATZ, J. (1962). The use of staggered spondaic words for assessing the integrity of the central auditory system. *Journal of Auditory Research* **2**, 327–337.

KORSAN-BENGTSEN, M. (1973). Distorted speech audiometry. *Acta Oto-Laryngologica Supplementum* 310.

LIDÉN, G. (1954). Speech audiometry. *Acta Oto-Laryngologica Supplementum* 114.

LUKAS, R.A. and GENCHUR-LUKAS, J. (1985). Spondaic word tests. In: Katz, J. (Ed.) *Handbook of Clinical Audiology*, 3rd edn, pp. 383–403. Baltimore: Williams & Wilkins.

LUNDBORG, T., ROSENHAMER, H., MURRAY, T. and ZWETNOV, N. (1975). Information abundance of speech and distorted speech testing in topical diagnosis within the CNS. *Scandinavian Audiology* **4**, 9–19.

MUELLER, H.G. (1985). Monosyllabic procedures. In: Katz, J. (Ed.) *Handbook of Clinical Audiology*, 3rd edn, pp. 355–382. Baltimore: Williams & Wilkins.

MUSIEK, F.E. (1985). Application of central auditory tests: an overview. In: Katz, J. (Ed.) *Handbook of Clinical Audiology*, 3rd edn, pp. 321–336. Baltimore: Williams & Wilkins.

MUSIEK, F.E. and BARAN, JA. (1987). Central auditory assessment: thirty years of challenge and change. *Ear and Hearing* **8**, Suppl., 22–35.

ÖDKVIST, L.M., ARLINGER, S.D., EDLING, C., LARSBY, B. and BERGHOLTZ, L.M. (1987). Audiological and vestibulo-oculomotor findings in workers exposed to solvents and jet fuel. *Scandinavian Audiology* **16**, 75–81.

PENROD, J.P. (1985). Speech discrimination testing. In: Katz, J. (Ed.) *Handbook of Clinical Audiology*, 3rd edn, pp. 235–255. Baltimore: Williams & Wilkins.

PFALTZ, C.R., PFALTZ, R. and SCHMID, P. (1975). Reconstructive surgery in chronic otitis media. Statistical analysis of long-term results. *Oto-Rhino-Laryngology* **37**, 257.

RASMUSSEN, A.T. (1940). Studies on the VIIIth cranial nerve in man. *The Laryngoscope* **50**, 67–83.

SCHILL, H.A. (1985). Thresholds for speech. In: Katz, J. (Ed.) *Handbook of Clinical Audiology*, 3rd edn, pp. 224–234. Baltimore: Williams & Wilkins.

STEVENS, K.N. and HOUSE, A.S. (1972). Speech perception. In: Tobias, J.V. (Ed.) *Foundations of Modern Auditory Theory*, Vol. II, pp. 1–62. New York: Academic Press.

THOMSEN, J. (1982). *Acoustic neuromas.* Copenhagen: FADL.

WILLEFORD, J.A. (1985). Sentence tests of central auditory dysfunction. In: Katz, J. (Ed.) *Handbook of Clinical Audiology*, 3rd edn, pp. 404–420. Baltimore: Williams & Wilkins.

WRIGHT, R. (1987). Basic properties of speech. In: Martin, M. (Ed.) *Speech Audiometry*, pp. 1–32. London: Taylor & Francis.

Chapter 7 Audiometry in Children

Indication

Special test methods are used to test the hearing in young children. Different methods are applicable from the neonatal period up to pre-school age. The child's psychomotor age determines which method to use and therefore, for developmentally handicapped patients, the methods are applicable over a wider range of biological age.

Early diagnosis of hearing loss and deafness is essential if the development of the child is not to be delayed. Therefore, in many countries, screening programmes are being carried out for special at-risk groups and also for certain age groups. The following risk factors which increase the probability of hearing loss should be considered as indications for hearing tests.

Prenatal risk factors

- Hereditary hearing loss in the family.
- Maternal rubella, cytomegalovirus infection and certain other infections during pregnancy.
- Malformation of the ears or face.
- Unclear syndromes.
- Chromosomal aberrations.

Perinatal risk factors

- Birth weight of less than 1500 grams.
- Severe asphyxia (10 min resuscitation time).
- Neonatal sepsis or meningitis.

Postnatal risk factors

- Meningitis.
- Parotitis.
- Trauma.

Screening tests of unselected groups of children may be performed at the age of 7–8 months by means of an informal test and around the age of 4 years by means of play audiometry.

Physiological and Psychoacoustic Background

Embryology (Figure 7.1)

The inner ear

At the end of the third gestational week, a thickening of the ectoderm at the rombencephalon occurs. Through an indentation which later separates from the ectoderm, a small cyst is created – the otocyst. In the otocyst the membranous labyrinth is developed which, during the sixth week, separates into the vestibular organ and the cochlea. During the sixth and seventh weeks, the membranous labyrinth becomes enclosed by cartilaginous tissue, and the space between the labyrinth and the cartilaginous part becomes filled with perilymph. In the sixteenth week all three cochlear cavities are present: scala vestibuli, scala tympani and scala media. At about the same time, inner and outer hair cells appear in the organ of Corti. During the period from the twenty-fifth to the thirtieth week, the cochlea becomes completely developed.

The middle ear and the eustachian tube

These begin to develop during the fourth week from the first branchial groove; the ossicles develop from the two first branchial arches. The stapes develops from the second branchial arch, and the malleus and incus from the first branchial arch.

The external auditory canal

This is formed from a tube which indents from the ectoderm into the first branchial groove. A protuberance from the middle ear appears in the direction of the indenting tube. The meeting place forms the eardrum, which consequently arises from all three germ layers (ectoderm, mesoderm and entoderm) and is fully developed during the seventh month of gestation.

The outer ear

This is formed from the first and second branchial arches.

During the seventh gestational month the development of the ear is complete (Langman, 1969; Northern and Downs, 1974).

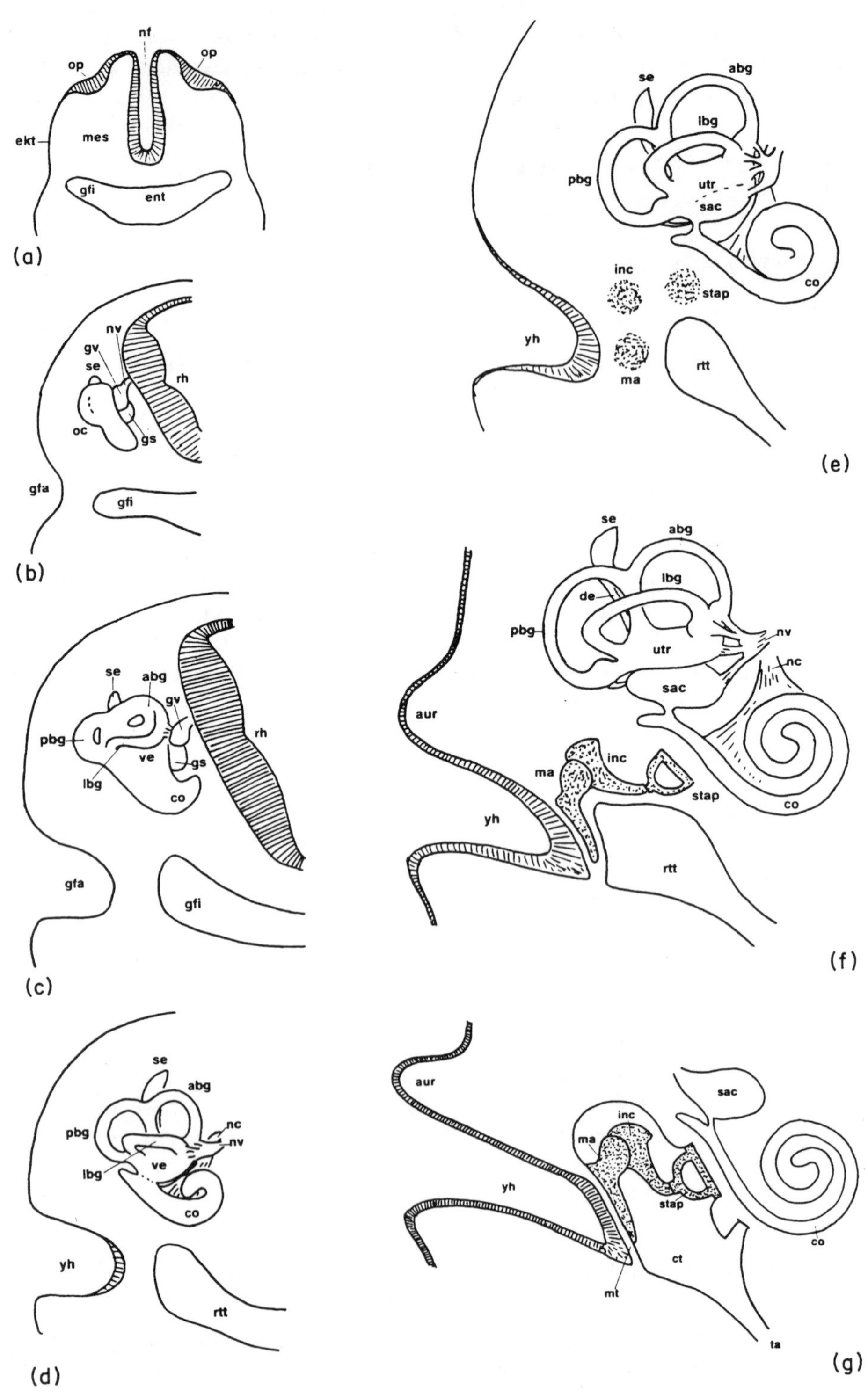
nf
op
op
ekt
mes
gfi
ent
(a)
nv
gv
se
rh
oc
gs
gfa
gfi
(b)
se
abg
gv
pbg
rh
ve
gs
lbg
co
gfa
gfi
(c)
se
abg
pbg
nc
nv
lbg
ve
co
yh
rtt
(d)
se
abg
lbg
pbg
utr
sac
inc
stap
co
yh
ma
rtt
(e)
se
abg
lbg
de
pbg
nv
utr
nc
sac
aur
inc
ma
stap
co
yh
rtt
(f)
aur
sac
inc
ma
yh
stap
co
ct
mt
ta
(g)

Knowledge in human embryology can provide understanding about why malformations often occur in several organs together. In the evaluation of auditory function, it is therefore important to examine if other malformations also occur, and vice versa since outer malformations may also indicate malformations in the ear. The ear is most sensitive to external influence during the first seven gestational months, i.e. during the period when it is developing.

The development of hearing

The fetus reacts to sound stimulation as early as during the twenty-fourth gestational week (Wedenberg, 1956). Immediately after birth, sound stimulation gives rise to recordable reactions by means of reflex mechanisms. The blinking reflex and the stapedius reflex can be recorded, as well as changes in cardiac and respiratory rates. In addition, effects on the child's motor activity can be observed. These reactions require nerve impulses from the auditory organ to be able to reach at least the superior olivary complex, but higher parts of the central auditory organ do not necessarily have to be fully developed.

At the age of about 3 months the auditory pathways up to the lateral lemniscus are fully developed. Sound stimulation now gives rise to a reflexive effort to localise the source of the sound. At about 5 months of age the child reacts to sounds by actively turning his or her head towards the source. From the age of 6 months, the child is capable of recognising meaningful sounds and begins to understand simple words.

The development of the normal child's reaction to sound can be summarised as follows:

Age	*Reaction*
Neonatal period	Reflex reactions to sudden loud sounds
4 weeks	Spontaneous activity ceases when the child detects speech or other sounds

Figure 7.1 Schematic illustrations of cross-sections of the head at the level of the first branchial arch in different stages of fetal development: (a) after 22 days, (b) after 36 days, (c) after 50 days, (d, e) after 2 months, (f) after 3 months and (g) after 6 months. Abbreviations: ekt=ectoderm, ent=entoderm, mes=mesoderm, op=optic placode, nf=neural fissure, gfi=first branchial groove, ac=otocyst, se=endolymphatic sac, rh=rhombencephalon, gv=vestibular ganglion, nv=vestibular nerve, gs=spiral ganglion, gfa=first branchial arch, co=cochlea, ve=vestibulum, abg=anterior semicircular canal, lbg=lateral semicircular canal, pbg=posterior semicircular canal, nc=cochlear nerve, yh=external auditory canal (first branchial groove), rtt=tubotympanic recess, utr=utricle, sac=saccule, ma=malleus, inc=incus, stap=stapes, de=endolymphatic duct, aur=auricle, mt=tympanic membrane, ct=tympanic cavity (middle ear), ta=eustachian tube.

3–6 months	Spontaneous activity ceases and the child turns his or her head towards the source of sound
7–12 months	The child can localise a sound source, imitates sounds and begins to recognise his or her name
1–1.5 years	The interest in repeated sounds decreases. The child can follow simple directives
1.5–2.5 years	The child begins to understand and to perform an increasing number of directives by increasingly complex messages

The development of language occurs on two levels. First, children gradually acquire the ability to understand speech, and secondly they acquire their own spoken language. The first sound production consists of reflexive activity such as babble and screams. At the age of about 5 months, children begin to imitate sounds and at the age of 10–14 months they start to say their own first words. By the age of 1.5 years they start to combine words into simple sentences.

Test Methods

Suprathreshold methods

Acoustic blink reflex (auropalpebral reflex, APR)

The test aims at the determination of the lowest sound level required to elicit the blink reflex. The normal reflex threshold range is 105–115 dB SPL in the frequency range 500–4000 Hz.

The test should be used as a complement to other test methods. A blink reflex which can be elicited suggests that the child can hear but it is not possible to say that the child has normal hearing. This is because the blink reflex can be elicited at normal levels in hearing-impaired children with recruitment (Wedenberg, 1956). The reflex may be absent in a normally hearing child either in a state of deep sleep or awake and crying, laughing or otherwise agitated.

In children up to 3 months of age, sudden loud sounds at levels above 75 dB SPL may give rise to a startle reflex in which the child bends the elbows and clenches the hands.

Waking audiometry

This method, where the lowest sound level at which a child can be awakened is determined, may be used on neonates (Wedenberg, 1956). A normally hearing child in a relatively light sleep stage wakes up with sound stimulation at levels around 70–75 dB SPL.

In the newborn child, waking audiometry is a relatively easy procedure, but in somewhat older children it may require considerable time because of the child spending longer and longer time awake. The method gives an approximate estimation of auditory function. A child with sensorineural hearing loss and recruitment may not wake up at the same sound level as a normally hearing child but is likely to need higher levels. In a child with a conductive hearing impairment, waking is expected to occur at levels that differ from normal by the magnitude of the conductive loss.

Methods for estimation of hearing thresholds

Respiration audiometry

In this method, the child's hearing is evaluated by studying recorded changes in respiration due to acoustic stimulation. The test provides a reliable estimate of hearing thresholds for air- or bone-conducted signals in the frequency range 250–4000 Hz (Kankkunen and Lidén, 1977). It can be used in the age range from birth up to about 4 months in normally developed children. A prerequisite for the test is that the child is relaxed and at ease. The lowest sound levels which evoke a change in the respiratory pattern should be considered as a type of reflex threshold and be somewhat higher than the true hearing thresholds.

Observation audiometry

In this test the child's hearing is evaluated by the observation of its motor reactions to unexpected sound stimuli. It is used up to the age of about a year and a half.

When interpreting the results it is important to recognise that the child may react in many different ways, e.g. hold the breath, look towards the sound source or at the tester.

The method provides a good estimate of the hearing thresholds for air- or bone-conducted sounds. A hearing loss of significant magnitude with regard to the development of speech and language can be diagnosed reliably. If the test signals are presented by means of loudspeakers, the child's binaural hearing is measured but unilateral hearing loss or deafness cannot usually be determined reliably. However, the use of insert earphones makes monaural auditory function assessable. In this method, a form of reflex threshold is actually measured which may be at a somewhat higher sound level than the true hearing threshold, particularly for younger children.

Visual reinforcement audiometry

The child's reactions to sound stimuli with visual reinforcement are evaluated; the optimum age range for this test is 1–3 years. The method is based on the child having understood the correlation between the test sound and the picture which follows immediately after. The response may vary: the child looks up from the toy he or she is playing with, starts laughing or points at the picture. The pictures should be simple and show well-known objects such as a ball, a chair, a spade etc. The test sounds may be presented by means of a loudspeaker, earphones or bone vibrator (Lidén and Kankkunen, 1969).

It is essential that a rapid judgement of the child's response is made. If the tester shows a new picture at the wrong moment, i.e. not directly after a sound which the child heard and responded to, the conditioning may be broken and the validity of the test is lost. In the hands of an experienced tester, the test gives reliable estimates of the child's hearing thresholds.

Play audiometry

This is a test where the child is actively listening for the test sounds. The child is taught to move a small object to a certain location to signal that a test sound has been heard. The method can be used both for determination of hearing thresholds and in a screening procedure. Depending somewhat on the child's age, hearing thresholds for air- and bone-conducted pure tones, and for older children with the use of contralateral masking if indicated, can be determined in the full frequency range from 125 to 8000 Hz. A normally developed child can usually cooperate in play audiometry by the age of about 3 years.

To explain the test procedure to a small child, a small electric bell may be used. The tester takes one of the objects to be moved in his or her hand, holds it against the bell, rings the bell and then moves the object to its given location. Then the child is given the object in his or her hand, the tester places the child's hand against the bell, rings the bell and moves the child's hand with the object. When the child has understood that the object is to be moved each time something happens, the actual test can be started.

When choosing objects for the child to move, it is essential not to mix too many colours, shapes or sizes. Simple cubes or bars made of wood or plastic are ideal. Too small or too large sizes should be avoided – such objects are difficult for the child to hold. It is essential that the child cannot see when the test stimulus is presented; the testers pressing the interrupter button should be invisible. A periodic presentation of the test sounds should also be avoided because the child may detect the rhythm and move the object accordingly without having heard the test sound.

Other methods

Informal tests

The purpose of the informal test is to provide a rough estimate of the child's auditory function. The test can be used from the neonatal period and is based on evaluating the child's spontaneous reactions to various sounds. Before the age of 3–4 months, the child reacts only by reflexes and eye movements. At a later age children can turn their heads towards the sound source.

The test can be performed by means of various informal sound sources, such as jingle bells, a cow-bell or a tambourine. If the characteristics of the sound (frequency contents, sound level at specified distances) are measured and known by the tester, both validity and reliability of the test increase (Stensland-Junker, 1972).

Conversation and whispering tests

Speech presented at normal conversational level and by whispering also provides possibilities for approximately estimating the auditory function.

Whispering provides more high frequency emphasis at a lower sound level than normal voiced speech. By varying the distance between the talker and the child, some variation in sound level can be obtained although the room acoustics may considerably influence the variation that is possible.

Small children can be tested while in bed. Preferably the test is performed from both sides without the child seeing the tester. When testing a child on the parent's lap, it is recommended that the child be allowed to play with a simple toy. A child usually recognises his or her name from the age of 9 months, and the test may use a brief sentence containing the child's name, e.g. 'Look David'. If the child does not react when the speaking distance is 2–3 metres reduce the distance and repeat the sentence. The test should be performed from both sides, especially if a unilateral loss is suspected.

From the age of about 2 years, the testing may be performed with the aid of pictures. A number of pictures are placed in front of the child and shown to him or her one at a time. The tester says what the picture shows and asks the child to point at the picture showing the object just mentioned. Words should be used that represent as large a variety of speech sounds from a spectral point of view as possible. A possible source of error is that the child may guess the spoken message from the limited contents of the pictures.

Special test methods

Often the methods mentioned above have to be complemented by special tests. This is particularly the case if the child is not capable of or willing to cooperate in conventional test methods. The special methods used mostly are impedance audiometry and electric response audiometry (ERA). In the future, the recording of evoked acoustic emissions may also become a clinically important complement (Johnsen et al., 1988).

Sources of Error and Test Accuracy

The emotional, psychological, physical and motor development of the child has a considerable influence on the child's ability to cooperate and respond to the various test sounds. In all tests except waking audiometry, the child has to be awake and thoroughly rested. In order to be able to perform the test and interpret the child's reactions, the tester must be good at handling children and be an experienced tester of children. This is of particular importance in observation audiometry.

The furniture and equipment in the test room should not attract the child's interest. Toys to be used in testing should not be stored in such a way that the child may discover them. The toys should be simple. The test itself is the important thing, and the toys are simply tools to be used to distract the child in between the presentations of test sounds – with the exception of play audiometry. The room illumination should be sufficient for observation of the child's reactions, but not unnecessarily bright. The test equipment must be placed within easy reach, but the child should not be able to see when a stimulus presentation occurs. It is always important to work rapidly to obtain as much information as possible before the child gets tired or bored by the test procedure. The test must be stopped as soon as the child is loosing attention and cannot be motivated to participate any longer.

Unfortunately, no quantitative information is available on the test accuracy of the various methods discussed.

References

JOHNSEN, N.J., BAGI, P., PARBO, J. and ELBERLING, C. (1988). Evoked acoustic emissions from the human ear. IV. Final results in 100 neonates. *Scandinavian Audiology* **17**, 27–34.

KANKKUNEN, A. and LIDÉN, G. (1977). Respiration audiometry. *Scandinavian Audiology* **6**, 81–86.

LANGMAN, J. (1969). *Medical Embryology.* Baltimore: Williams & Wilkins.

LIDÉN, G. and KANKKUNEN, A. (1969). Visual reinforcement audiometry. *Acta Oto-Laryngologica* **89**, 865–872.

NORTHERN, J.L. and DOWNS, M.P. (1974). *Hearing in Children.* Baltimore: Williams & Wilkins.

STENSLAND-JUNKER, K. (1972). Selective attention in infants and consecutive communicative behavior. *Acta Paediatrica Scandinavica Supplementum* 231.

WEDENBERG, E. (1956). Auditory test on new-born infants. *Acta Oto-Laryngologica* **46**, 446–461.

Chapter 8
Acoustic Impedance Audiometry

Physical and physiological background

Impedance is a measure of resistance against motion. The acoustic impedance of an ear is a measure of the sound pressure that is required to make the air molecules in the external auditory canal, the middle ear, the eardrum and the ossicles vibrate with a certain volume velocity. The acoustic impedance is defined as the ratio between sound pressure and volume velocity and is expressed in the unit Pa·s/m^3 (SI units).

The acoustic impedance of the middle ear itself is of diagnostic interest, as well as changes in this impedance caused by reactions in the ear to certain external stimuli.

The aural acoustic impedance is usually measured by means of a tone – a carrier – transmitted from a small earphone into the external auditory canal by means of a probe (Figure 8.1) (Wiley and Block, 1985). The earphone produces a sound that gives rise to a certain volume velocity in the air of the auditory canal. If the middle-ear impedance is high, the sound pressure in the auditory canal is relatively high. If the impedance is low, the sound pressure becomes relatively low. The sound pressure is recorded by means of a microphone, which is also connected to the probe. The signal from the microphone is analysed with regard to its magnitude and, in some types of equipment, also with regard to phase in relation to the emitted sound. The probe is also connected to a device by means of which the air pressure in the external auditory canal can be varied.

Admittance is the opposite of impedance, i.e. a measure of mobility, and therefore admittance is the inverted value of the impedance. High impedance means low admittance and vice versa. The acoustic admittance is thus defined as the ratio between volume velocity and sound pressure and is expressed in the unit m^3/Pa·s.

Sometimes the term 'immittance' is used as a general term, referring to both impedance and admittance. Immittance is therefore not a physical

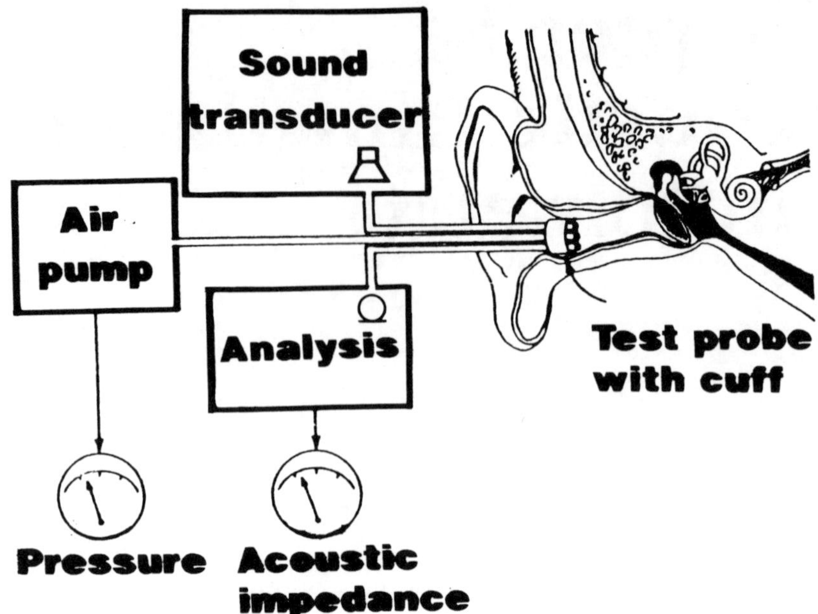

Figure 8.1 The main parts of an impedance audiometer and their interconnections.

characteristic but only a term. The reason for introducing such a term is that, from a clinical point of view, acoustic impedance and admittance contain the same information.

If impedance measurements are performed by means of a probe tone with low frequency (the standardised low frequency value is 226 Hz), the middle-ear acoustic impedance is determined mainly by the acoustic stiffness of the eardrum and the ossicular chain. This characteristic is referred to as the acoustic compliance.

A membrane, a spring or an enclosed air volume can be characterised by how much each yields when loaded by a certain pressure. The acoustic compliance expresses this characteristic and is defined as the ratio between a change in volume and the change in pressure required to give rise to this change in volume. It is expressed in the unit m^3/Pa.

A high value of the middle-ear acoustic compliance thus means that the vibrational movement of the eardrum covers a larger volume than in an ear with a lower compliance for the same applied sound pressure.

A certain volume of enclosed air at a certain barometric pressure always has a certain compliance. Therefore, the equivalent volume of the middle ear is defined as that volume of air at normal barometric pressure which has the same acoustic compliance as the ear under test. The equivalent volume is usually expressed in cm^3. At the frequency 226 Hz, an equivalent volume of 1 cm^3 corresponds to the acoustic admittance 10^{-8} $m^3/Pa{\cdot}s$.

The SI unit for pressure is the pascal (Pa). In impedance audiometry, the static pressure in the external auditory canal is most often expressed in decapascals (1 daPa = 10 Pa). Older types of equipment often show static pressure in the unit millimetres of water (mmH_2O) which is almost equal to a decapascal (1.02 mmH_2O = 1 daPa). Normal barometric pressure is around 100 kPa (or 10 000 daPa).

The acoustic impedance of the middle ear essentially consists of three physical phenomena (Figure 8.2):

1. Acoustic resistance related to friction in the middle-ear tissues and absorption of energy in air-filled cavities and in the cochlear fluids.
2. Acoustic mass, i.e. inertia: this is caused by the mass of the moving air, eardrum and ossicles. Each object with a mass needs an external force in order to change its velocity.
3. Acoustic compliance, i.e. spring action: this is caused by the elastic properties of the eardrum, ossicles and the enclosed air.

These three components are basic in all mobile mechanical systems. Whatever the complexity of the system, the three components interact in a specific way. At a given frequency, the system seems to move as if determined by two components: one is the friction component; the other is either a mass or a spring component. Thus the impedance can be described by two values at each frequency. When in resonance, the motion of the system is determined only by the friction component. The total impedance of the system then has a minimum value.

The impedance due to friction is called resistance whilst that due to mass and spring components is called reactance. At frequencies where the elasticity dominates (low frequencies), the reactance has a negative value. When inertia dominates (at high frequencies), the reactance is positive. At resonance the reactance is zero. Impedance is often denoted by the letter Z, resistance by R and reactance by X.

Correspondingly, the admittance of the system can be described by two terms at each frequency. The component related to friction is known as conductance and the component related to mass and elasticity as susceptance. If the conductance and susceptance of a system are known, its resistance and reactance can be calculated and vice versa. Admittance is often denoted by the letter Y, conductance by G and susceptance by B.

Separate determination of the two components of impedance or admittance of the middle ear is of importance mainly for scientific purposes, and this is usually in the frequency range 500–1000 Hz.

The acoustic impedance of the normal ear is strongly frequency dependent (Figure 8.3) (Moller, 1974; Shaw, 1974). At low frequencies, it is mainly determined by the acoustic compliance of the ear. The middle-ear resonance frequency is normally in the range 800–1500 Hz. At the

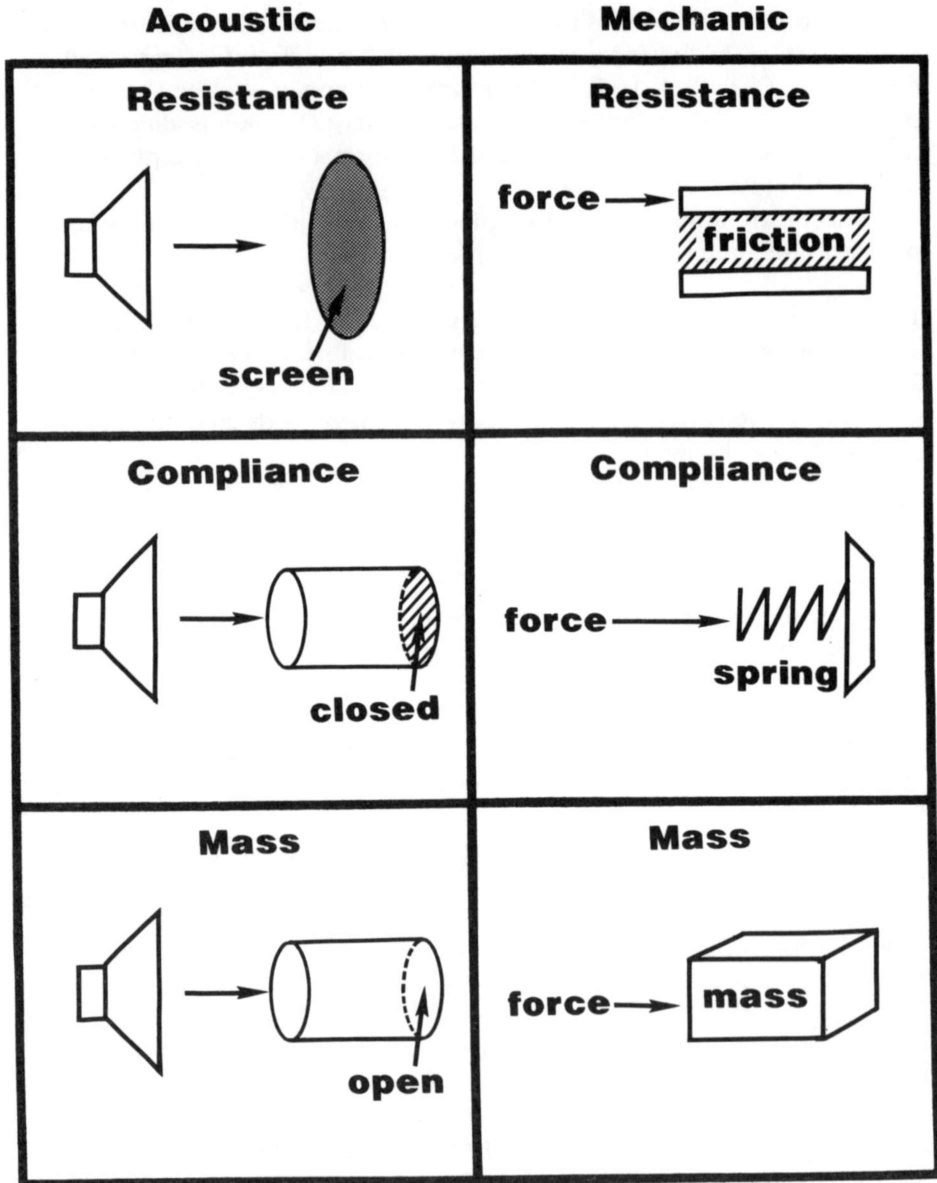

Figure 8.2 The three components of acoustic or mechanical impedance: friction gives rise to resistance. Mass and compliance give rise to reactance.

resonance frequency the impedance has its minimum value and the admittance its maximum. At higher frequency, the acoustic mass of the ear dominates the reactance and the impedance.

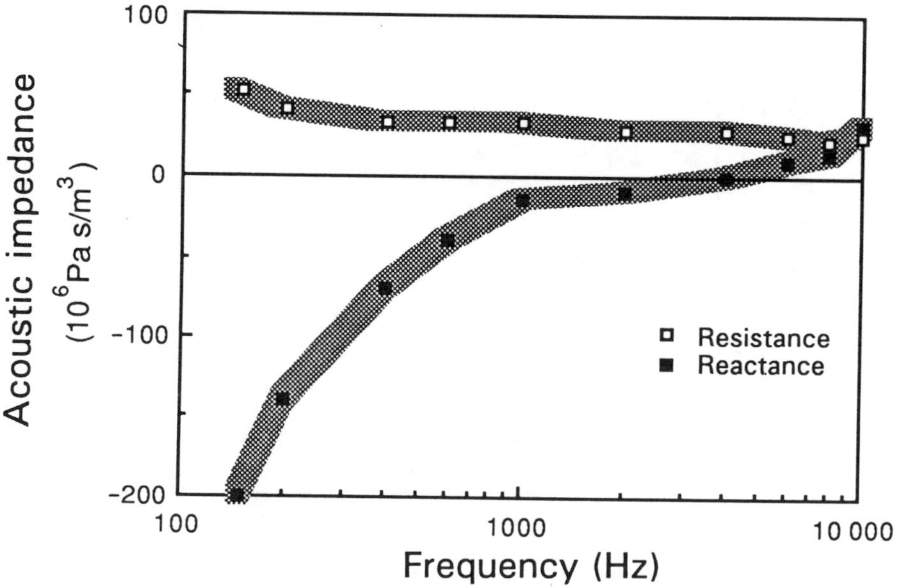

Figure 8.3 The normal acoustic resistance and reactance of the middle ear as measured in the plane of the tympanic membrane (according to Shaw, 1974). The values are approximate and large individual variations occur. Negative reactance means that the acoustic compliance dominates over the acoustic mass.

Tympanometry

Tympanometry is the recording of tympanograms, middle-ear pressure or middle-ear compliance.

Indication

These tests are used in the study of conductive hearing disorders and in the evaluation of the function of the eardrum and the middle ear. The recording of the middle-ear pressure may be of importance when repeated determinations of hearing thresholds are to be made on the same patient with the highest possible accuracy.

Physiological and physical background

Tympanometry is a test method where the middle-ear admittance or impedance is measured when the air pressure in the external auditory canal is being varied. A graphical recording of the test result is called a tympanogram (Figure 8.4). When using a low probe tone frequency (e.g. 226 Hz), the admittance or impedance measured is primarily determined

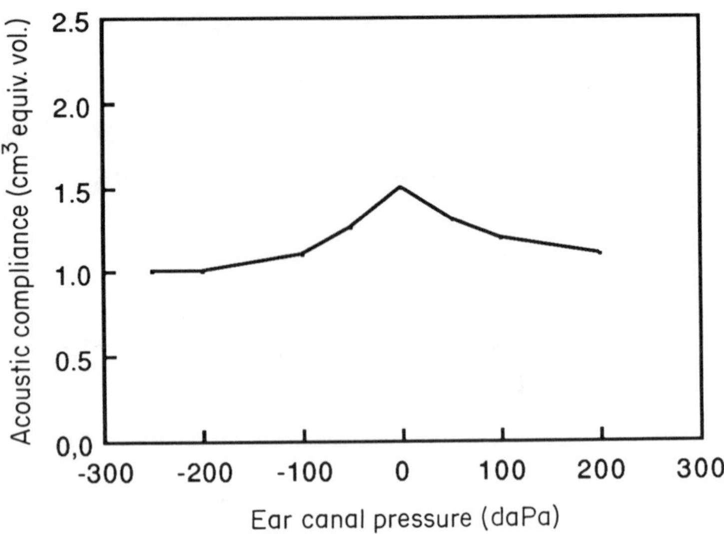

Figure 8.4 A normal tympanogram: the acoustic admittance has been recorded as a function of the ear-canal air pressure at a probe frequency of 220 Hz. At this frequency the admittance is mainly determined by the middle-ear compliance. The middle-ear pressure is approximately equal to the ambient pressure. The maximum compliance is 1.5 cm^3 equivalent volume. This value includes the ear canal volume of about 1 cm^3. Thus, the middle-ear compliance equals the difference between these two values – about 0.5 cm^3 equivalent volume.

by the acoustic compliance of the eardrum, ossicular chain and the enclosed air in the auditory canal, middle ear and cell system.

When an over- or under-pressure is created in the auditory canal, the eardrum will become pressed inwards or outwards. This usually reduces its mobility. When the air pressure in the auditory canal corresponds to that in the middle-ear cavity, the eardrum has its highest mobility. This corresponds to maximum compliance. This maximum compliance is the sum of the compliance of the middle ear and that of the air volume in the auditory canal inside the probe.

When the air pressure in the auditory canal is much higher or much lower than the middle-ear air pressure, the eardrum becomes almost completely immobile. The acoustic compliance recorded, expressed as equivalent volume, then corresponds approximately to the physical volume of the auditory canal. Thus, the middle-ear compliance can be determined by subtracting this compliance value for the auditory canal from the total compliance measured when the middle-ear and the auditory canal pressures are equal, i.e. the maximum compliance value recorded.

If the middle ear is filled by fluid, its compliance is close to zero. In addition, the compliance recorded does not change significantly when the air pressure in the auditory canal is varied.

Also if the eardrum has a perforation, the compliance does not change when the canal air pressure is varied. The compliance recorded is mainly determined by the physical volume of air in the auditory canal, middle-ear cavity and cell system. The compliance measurement in this case becomes an indirect determination of physical volume.

When tympanometry is performed by means of a probe tone with a higher frequency (500–1000 Hz), the variations in the admittance recorded can be interpreted only by analysis of the complex interaction of the three components: friction, inertia and elasticity. Such a tympanogram sometimes shows two maxima, i.e. it has a W-shape. Lutman (1984a,b) showed that the main results can be explained by describing the eardrum as consisting of two (or three) separate parts which are able to move independently of each other. The movement of one part is mainly determined by the mechanical impedance of the ossicular chain and that of the other part by the elasticity of the eardrum and the compliance of the enclosed air volume in the middle-ear volume.

A W-tympanogram can be caused by the resonance frequency of the middle ear being lower than the probe tone frequency when the pressure is equal on both sides of the eardrum, but higher than the probe tone frequency at over- or under-pressures (Figure 8.5). Normally, the mass and the elasticity of the middle ear cooperate to give a resonance frequency which is considerably higher than the probe tone frequency over the whole pressure range used in tympanometry. But if the middle ear has an abnormally high acoustic compliance (elasticity), the resonance frequency may become lower than the probe tone frequency during parts of the pressure sweep. This may occur in ears with ossicular discontinuity and sometimes, although rarely, in normal ears.

If only a small part of the eardrum is very mobile, e.g. because of a scar after a healed perforation, another type of W-tympanogram may arise (see Figure 8.7). This result may be explained by describing the very mobile part of the eardrum as a third separate part (Lutman, 1984a). The resonance frequency of this part may vary in relation to the probe tone frequency and influence the total admittance in the way illustrated in Figure 8.5, although the resonance frequency of the rest of the system is clearly higher than the probe tone frequency. If the two admittance components (conductance and susceptance) are recorded separately, two or more maxima may also occur in one or both of the recorded curves (Vanhuyse, Creten and Van Camp, 1975).

Equipment

An international standard (IEC 1027, 1991) regarding technical requirements on impedance audiometers has recently been published. All impedance audiometers are based on the principle of a probe sound,

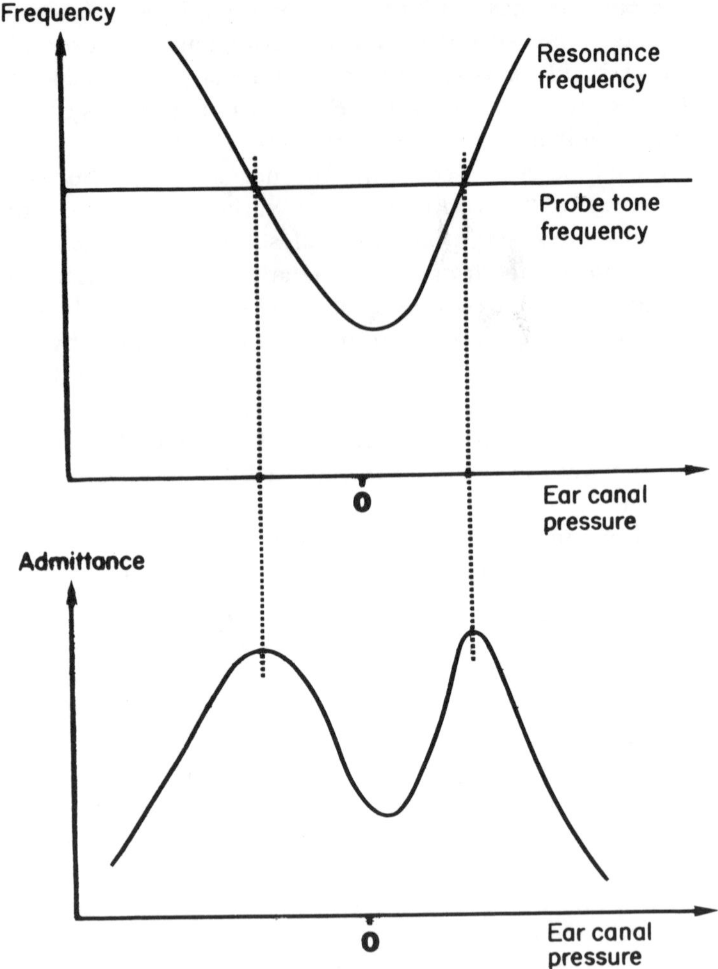

Figure 8.5 The origin of a W-tympanogram. A hypermobile tympanic membrane may give rise to a middle-ear resonance frequency that is lower than the probe tone frequency at pressures close to atmospheric (upper part) but higher for other pressures where the tympanic membrane becomes stiffer. The admittance recorded (lower part) shows two maxima, corresponding to the positive and negative pressures where the resonance frequency equals the probe frequency.

usually a pure tone, transmitted into the auditory canal by means of a probe tube. The sound pressure in the auditory canal is recorded by means of a microphone connected to the probe. The principle of the equipment is illustrated in Figure 8.1.

Some types of equipment present the test result (compliance, admittance or impedance) more or less automatically. In other types the equipment has to be balanced manually. The sound pressure of the probe tone is then adjusted to a certain value in the ear canal. The result is often recorded on paper, although the mode of graphic presentation is not standardised. Depending on the type of equipment, an admittance maximum may be recorded either upwards or downwards on the recording paper.

Certain impedance audiometers can show the two impedance or admittance components separately. However, most types show only the total admittance value. Since this is determined mainly by the middle-ear compliance at low probe tone frequencies, the instrument is often calibrated in compliance units, most commonly in an equivalent volume of air. The compliance scale of the instrument is then calibrated by performing a measurement with the probe placed in hard-walled test cavities with known volumes.

The static air pressure in the auditory canal can be varied manually or automatically at fixed rates of change. The instrument is always equipped with an air pump and a calibrated manometer connected to the probe.

Sources of error and test accuracy

Repeated measurements of the middle-ear pressure on the same individual by means of tympanometry have shown a test accuracy of about 6 daPa, i.e. one standard deviation, when using a pressure sweep from over- to under-pressure in the ear canal and about 9 daPa using the opposite sweep direction (Ivarsson et al., 1983).

Repeated measurements of the middle-ear compliance on the same individual by means of tympanometry have shown a test accuracy of about 0.16 cm^3 (s.d.) (Jerger, Jerger and Mauldin, 1972). This means that the results from two tests on the same individual should differ by at least 0.44 cm^3 to indicate a statistically significant change ($P<0.05$).

The results of tympanometry are influenced by both the rate and the direction of change of ear-canal air pressure. These effects are due partly to limitations of the equipment, partly to characteristics of the middle ear. Results of determination of the middle-ear pressure may differ by up to 30 daPa due to differences in direction and rate of change of ear-canal air pressure (Ivarsson et al., 1983). One way to avoid this error is to use pressure sweeps in both directions and take the average of the two results.

In some impedance instruments, the air pressure is recorded by means of a transducer placed close to the air pump in the instrument. The pressure changes are transmitted by means of a thin tube to the probe in the ear canal. This causes a time delay for pressure changes to pass through the tube. If the pump changes the pressure too fast, the manometer may record a pressure which has not yet reached the ear canal. The compliance maximum naturally occurs when the true ear-canal air pressure equals that of the middle ear. Such a delay in the pressure system will, however, cause the recording to indicate compliance maximum at a lower pressure than the true pressure when using a pressure sweep in negative direction (from over- to under-pressure) and a higher pressure than the true one when sweeping in the positive direction.

Additionally, the eardrum and the middle ear have plastic characteristics, i.e. they yield gradually when subjected to a static over- or under-pressure (Elner, Ingelstedt and Ivarsson, 1971). This causes the ear-canal pressure at admittance maximum to differ somewhat from the middle-ear pressure, independent of which admittance component is recorded (Decraemer, Creten and Van Camp, 1984). This may also explain why the middle-ear compliance seems to be higher when determined by a high rate of change of air pressure than by a low rate (Ivarsson et al., 1983).

Some types of impedance audiometers automatically check that the probe fit in the ear canal is airtight before the test can start. It is of course important that the probe is not permitted to move during the course of the test once this check has been made.

Clinical interpretation

A tympanogram can be interpreted with regard to the following:

- The pressure at compliance maximum.
- The compliance value at the maximum.
- The shape of the curve.

The middle-ear pressure and compliance can be determined reliably only if the tympanogram shows a clear compliance maximum (Figure 8.6).

Middle-ear pressure

The ear-canal air pressure which corresponds to the compliance maximum at a low probe tone frequency (e.g. 226 Hz) can be interpreted as an approximate value of the middle-ear pressure. In a W-tympanogram, the line of symmetry of the W is the best indicator of the middle-ear pressure. A normal value is about ±25 daPa relative to the air pressure of the environment for adults (Margolis and Shanks, 1985; Wiley, Oviatt and Block, 1987). In children under-pressures of down to about −150 daPa are not uncommon.

Middle-ear compliance

The adult middle-ear compliance is normally 0.7 cm^3 equivalent volume (median value) with individual variations between about 0.4 and 1.3 cm^3 (10th and 90th percentiles) (Jerger, Jerger and Mauldin, 1972; Jerger et al., 1974; Wiley, Oviatt and Block, 1987). In children below the age of 13

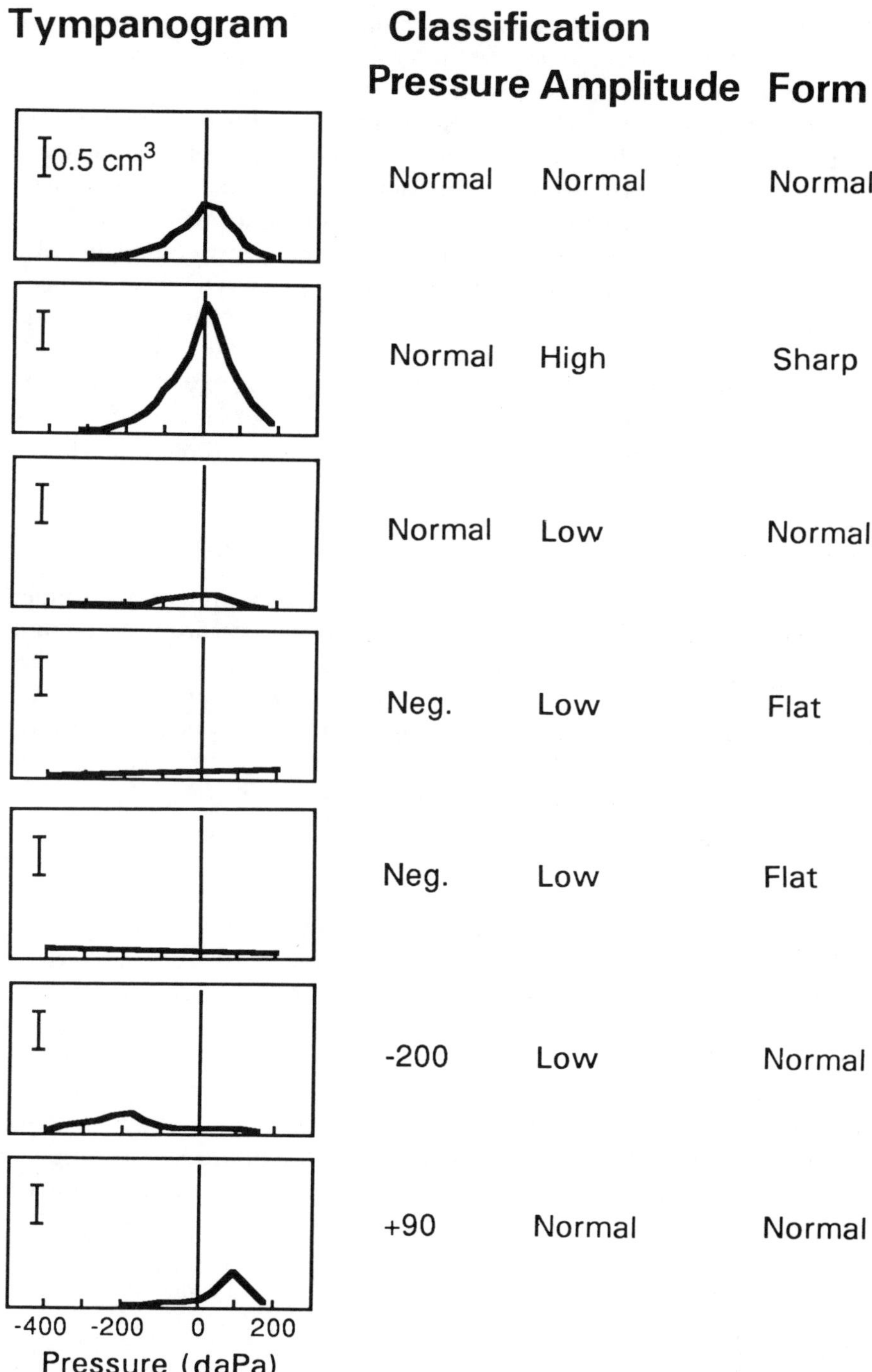

Figure 8.6 Classification of common tympanogram types based on the pressure that gives compliance maximum, the compliance value at maximum and the shape of the tympanogram.

years, the median compliance value is about 0.5 cm^3 equivalent volume with somewhat larger variability (Jerger, 1970; Jerger et al., 1974a; Bylander, 1983). Note that these values refer to the middle-ear compliance alone; the ear-canal volume has been subtracted from the total compliance.

A tympanogram with abnormally large maximum compliance indicates a scarred eardrum with atrophic parts or luxation of the ossicular chain (Figure 8.6). In both cases the eardrum becomes abnormally mobile and the compliance value higher than normal. Abnormally low compliance also indicates some kind of conductive disorder (Figure 8.6). The reduced mobility may be due to fixation of the ossicular chain, otosclerosis, adhesive otitis media or a calcified eardrum. However, a considerable overlap exists in the results obtained by tympanometry on groups of subjects with different types of middle-ear disorder and with normal middle ears. Therefore, the maximum compliance is of limited diagnostic value as a test result on its own (Jerger et al., 1974b).

Flat tympanogram – determination of physical volume

If the eardrum is very stiff, the total compliance measured is determined by the volume of enclosed air between the probe and eardrum. A common value for this is 0.8 cm^3 (Lindeman, 1982). A fluid-filled middle ear makes the eardrum stiff and no compliance maximum can be recorded. Tympanometry will show a flat line at a low compliance value (Figure 8.6). The total compliance value at atmospheric pressure, expressed as equivalent volume, can then be interpreted as a measure of the physical volume of the enclosed air.

A perforated eardrum will also give rise to a flat tympanogram but with higher total compliance. The compliance recorded is then determined by the total volume of air in the auditory canal, middle ear and cell system. This volume varies considerably between individuals. Volumes in the range 4–8 cm^3 are common (Lindeman, 1982). Since the measurement range of the impedance instrument is often limited to 5 cm^3 the larger volumes cannot be measured.

In order to differentiate between these two types of flat tympanograms, it is important to know how the test result is presented by the impedance audiometer. Some types of instrument show a graphic representation of the total impedance, whilst others only show the variation in middle-ear compliance with the total compliance indicated digitally or by other means. In the latter type the two kinds of flat tympanograms may look the same. The difference in total compliance then has to be noted.

W-tympanogram

Tympanometry with a high probe tone frequency (500–1000 Hz) may give rise to two admittance maxima, one at over-pressure and one at under-

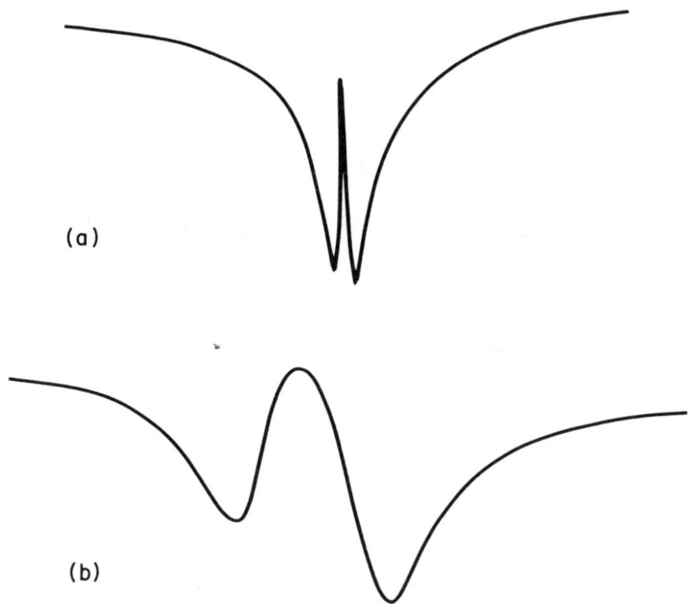

Figure 8.7 Two examples of W-tympanograms obtained at 625 Hz probe tone frequency. In this recording increasing admittance is shown downwards. (a) An eardrum with atrophic scars gives rise to sharp maxima; (b) an ossicular discontinuity produces broader maxima.

pressure in the ear canal, and between them a minimum (Figure 8.7). This indicates abnormally high mobility of the eardrum or the ossicular chain, but may also occur in middle ears which lack any other signs of abnormality (Alberti and Jerger, 1974). Small atrophic scars on the eardrum may give rise to very sharp admittance maxima while ossicular luxation may cause flatter and smoother maxima.

Stapedius Reflex Thresholds

Indications

Recording of the stapedius reflex aims at the diagnosis of lesions engaging one or several of the three parts of the reflex arc:

1. The afferent pathway.
2. The interneurons in the brain stem.
3. The efferent pathway

The afferent function is of main interest in the evaluation of sensorineural hearing loss to differentiate cochlear from retrocochlear lesions, to identify carriers of genes for hereditary hearing loss, and possibly also for a coarse estimation of hearing thresholds. The efferent pathway may be affected by facial paresis, certain muscular diseases and by conductive disorders (ossicular fixation or discontinuity).

Anatomical, physiological and physical background

The afferent part of the reflex arc consists of the cochlea and the auditory nerve (nervus cochlearis). In the brain stem, connections are made to the next neuron in the cochlear nuclei. From there, nerve impulses continue to the facial nuclei via interneurons. Most of the connections make use of two successive interneurons. Interneurons thus connect the ventral cochlear nucleus with both ipsi- and contralateral nuclei in the superior olive, and the superior olive then connects with the facial nuclei through yet another neuron. There is also a connection between the ventral cochlear nucleus and the ipsilateral facial nucleus via a single interneuron (Borg, 1973) (Figure 8.8). The right and left cochlear nucleus complexes thus each connect with both the ipsilateral and the contralateral facial nucleus. The reflex arc is double sided.

The facial nuclei are situated in the pons which is part of the brain stem. They contain nerve cells, the axons of which extend to the facial nerve. The neurons which are part of the reflex arc are situated in the medial part of the facial nucleus according to Borg (1973), but later studies have shown that these neurons are located just outside the medial part of the facial nucleus (Lyon, 1978; Strutz, Munker and Zöllner, 1988).

The efferent part of the reflex arc consists of the neurons in the facial nerve. These neurons leave the facial nerve in the middle ear and constitute the stapedial nerve which ends at the stapedius muscle. This little muscle is situated within a conical cavity – the pyramidal process – in the rear wall of the middle-ear space below the facial nerve. The stapedius muscle has a tendon which extends into the middle ear and is attached to the tip of the stapes. When the stapedius muscle contracts, the stapes is pulled backwards and the ossicular chain becomes stiffer, thus losing part of its mobility. In this way the sound which is conducted to the cochlea via the ossicles is attenuated. When impedance audiometry is performed, this reduced ossicular mobility appears as an increased acoustic impedance or reduced compliance.

Since the reflex arc is double sided, the stapedius reflex will be activated in both ears if only one ear is exposed to loud sound. For pure tones, sound levels in the range 75–95 dB HL will be needed to activate the reflex. The muscle contraction normally increases in force when the sound level is increased up to about 15 dB above the reflex threshold (Anderson, 1969).

The stapedius reflex attenuates loud sounds before they reach the cochlea. Thereby the risk for noise-induced hearing loss is reduced (Nilsson, 1983). The reflex protects mainly against sounds in the low

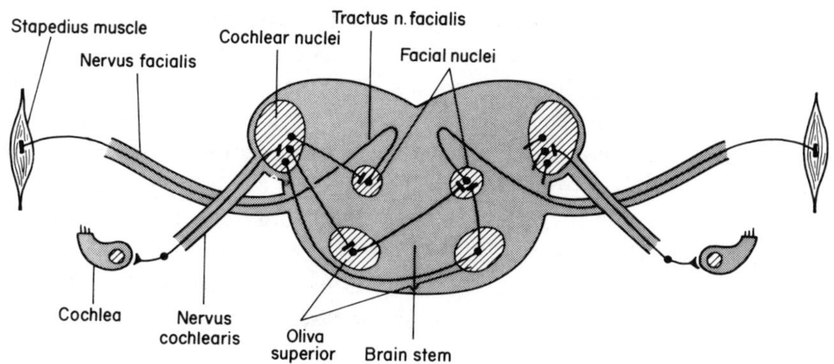

Figure 8.8 Schematic illustration of the stapedius reflex arc. The afferent part consists of the cochlea and the auditory nerve. Connection to the next neuron occurs in the cochlear nucleus in the brain stem. The impulses are led to the facial nuclei via two (or sometimes one) interneurons. The reflex is bilateral. From one ear both facial nuclei are activated. The efferent part of the reflex arc consists of neurons in the facial tract and the facial nerve. The stapedial nerve innervates the stapedius muscle.

frequency range, whilst sounds at frequencies above 2 kHz are negligibly affected. At a maximum contraction of the stapedius muscle, the attenuation provided is around 20 dB at low frequencies (Borg and Zakrisson, 1974).

The contraction of the muscle does not appear immediately when a loud sound occurs, but with a latency of at least 10–20 ms (Moller, 1974). The reflex therefore provides no protection against a sudden impulsive noise. It often takes up to a couple of hundred milliseconds before an impedance change can be recorded acoustically (Moller, 1974; McPherson and Thompson, 1977; Clemis and Sarno, 1980; Borg, 1982). The delay is longer at stimulus levels close to the reflex threshold and also clearly prolonged in subjects with retrocochlear lesions. The major part of the acoustically detectable reflex latency thus depends on the slow reaction of the muscle, the ossicular chain and the test equipment, and only a minor part consists of the time needed for the nerve impulses to travel through the auditory nerve, pass the interneurons in the brain stem and down the facial nerve.

When stimulating with pure tones in the low frequency range (up to about 1 kHz), the reflex has considerable persistence. The muscle remains contracted as long as the eliciting sound remains. At higher stimulus frequencies, a considerable fatigue is seen – the reflex decay. The reflex decay is faster the higher the stimulus frequency. However, when exposed to loud noise with considerable variations in level and spectrum, very little reflex decay is seen (Nilsson, 1983).

The duration of the stimulus sound is of considerable importance for the reflex. For pure tones in the low frequency range with durations shorter than about 80 ms, the detectable reflex threshold increases by 20–25 dB for a ten-fold decrease of the stimulus duration (Djupesland et al., 1973). For higher stimulus frequencies, this relation holds for durations of less than 500–600 ms. At durations longer than these values, the reflex threshold is influenced much less. However, later studies indicate a more complex relationship. Jerger, Mauldin and Lewis (1977) interpret the test results as the initial muscle reflex depending only on the stimulus level, independent of duration, whereas the subsequent reflex growth is influenced by a summation with a time constant of the order of 100 ms for loud stimuli and somewhat longer for stimuli just above the reflex threshold.

Equipment

An international IEC standard (IEC 1027, 1991) concerning the technical requirements for impedance audiometers has recently been published. All instruments make use of a probe tone being presented in the auditory canal by means of a probe. The sound pressure in the ear canal is recorded by means of a microphone connected to the probe. The principles of the equipment are shown in Figure 8.1.

When recording the stapedius reflex, only changes in middle-ear acoustic impedance or compliance are of interest, not the absolute impedance value.

In contralateral reflex measurements, the stimulus tone is usually presented by means of a conventional audiometer earphone. The stimuli are calibrated in the same way as for a pure-tone audiometer. The earphone is placed on an acoustic coupler or artificial ear. The pure-tone level is

Table 8.1 Examples of conversion of ipsilateral stapedius reflex thresholds from dB SPL to dB HL*

Stimulus frequency (Hz)	Conversion factor	
	Grason-Stadler 1723	IEC 118-10
500	−14	−8
1000	−8	−5
2000	−5	−7
4000	+3	−2

Example: If an ipsilateral reflex threshold has been obtained at 90 dB SPL (as measured in a 2 cm^3 coupler) at 1000 Hz this corresponds to 82–85 dB HL.

*Reference values for the impedance audiometer Grason-Stadler 1723 are as specified by the manufacturer. The values are approximate and based on the difference between sound pressure levels at the eardrum and in the acoustic coupler (IEC 118-10) and on the lowest detectable sound pressure level at the eardrum (Killion, 1978).

calibrated in decibels hearing level (dB HL) according to the same international standard as is used for pure-tone audiometers (ISO 389, 1985).

In ipsilateral reflex measurements, the stimulus tone is presented via the probe. For calibration the probe is placed on a 2 cm^3 coupler according to IEC 126 (1961). The stimulus level is expressed as decibels sound pressure level (dB SPL), determined on this coupler. There are as yet no standardised reference values to express ipsilateral stimulus level in terms of dB HL. The 2 cm^3 coupler has mainly been used for measurements on hearing aids. However, the sound pressure recorded in this coupler is not the same as that obtained at the eardrum of an ear being tested. The difference is significantly influenced by the equivalent volume of the tested ear (Laukli and Mair, 1980). An ipsilateral reflex threshold in dB SPL can therefore be converted to dB HL only in approximate terms by use of Table 8.1. The normal variation between individuals is large (± 10 dB). For ears with abnormal impedance the variation may be even larger. If an ipsilateral stapedius reflex threshold is expressed in dB HL the reference values used have to be clearly specified.

The stimulus level can also be calibrated individually in decibels sensation level (dB SL) by first determining the hearing threshold levels for the stimulus tones as presented by means of the probe with the probe tone switched off (Laukli and Mair, 1980). The stimulus generator of the impedance audiometer may have to be modified in order to permit sufficiently low stimulus levels.

Sources of error and test accuracy

In ipsilateral reflex testing at high stimulus levels, the attenuation of the stimulus tone by the filtering circuits in the impedance recording system may be insufficient. This may give rise to a reflex response-like change that is caused by the stimulus tone picked up by the probe microphone, a stimulus artefact. To evaluate the risk of stimulus artefacts in a particular instrument, the probe can be placed in a calibration test cavity and stimulus tones presented at increasing level until the instrument shows a change in probe microphone signal level, i.e. an artefact. In contralateral stimulation, similar artefacts may occur at high stimulus levels and low frequencies and this risk can be estimated roughly by placing the probe in a test cavity and holding the contralateral earphone close to the probe.

According to Kunov (1977), another possible source of error when using ipsilateral stimulation may be a non-linear interaction between the stimulus tone and the probe tone, which varies with the eardrum position within each vibration period of the low frequency probe tone.

The reflex threshold is usually determined as the lowest stimulus level at which a change in middle-ear acoustic impedance can be detected.

Difficulties sometimes arise as to whether a small change is a response or just a random disturbing event. Therefore, the threshold may be defined as the stimulus level at which the reflex response magnitude is for example 10% of its maximum value. When maximum accuracy is desired it is necessary to have an exact and reproducible threshold definition.

The step size of the stimulus level is also of importance. When threshold is defined as the lowest level where a response can be detected, a step size of 2 dB usually gives somewhat better thresholds than a step size of 5 dB. However, if the lower step size is used, the impedance change may become very small and less reliable at the lowest stimulus levels close to threshold. This may increase the difficulty in identifying at which of the low levels a response occurs (Laukli and Mair, 1980).

The time course of the impedance change recorded is influenced by the response characteristics of the impedance recording system. When reflex latency is to be determined, the temporal response characteristics of the impedance instrument therefore have to be determined separately in order to make sure that the instrument can be used for such measurements.

Weak responses may sometimes be difficult to identify due to disturbances caused by the test subject's breathing or by pulse-synchronous volume changes caused by the blood circulation in the ear canal wall. In such cases the identification of responses may become easier if a small over- or under-pressure is applied in the ear canal.

Certain drugs, e.g. sedatives or alcohol, may cause an increased reflex threshold (Northern, Gabbard and Kinder, 1985).

When testing children the reflex threshold can be determined reliably more often if a higher probe tone frequency is used, e.g. 660 Hz. The reflex threshold recorded is often somewhat better at such a higher probe frequency (Northern, Gabbard and Kinder, 1985).

Sometimes the reflex threshold, determined by a stepwise increasing stimulus level, is somewhat worse than when using a stepwise decreasing stimulus level – a hysteresis phenomenon. The threshold should then be defined as the lowest (best) of the two values obtained from the ascending and descending series.

When testing, the middle-ear pressure has to be compensated by applying a corresponding pressure in the ear canal. Therefore, the middle-ear pressure always has to be determined before the stapedius reflex test. If the middle-ear pressure is abnormal, the patient can be asked to try to equalise the pressure by means of the Valsalva or Toynbee manoeuvre before the ear-canal pressure is adjusted to correspond to the middle-ear pressure.

A collapsing ear canal on the stimulus ear may cause a false increase in contralateral reflex thresholds. If this is suspected, a piece of rubber or plastic tubing may be placed in the ear canal to keep it open.

Repeated measurements of the stapedius reflex thresholds on normally hearing subjects indicate a test accuracy of 4.5 dB (standard deviation in single measurements) if the step size of the stimulus tone level is 5 dB (Jerger, Jerger and Mauldin, 1972). This implies that two measurements on the same subject should differ by at least 15 dB to be statistically significant ($P<0.05$).

Clinical interpretation

Reflex threshold levels for normally hearing subjects have been determined in several studies (Jepsen, 1951; Metz, 1952; Anderson and Wedenberg, 1968; Lidén, 1970; Colletti, 1974; Chiveralls, 1977; Jerger et al., 1978; Wiley, Oviatt and Block, 1987). Normal values for contralaterally elicited reflex thresholds using pure tones in the range 250–4000 Hz are found in the range 75–95 dB HL, with mean values around 85 dB HL.

Anderson and Wedenberg (1968) base their results on 100 ears from 50 subjects with normal hearing. They placed the upper limit for normality at the 90th percentile and the lowest pathological reflex threshold level at the next highest 5-dB step. Lidén (1970) applied similar criteria and based his results on 88 normally hearing subjects. Both studies result in the lowest pathological level for the reflex threshold being at 95 dB HL in the frequency range 250–4000 Hz. Laukli and Mair (1980) also found mean values for contralateral reflex thresholds at 84–85 dB HL in the frequency range 500–2000 Hz. The standard deviation in their study was around 6 dB. This means that, if a pathologically elevated reflex threshold is defined as the mean plus two standard deviations, the lowest pathological value is at 96–97 dB HL.

The ipsilateral stapedius reflex is elicited at lower levels than the contralateral according to Moller (1961), Borg and Zakrisson (1974) and Reker (1977). Reker found ipsilateral reflex thresholds at levels 9–14 dB below the contralateral thresholds. However, Laukli and Mair (1980) found ipsilateral reflex thresholds on approximately the same levels as the contralateral ones. They found no significant difference between ipsi- and contralateral thresholds. The mean values for the ipsilateral thresholds were 86–88 dB SL (sensation level) with a standard deviation of about 7 dB in the frequency range 500–2000 Hz.

Broad-band sounds normally elicit the reflex at a lower total sound pressure level than narrow-band sounds or pure tones (Deutsch, 1972; Djupesland and Zwislocki, 1973; Popelka, Margolis and Wiley, 1976). This phenomenon corresponds qualitatively to the auditory critical bandwidth as shown in studies of loudness summation. However, later results indicate no definite bandwidth limit at which the reflex threshold starts to decrease. If the bandwidth is expressed in octaves, a linear correlation is obtained between reflex threshold and bandwidth (Green and Margolis, 1983).

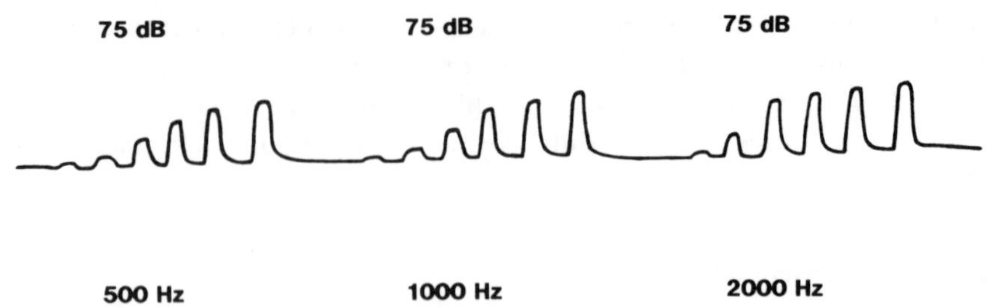

Figure 8.9 Example of a normal recording of the stapedius reflex. The reflex threshold is 75 dB HL at all test frequencies. The stimulus level is increased in 5-dB steps, causing increasing response amplitude up to saturation.

Bone-conduction stimulation may also be used to elicit a stapedius reflex (Djupesland et al., 1973). However, the reflex thresholds may differ from those using air conduction. This may be due to a possible binaural stimulation. Most bone vibrators in clinical use will not be capable of producing sufficiently high stimulus levels to make bone-conduction stimulation a practical clinical method.

The amplitude of the reflex response normally grows with increasing stimulus levels up to about 15 dB above the reflex threshold (Figure 8.9) (Anderson, 1969; Jerger, Mauldin and Lewis, 1977). Sometimes no stapedius reflex can be elicited without any evident organic reason. At the stimulus frequency 4000 Hz, this is found in about 4% of otherwise evidently normal ears (Jerger, Jerger and Mauldin, 1972).

A reliable interpretation of the results of stapedius reflex testing presumes that the response ear has a whole eardrum without severe scar tissue and, in addition, that the middle-ear pressure must have been balanced by the ear-canal pressure so as to provide an eardrum with maximum mobility. If the middle-ear pressure of the response ear were significantly different from the atmospheric pressure, the test results would have to be interpreted with caution because it is sometimes difficult to keep the pressure balanced during the full course of testing.

Conductive lesions

The stapedius reflex is usually affected by conductive disorders that engage the ossicular chain. When stimulating the ear with a conductive loss, the reflex threshold is elevated and sometimes cannot be reached at the maximum stimulus level available. A conductive loss usually also prevents a contraction of the stapedius muscle causing any recordable change in acoustic impedance. This is of course independent of whether ipsi- or contralateral stimulation is used.

A fixation of the ossicular chain prevents the activity of the stapedius muscle reaching the eardrum because of the immobile chain. The fixation usually engages the stapes and the most common cause is otosclerosis (Figure 8.10). In early otosclerosis, when the mobility of the stapes is only moderately reduced, a reflex response may still be recordable. The

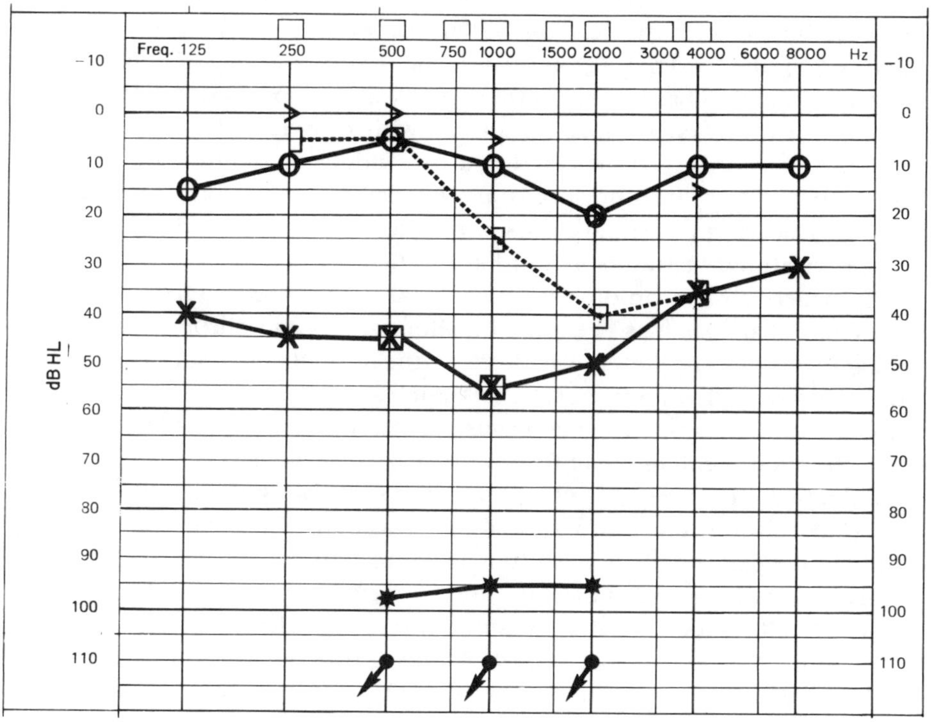

Figure 8.10 An audiogram from a patient with left-sided otosclerosis. No reflex response can be recorded when the right ear is stimulated and the probe is placed in the left ear. Stimulating the left ear gives rise to reflex responses at relatively low sensation levels (conductive recruitment).

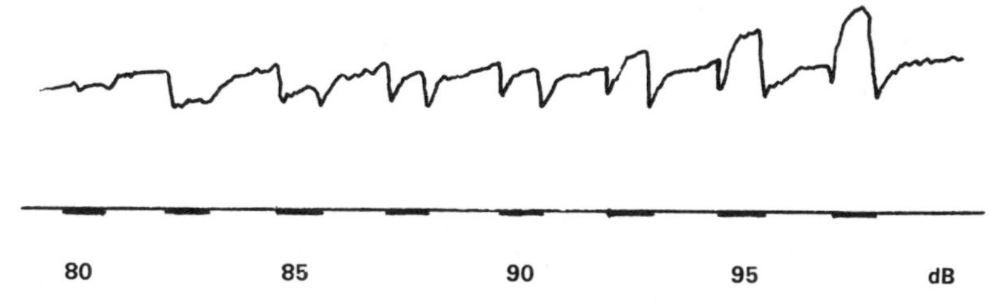

Figure 8.11 Example of a recording of diphasic stapedius reflex responses.

response could then occur in the abnormal direction at the beginning and end of the stimulus, i.e. shows a reduced impedance, often with an increased impedance in between. This diphasic inverted reflex is illustrated in Figure 8.11 and may sometimes be seen in early otosclerotic cases before any significant hearing loss occurs (Flottorp and Djupesland, 1970; Djupesland and Kvernbold, 1975). The reason for this would be a reduced mechanical contact between the cochlea and the middle ear, caused by otosclerosis leading to an abnormal position and vibratory pattern of the ossicles (Djupesland and Kvernbold, 1975). When the extent of fixation has increased the reflex will disappear completely in the diseased ear. When stimulating an ear with otosclerosis, a contralateral reflex can be observed provided that the middle ear on the opposite side is normal. The reflex thresholds are typically elevated but often less so than the hearing thresholds. This phenomenon has been termed 'conductive recruitment' (Anderson and Barr, 1966).

Disorders other than otosclerosis may also give rise to a fixation of the ossicular chain, such as congenital malformations and chronic middle-ear inflammations. The latter may lead to the growth of tissue around the ossicles – so-called tympanosclerosis. Such growth is often situated in the upper part of the middle ear and causes a fixation of the head of the malleus and the incus (epitympanic fixation or frozen malleus). In such cases no conductive recruitment can be seen when stimulating the diseased ear. In addition to the absence of a normal reflex response in an ear with fixation, the middle-ear compliance is often abnormally low.

In ears with ossicular discontinuity, reflex responses are absent if the discontinuity is located laterally relative to the attachment of the stapedius tendon on the neck of the stapes. The long process of the incus may be missing, which often occurs in chronic otitis media. Another possibility is a dislocation of the incus away from its normal position. However, if connective tissue forms a bridge from the stapes to the eardrum, a reflex response is often present.

If the discontinuity is situated medial to the attachment of the stapedius tendon, a recordable response is usually present in the diseased ear (Figure 8.12). The crura of the stapes may be fractured due to trauma to the skull or ear. They may also be abnormally soft because of a congenital malformation. In such cases the stapedius reflex often shows an abnormally large amplitude because the ossicular chain lacks its normal stiffness. For the same reason, the tensor reflex is also of abnormally large amplitude. When the diseased ear is stimulated, the reflex threshold is increased. The difference between reflex thresholds and hearing thresholds is within normal range. Thus, in contrast to cases with otosclerosis, no conductive recruitment is present in ears with an ossicular discontinuity. The audiogram often has a very typical pattern if a partial discontinuity is present with a larger conductive loss at higher frequencies. The evaluation

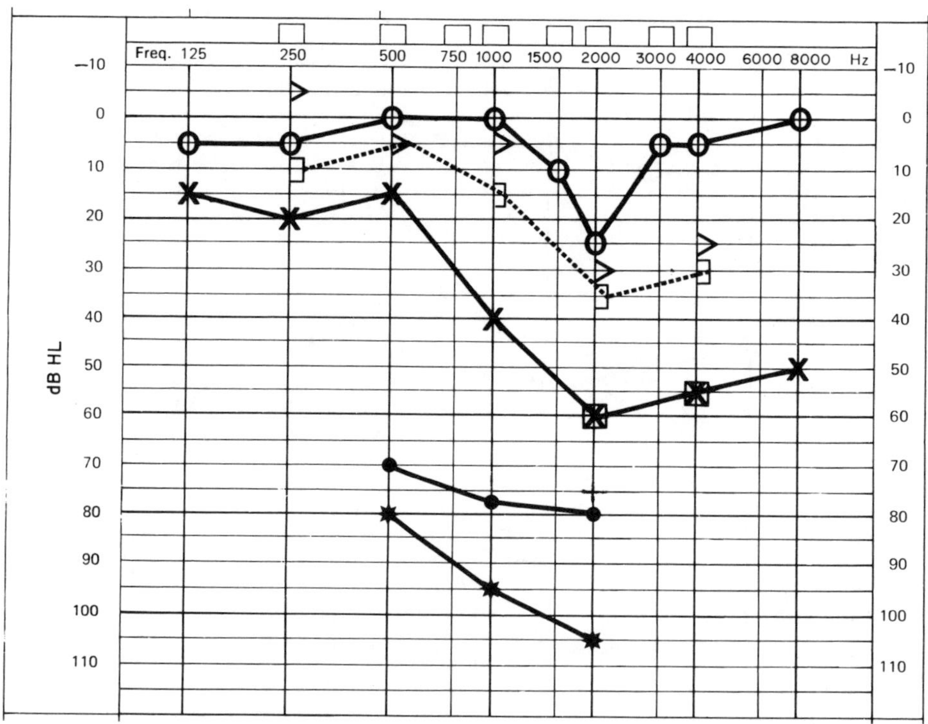

Figure 8.12 An audiogram from a patient with partially broken ossicular chain after a motor-cycle accident. Since the fracture is at the crura of the stapes, reflex responses are present on both ears. (The tympanogram of the same patient is shown in Figure 8.7b.)

of such cases should also include tympanometry with high probe tone frequency.

Sensorineural hearing loss

When evaluating sensorineural hearing loss the reflex threshold obtained in the diseased ear is of value. Recording of the reflex response may be undertaken either contra- or ipsilaterally.

In cochlear hearing loss of moderate degree, the reflex thresholds for pure tones are normally found at the same levels as in normal ears (Figure 8.13). This means reflex thresholds are in the range 75–95 dB HL in spite of increased hearing thresholds. Thus, the difference between hearing thresholds and stapedius reflex thresholds is less than normal. This phenomenon is correlated to the presence of recruitment. Whilst the normal range shows a difference in the range 75–95 dB, an ear with cochlear hearing loss may show a difference as small as 20 dB (Hayes and Jerger, 1978). When the cochlear loss is severe, however, the stapedius

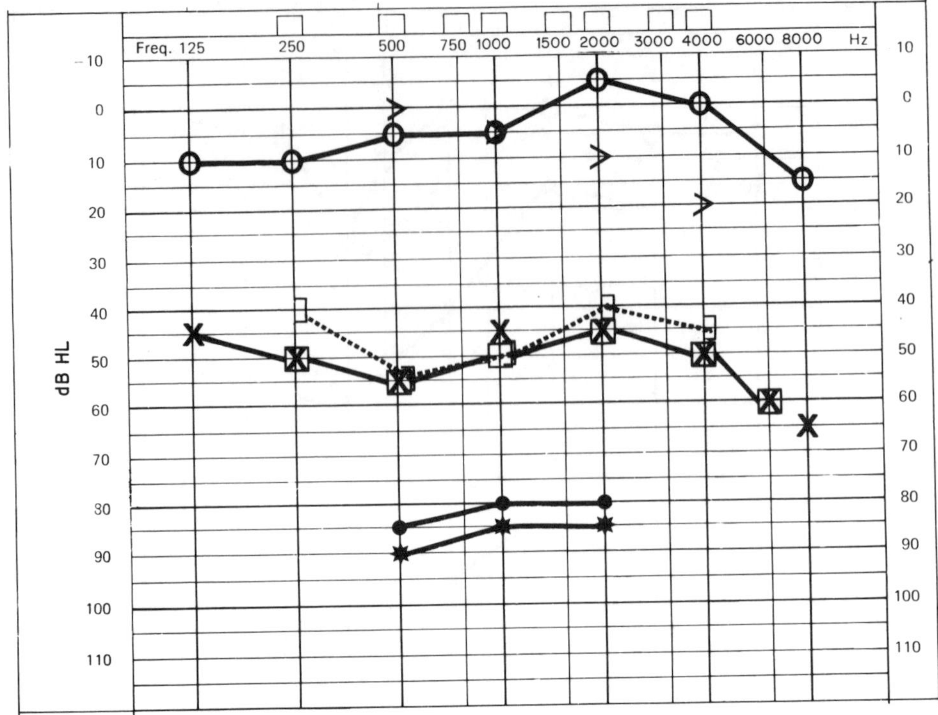

Figure 8.13 An audiogram from a patient with cochlear hearing loss and recruitment (Menière's disease). The reflex thresholds are obtained at normal levels when stimulating the diseased ear.

reflex thresholds will be outside the normal range, although the elevation is always less than the change in hearing thresholds.

Stapedius reflex thresholds which are equal to or better (lower) than the hearing thresholds indicate a non-organic hearing loss.

A retrocochlear lesion is a disorder affecting the auditory nerve (the first order neuron). Often, the difference between hearing thresholds and stapedius reflex thresholds is within normal range but sometimes the difference is larger than normal. A slight or moderate retrocochlear hearing loss will thus cause elevated stapedius reflex thresholds. It is not uncommon, particularly with a somewhat more substantial hearing loss, that the stapedius reflex cannot be elicited within the stimulus range available in the impedance instrument (Figure 8.14). A subject with retrocochlear hearing loss usually lacks recruitment and does not perceive uncomfortable loudness when exposed to sounds of high level.

Therefore, an ear with retrocochlear hearing loss either shows elevated reflex thresholds or lacks measurable reflexes in both ipsi- and contralateral stimulation of the diseased ear. Usually a normal reflex response can

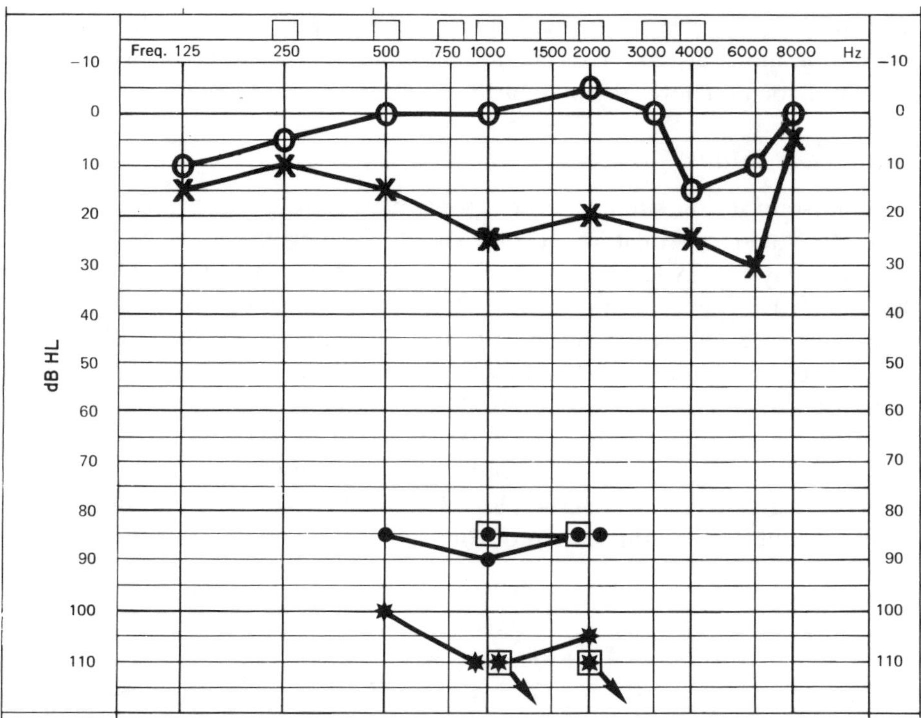

Figure 8.14 An audiogram from a patient with retrocochlear lesion (acoustic neuroma on the left side). The reflex thresholds are pathologically elevated when the left ear is stimulated and response recording is contralateral. No ipsilateral reflex is present in the left ear.

be recorded in that ear when contralateral stimulation is used. A rare exception to this is a large acoustic neuroma that may give rise to facial paralysis; this will also paralyse the stapedius muscle.

Another common finding in retrocochlear lesions is an abnormal fatigue of the stapedius reflex which will be discussed further in the section on stapedius reflex decay.

The sensitivity of the stapedius reflex threshold test in identifying retrocochlear lesions has been determined as 85% and a specificity of 80% found in 20 cases each of retrocochlear and cochlear lesions (Jerger and Jerger, 1983). Hirsch and Anderson (1980b) reported a sensitivity of 98% in the specific diagnostic question of acoustic neuroma, Lidén and Rosenhall (1985) found 93% and Reimer (1987) reported a sensitivity of 80% and specificity of 75%.

The reflex latency is typically prolonged to about 300 ms at 2 kHz and 200 ms at 1 kHz in retrocochlear lesions, as compared to the latency of about 100 ms found in normally hearing subjects and in cochlear lesions (Clemis and Sarno, 1980). The latter authors suggest pathological limits of

142 ms at 2 kHz and 123 ms at 1 kHz; an interaural latency difference of 40 ms or more at 2 kHz or 32 ms or more at 1 kHz is an alternative indicator for unilateral retrocochlear disorder.

Brain-stem lesion

A brain-stem lesion situated in the pons may disturb the stapedius reflex. Both ipsi- and contralateral testing should be performed as well as the reflex decay test. A lateral lesion in the brain stem in the boundary area between the pons and medulla oblongata may cause the same reflex abnormality as a retrocochlear disorder. Thus the reflex thresholds may be elevated or the reflexes absent when stimulating the ear on the diseased side for ipsilateral as well as contralateral stimulation. When stimulating the other ear, normal reflex characteristics will be present.

A lesion which is situated centrally close to the medial line within the pons may give rise to threshold elevation or absence of the contralaterally elicited reflexes on stimulation of the right as well as the left ear (Figure

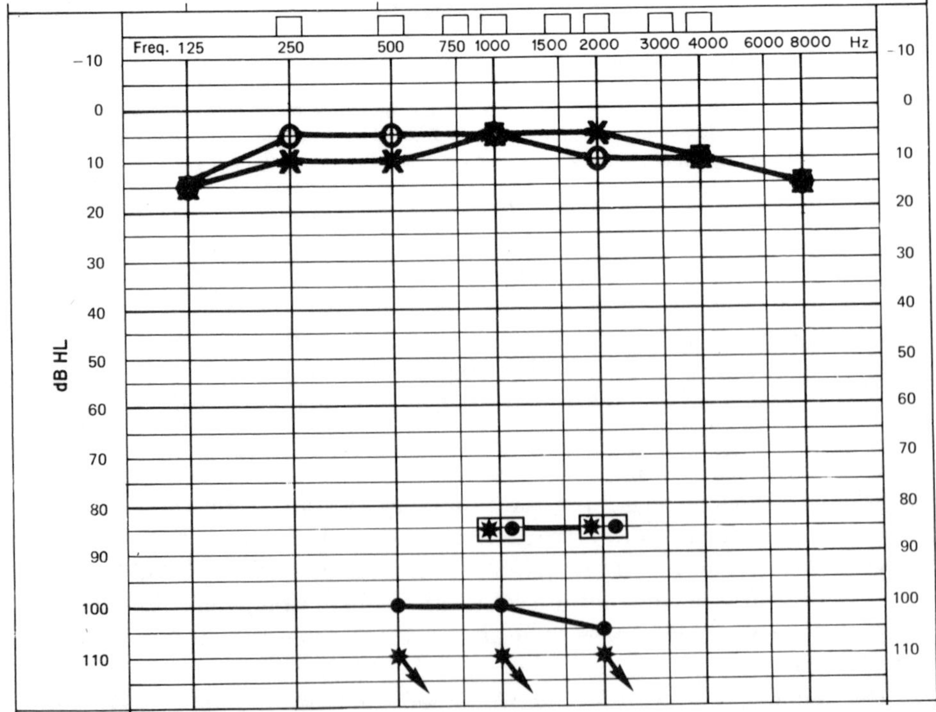

Figure 8.15 An audiogram from a patient with a central brain-stem lesion. The ipsilateral reflexes are present. The interneurons for the contralateral reflexes pass the midline in the pons and the contralaterally evoked reflexes are absent or present but with elevated thresholds.

8.15). However, the ipsilaterally elicited reflexes are often normal in such cases (Jerger and Jerger, 1977).

A lesion within the pons, which engages the facial nucleus and/or the facial nerve tract (the facial nerve pathway within the pons) on one side, often results in an absent reflex or elevated reflex thresholds when trying to record the reflex response in the ear on the side of the lesion. This holds for both ipsi- and contralateral stimulation. Often, but not always, a facial paralysis is present in cases with brain-stem lesions of this location.

Thus, stapedius reflex testing may provide valuable topographic information in cases with neurological disorders in the brain stem. Different combinations of the patterns described above may occur. It is also quite common in brain-stem disorders for the stapedius reflex to show completely normal characteristics. In order for the reflex to show any abnormality, the lesion has to involve some part of the reflex arc in the brain stem.

Facial paralysis

When a facial paralysis is present normally, the stapedius reflex cannot be recorded in the ear on the paralysed side, independent of whether the stimulation is ipsi- or contralateral. On the non-paralysed side a normal reflex response is present for both ipsi- and contralateral stimulation. If another pattern of reflex abnormality is found, this may indicate a brain-stem lesion (see above). If the lesion is situated distal to the point where the stapedius nerve leaves the facial nerve, it will have no influence on the stapedius reflex. Stapedius reflex testing can, therefore, be used to determine the site of a lesion that causes facial paralysis. In addition, the test can be used to follow the recovery process in cases where the reflex was affected.

Muscular diseases

Certain muscular diseases, e.g. myasthenia gravis, may also influence the function of the stapedius muscles. This can be shown by the stapedius reflex decay test which then shows pathological results.

Carriers of genes for hereditary hearing loss

A person who is a carrier of genes for hereditary hearing loss may have bilaterally elevated stapedius reflex thresholds in the high frequency range (Anderson and Wedenberg, 1968, 1970). The reflex decay test is normal in these cases. When testing children with hearing loss of unknown origin, it may, therefore, be recommended that the stapedius reflex thresholds of the child's parents are also determined. The presence of bilaterally elevated reflex thresholds in one or both of the parents indicates a hereditary hearing loss in the child.

Estimation of hearing thresholds

The difference in stapedius reflex thresholds obtained when stimulating with pure tones and with a broad-band noise has been suggested as a possible basis for an approximate estimation of the degree of sensorineural hearing loss (Jerger et al., 1974c; Niemeyer and Sesterhenn, 1974). However, later studies have failed to confirm this as a procedure to be recommended (Hyde et al., 1980; Kankkunen and Lidén, 1984).

Stapedius Reflex Decay Test

Indication

The test is used for the diagnosis of retrocochlear lesions, lesions in the brain stem and certain muscular diseases.

Physiological background

The fact that the stapedius reflex is subject to fatigue or adaptation had been demonstrated before impedance audiometers were available (Luscher, 1930; Kobrak, Lindsay and Perlman, 1941) and was later confirmed by impedance audiometry (Metz, 1951). This phenomenon is not normally due to fatigue of the stapedius muscle but the cause is to be found in the afferent part of the reflex arc (Jepsen, 1963). Thus, Wersäll (1958) showed that an additional acoustic stimulus can reactivate an already fatigued reflex, provided that the new stimulus is of a different frequency from the original.

The reflex adaptation depends on the characteristics of the sound stimulus, e.g. the sound level is of importance (Dallos, 1964). Another factor of great importance is the stimulus frequency. When stimulating with pure tones of low frequencies (1 kHz or lower), the stapedius reflex is quite persistent (Anderson, Barr and Wedenberg, 1969). The muscle remains contracted as long as the low frequency stimulus remains on. At higher stimulus frequencies a considerable reflex decay is normally seen (Anderson, Barr and Wedenberg, 1969). The reflex decays faster at higher stimulus frequencies. However, on exposure to high level noise with considerable variation in sound level and spectrum, no decay is evident (Nilsson, 1983).

Anderson, Barr and Wedenberg (1969, 1970) showed that, in retrocochlear hearing loss caused by acoustic neuromas, an abnormal reflex decay is present also at low stimulus frequencies. Further studies on patients with cerebellopontine angle tumours as well as brain-stem lesions have later confirmed this observation (Fisch and Wegmuller, 1974; Jerger et al., 1974d; Colletti, 1975; Thomsen and Terkildsen, 1975; King, Gibson and Morrison, 1976; Hall, 1977; Hirsch and Anderson, 1980a).

In subjects with retrocochlear hearing loss (acoustic neuroma), reflex decay is shown when the stimulus is presented to the ear on the tumour side which again confirms that the phenomenon is localised to the afferent part of the reflex arc. A possible explanation for the reflex decay in retrocochlear lesions has been proposed by Anderson, Barr and Wedenberg (1970). Normally, a low frequency tone stimulates a larger number of neurons than a high frequency tone (Wever, 1949), which may explain why the reflex normally decays at higher frequencies. In a retrocochlear lesion, therefore, a reduction of the number of normally functioning nerve fibres might lead to reflex decay also at low stimulus frequencies.

Equipment

For reflex decay testing, a normal clinical impedance audiometer can be used, equipped with recorder or other suitable means of displaying the reflex response for a sufficient period. The criteria for evaluation of the results are based on measurements using logarithmic recording of the impedance change. These criteria should be applied with some caution to results obtained by means of other types of equipment.

Sources of error and test accuracy

The applicability of the reflex decay test in the diagnosis of retrocochlear lesions has been subject to some questioning (Chiveralls, 1977) due to false positive test results occurring quite frequently. Also in normal ears a small reflex decay is present at low frequencies (Chiveralls and FitzSimons, 1973; Rosenhall, Lidén and Nilsson, 1979). With the criteria for pathological reflex decay specified by Anderson, Barr and Wedenberg (1969), the incidence of false positive test results is about 3% in normally hearing subjects (Rosenhall, Lidén and Nilsson, 1979), but about 9% in subjects with sensorineural hearing loss (Chiveralls, 1977).

Sometimes the reflex response is difficult to analyse because of the low amplitude or irregular form due to disturbances in the recording. A gradually changing baseline during the test time must be taken into account and such a change could make the decay test less reliable.

Another limitation is that, in retrocochlear cases with elevated reflex thresholds, a stimulus level of 10 dB above reflex threshold may be above the range of the instrument used.

During the reflex decay test, the patient is exposed to very loud sounds for several tens of seconds. Therefore, the test must always be carried out with great care and be stopped immediately if the patient indicates discomfort. It is important to note that a patient with a retrocochlear hearing loss does not always perceive uncomfortable loudness, although high stimulus levels may still constitute a risk for cochlear damage.

Differences can occur in the test results depending on whether the impedance instrument records the reflex response in a linear or logarithmic mode. Other instrument characteristics may also influence the results, e.g. its response time (Jerger, Oliver and Stach, 1986; Thompson and Robinette, 1988). Karlsson and Hagerman (1984) found a rather low correlation between reflex decay recorded by means of an impedance audiometer-type Grason-Stadler 1723 and by laboratory equipment built according to Anderson (1969) when the Grason-Stadler instrument had been modified for logarithmic recording.

Clinical interpretation

The reflex decay test is performed at the stimulus frequencies of 500 and 1000 Hz at 10 dB above the reflex thresholds. If the reflex response amplitude decreases by 50% or more within 5 s after the maximum initial amplitude, a pathological decay is considered present (Anderson, Barr and Wedenberg, 1969). This result is a sign of a retrocochlear disorder, e.g. an acoustic neuroma (Figure 8.16). However, due to the high stimulus levels often required, difficulties frequently arise when trying to obtain reliable results. This is probably the reason why the reflex decay test is considered to add only limited new information to that already obtained by the determination of stapedius reflex thresholds (Bergenius, Borg and Hirsch, 1983; Lidén and Rosenhall, 1985; Reimer, 1987).

The test can also be applied in cases with muscular disease, e.g. myasthenia gravis. An abnormal muscular weakness will often be shown by the reflex decay test in such cases. The test may provide diagnostic information and can also be of value when following the course of the disease and evaluating the effect of medical treatment (Blom and Zakrisson, 1974).

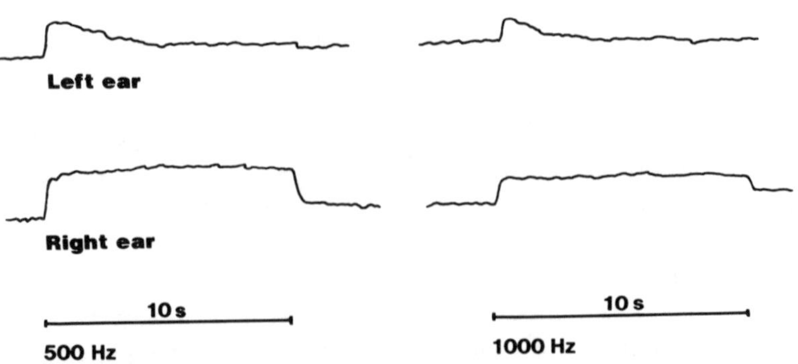

Figure 8.16 Pathological reflex decay in a patient with retrocochlear hearing loss – a left-sided acoustic neuroma. When the normal right ear is stimulated the reflex decay test yields normal results.

Tensor Reflex Test

Indications

The tensor reflex test may be used in the diagnosis of otosclerosis and discontinuity of the ossicular chain (Klockhoff, 1961).

Anatomical and physiological background

The tensor tympani muscle is a small fusiform muscle about 2 cm long which is located in a bony canal above the eustachian tube. These two canals, which run in parallel, are separated by a thin wall. The muscle fibres, which are arranged in a feather-like shape, are attached to the wall of the bony canal, the sphenoidal bone and the cartilaginous wall of the eustachian tube. The tendon from the muscle extends into the middle-ear cavity and passes a bony process (processus cochleariformis) in the medial wall of the middle ear. The tendon runs laterally and is attached to the handle of the malleus close to the head (Schuknecht, 1974). The tensor tympani muscle is innervated by motor fibres from the mandibular branch of the trigeminal nerve. When the muscle contracts the malleus is pulled medially, thereby increasing the tension of the eardrum.

In many animals, e.g. cat, dog, rabbit and guinea-pig, it has been shown that the tensor tympani is engaged in an acoustic reflex in the same way as the stapedius muscle. Contractions of the tensor muscle can also be elicited by tactile stimulation of the pinna in animals.

In humans, the tensor reflex is normally not elicited by acoustic stimuli (Lidén, Peterson and Harford, 1970). The function of the tensor muscle in humans is unclear. A surprising tactile stimulation of areas innervated by the trigeminal nerve may give rise to a brief tensor contraction (Figure 8.17). An example of such stimulation is a sudden unexpected puff of air directed towards the eye. In humans the tensor reflex is considered to be a component of a startle reaction (Klockhoff, 1961).

Equipment

The test is performed by means of an impedance audiometer. In principle, the reflex response is recorded in the same way as for the stapedius reflex. One specific requirement is that the instrument must have provision for continuous graphic recording of impedance changes.

Clinical interpretation

The tensor reflex may be used for the diagnosis of various middle-ear disorders. A whole eardrum is a prerequisite. In cases with ossicular discontinuity, a recordable tensor reflex is usually found with abnormally large amplitude because of the increased mobility of the malleus. In cases

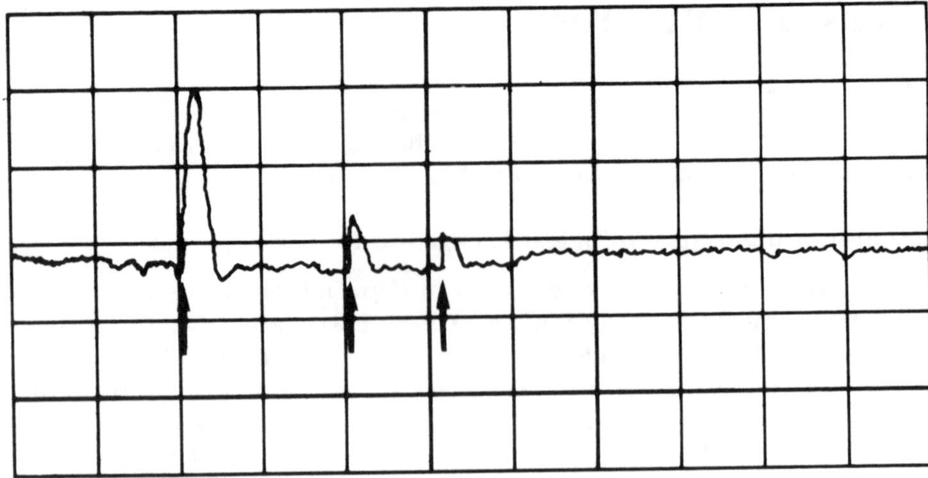

Figure 8.17 Tensor reflexes elicited by air puffs (marked by arrows) directed towards the eye.

with otosclerosis, a normal tensor reflex can typically be recorded in the diseased ear in contrast to the stapedius reflex which is typically not recordable or abnormal. In cases with epitympanic fixation the tensor reflex cannot normally be recorded.

The tensor tympani syndrome

In some people, an increased spontaneous middle-ear activity is present which has been interpreted as caused by the tensor tympani muscle – the so-called tensor tympani syndrome (Klockhoff, 1961, 1981). The phenomenon can be recorded by means of an impedance audiometer with facilities for continuous graphic impedance recording. Slow irregular fluctuations in the baseline can be seen (Figure 8.18). There is also typically a regular pulse-synchronous activity, the relation of which to the tensor tympani muscle is unclear. The phenomenon may come and go and can often be provoked by pressure changes in the ear canal.

According to Klockhoff, the tensor tympani syndrome is often seen in patients with stress-induced headache. Other symptoms often found in connection with the syndrome are feelings of pressure in the ear, otalgia, tinnitus, slight hearing loss and vertigo. The generating mechanism may be a state of muscular and/or psychic stress.

Continuous impedance recording may also be useful in the evaluation of other neuromuscular disorders in the face or throat. Such disorders are palatal myoclonus, facial tics and hemifacial spasms.

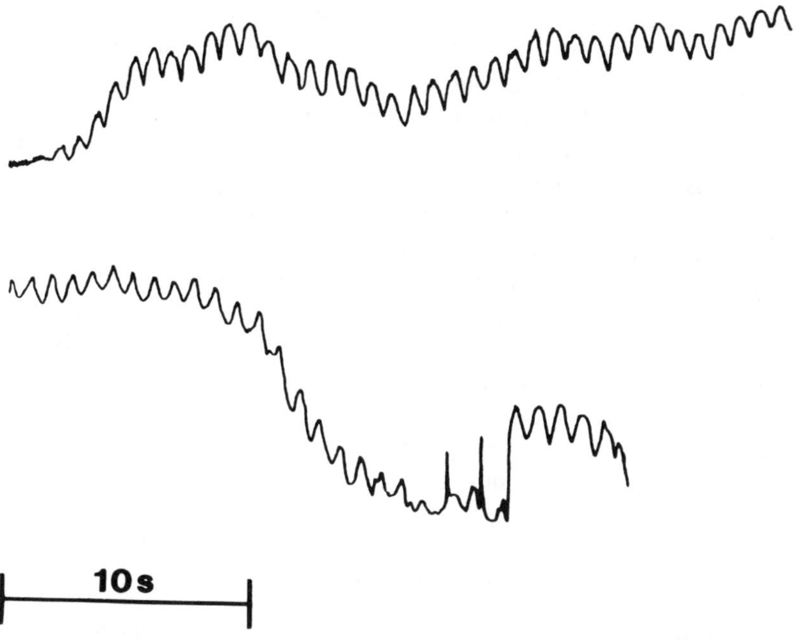

Figure 8.18 Example of recordings from a patient with the tensor tympani syndrome. Slow irregular fluctuations in impedance are seen in the recording and, in addition, a pulse-synchronous activity.

Tubal Function Tests

Indications

Tubal function tests are used to study the capacity of the eustachian tube to equilibrate over- or under-pressure in the middle ear. Different methods are used depending on whether the eardrum is whole or perforated.

The tests are used in the evaluation of disorders in the middle ear and/ or the eustachian tube. The tubal function may also have to be tested if a patient with a whole eardrum experiences problems with feeling of pressure or difficulty in equalising middle-ear pressure when the ambient air pressure changes. The ability to equalise middle-ear pressure may be of particular interest in people involved in aviation or diving.

Physiological and physical background

The eustachian tube connects the middle ear with the epipharynx, the cavity between the nose and throat. The tube runs from the middle ear forwards–downwards with a slope of about 30–40 degrees relative to the horizontal plane. In children its course is more horizontal with a slope of about 10 degrees. Its length is 35–40 mm in adults. The anterior two-thirds of the canal wall is cartilaginous whilst the rest is bony. The inner wall is covered by a ciliated mucous membrane. The narrowest part of the tube (the isthmus) is situated at the borderline between the bony and cartilaginous walls. The diameter here is 1–2 mm. The cross-section of the tube is long and narrow. At rest the walls rest against each other and the tube is then closed. It opens momentarily during swallowing, yawning and other jaw movements. It is actively opened by a muscle – the tensor veli palatini. When this muscle relaxes, the tube returns spontaneously to the closed resting state. In addition, the tube can be opened passively by over-pressure in the middle ear and by over-pressure in the nose, such as when sneezing, but also by under-pressure in the nose. The under-pressure may arise by sniffing, when the patient rapidly inhales air through the nose. A review of the anatomy, function and pathophysiology of the eustachian tube is given by Bluestone (1980).

The functions of the eustachian tube are equalisation of pressure difference and drainage of the middle ear.

Equalisation of pressure difference (over- or under-pressure)

This may arise in the middle ear. The mucous membrane of the middle ear constantly absorbs air. This may lead, at least in some persons, to the middle-ear pressure falling by 0.3–0.5 kPa/hour if the tube is closed (Elner, Ingelstedt and Ivarsson, 1971). The tube normally opens at swallowing about once per minute; the air pressure is then equalised to the ambient pressure. The same mechanism also takes care of the discomfort from external pressure changes, e.g. when flying and diving. However, the practical importance of this mechanism has been questioned by Magnuson (1980). Some people produce an under-pressure in the middle ear by sniffing, either consciously or unconsciously. For these people the absorption of air by the mucous membrane is probably of less importance for the pressure variations in the middle ear.

Drainage of the middle ear

Secretion produced in the middle ear is transported by ciliary movement in the eustachian tube to the epipharynx. This flow of secretion reduces the risk of upper respiratory infections spreading to the middle ear.

The actual existence of the eustachian tube constitutes certain problems. The tube has to protect the middle ear from the respiratory pressure variations in the epipharynx. Further, loud speech sounds have to be prevented from reaching directly to the middle ear. Prevention of infected secretions reaching the middle ear from the nose and throat is also important.

The tubal function may be abnormal in two ways: opening insufficiency (tubal obstruction) or closing insufficiency (tuba aperta). Both conditions can lead to middle-ear diseases.

Tubal obstruction may depend on muscular dysfunction. This is common in children with cleft palate and with recurrent secretory otitis media (Bylander, 1983). The eustachian tube may also be squeezed by an enlarged adenoid or by a tumour in the epipharynx. A further reason for obstruction could be a swollen mucous membrane due to upper respiratory infection or allergy.

A closing insufficiency may be more or less permanent. A patient whose tube is always wide open has usually adjusted to this state and does not perceive any problems. However, if the tube is open only for limited periods the patient may find it very annoying. His or her own voice will sound distorted and strange due to the direct acoustic path from the throat to the ear (autophony); also the respiratory pressure variations may be disturbing. Some patients find these effects too unpleasant and develop an unconscious sniffing behaviour, whereby a brief under-pressure is created in the nose and the middle ear. This under-pressure will keep the tube closed for some time, relieving the patient from the symptoms of an open eustachian tube. Thus these patients continually have a certain under-pressure in the middle ear which may increase the risk of middle-ear disease (Magnuson, 1980).

The ability of the eustachian tube to equalise the middle-ear pressure is tested with different methods, depending on whether the eardrum is whole or perforated. With a whole eardrum, the tubal function is tested by means of impedance audiometry, the middle-ear pressure being determined by tympanometry. Repeated tympanometry will reveal whether any pressure change has occurred after the Toynbee or Valsalva maneouvres (Holmquist, 1969a). This test shows the capacity of the tube for active pressure equalisation.

If the tube is constantly open, impedance variations which are synchronous with the patient's breathing can be seen in a continuous recording. If the patient is asked to hold his or her breath for a brief time, these rhythmic impedance variations will cease. In this way the diagnosis of tuba aperta can be confirmed.

If the eardrum has a perforation, no normal tympanogram can be recorded but the pressure of the middle ear is measured directly, usually by means of the pressure transducer incorporated in the impedance audiometer. The pressure in the auditory canal is varied gradually by means of the pump of the instrument to over-pressure (the deflation method) or under-pressure (the aspiration method). A simultaneous recording is made of the sudden pressure changes due to the tubal opening, whether spontaneous or induced by swallowing. This test will show the tubal capacity for passive pressure equalisation (Holmquist,

1969b). Also a tuba aperta will show up by this method as respiration-synchronous variations, but not as variations of the recorded pressure.

Sonotubometry is a special test which has been proposed for the testing of tubal function (Virtanen, 1977). A sound is transmitted into the patient's nose and the level of this sound is measured in the auditory canal, being conducted from the nose via the tube and the middle ear. A tubal opening is expected to give an increase in sound level. However, the specificity of this method seems quite poor because 40–50% of normal healthy subjects do not show any change in test sound level in the ear canal on swallowing (Holmquist and Olén, 1981).

The ability of the eustachian tube to drain the middle ear can only be evaluated indirectly by the methods mentioned. For direct evaluation other methods must be used, e.g. using X-ray with contrast.

Equipment

The test is usually performed by means of an impedance audiometer. The ear-canal pressure should be variable within at least the range +2 to −4 kPa relative to ambient pressure. When testing ears with a perforated eardrum, a pressure range of from +6 to −4 kPa is preferable. Types of pressure recording instruments other than an impedance audiometer may then be used.

Sources of error and test accuracy

When testing an ear with perforated eardrum, the opening pressure is influenced by the rate of change of pressure. At higher rates, higher pressure is required before the tube will be passively opened (Bluestone, 1980).

A sudden pressure change in the middle ear is not a normal physiological event. The creation of a sudden under-pressure in the middle ear at testing may make the eustachian tube clasp, preventing a reliable evaluation of tubal function (Bluestone, 1980).

When testing ears with a whole eardrum by means of the Valsalva and Toynbee maneouvres, then clearly measurable pressure changes are usually found if the tubal function is normal (Riedel, Wiley and Block, 1987). However, large variations occur with regard to the over-pressure that can be created in the middle ear by means of the Valsalva maneouvre, and these may depend on individual variations in ability and motivation.

Clinical interpretation

Whole eardrum

If tympanometry shows an under-pressure in the middle ear of more than 1.5–2 kPa (150–200 daPa), a tubal dysfunction should be suspected.

However, a normal middle-ear pressure does not exclude tubal dysfunction.

The Toynbee test can be considered positive if a patient with a whole eardrum can produce a middle-ear pressure change (increase or decrease) by keeping his or her nose closed and swallowing. A positive result indicates a normal tubal passage and a negative result indicates tubal passage dysfunction. In healthy normal subjects pressure equalisation in the Toynbee test has been found in 97% of the cases by Elner, Ingelstedt and Ivarsson (1971), in 96% by Riedel, Wiley and Block (1987) and in 80% by Jörgensen and Holmquist (1987). Thus, the specificity is good, but the sensitivity is poorer. According to Jörgensen and Holmquist (1987), 50% of patients with chronic otitis media could equilibrate their middle-ear pressure.

The Valsalva test is considered positive if a patient with a whole eardrum can produce an increase in the middle-ear pressure by keeping his or her nose closed and trying to press air out through it. A negative result indicates tubal passage dysfunction, but a positive result does not prove a normal function (Bluestone, 1980). Elner, Ingelstedt and Ivarsson (1971) found that 28% of normal healthy subjects had certain problems in equalising an over- or under-pressure or both, but fully 82% of these had positive results in the Valsalva test. Thus, the sensitivity is poor concerning the ability to prove a minor tubal dysfunction. Riedel, Wiley and Block (1987) found a positive result in 94% of normal healthy persons. Thus, the specificity must be considered to be good.

Perforated eardrum

In patients with a perforated eardrum, the evaluation of tubal function is based on the measurement of air pressure in the ear canal and middle ear (Holborow, 1962; Flisberg, Ingelstedt and Örtegren, 1963; Ingelstedt and Örtegren, 1963; Flisberg, 1966; Holmquist, 1969b). The opening pressure, i.e. the over-pressure in the ear canal and middle ear which makes the eustachian tube open passively, is of the order of 4 kPa (400 daPa). In a group of subjects with eardrum perforations caused by trauma but with otherwise healthy ears, an average opening pressure of 3.3 kPa was found (Cantekin et al., 1977). The closing pressure, i.e. the over-pressure that remains in the middle ear after the tube has closed again, is usually of the order of 1 kPa (Holmquist and Olén, 1980). The remaining over-pressure, which remains after the subject has swallowed a number of times, is normally close to zero as is the remaining under-pressure, i.e. the pressure which remains in the middle ear after the subject has equalised an induced under-pressure.

The measurement of tubal function in patients with a perforated eardrum may be of some importance in the evaluation of the prognosis of middle-ear surgery. An abnormal tubal function may reduce the probability of successful surgery because of recurrent middle-ear inflammations (Bluestone, 1980). However, the sensitivity of tubal function testing for this type of risk evaluation is rather poor. This is especially true for children, in whom tubal function tests could not provide a reliable prognosis for the results of middle-ear surgery (Bluestone, 1980). Other results from 162 operated ears indicate a certain correlation between poor healing and poor preoperative tubal function (Holmquist and Lindeman, 1987).

Recurrent eardrum perforations following myringoplastic surgery may sometimes be due to the absence of a tubal passage. This can be recorded preoperatively by means of tubal function tests, and at surgery the tubal ostium should be carefully inspected.

References

ALBERTI, P.W. and JERGER, J. (1974). Probe tone frequency and the diagnostic value of tympanometry. *Archives of Otolaryngology* **99**, 206–210.

ANDERSON, H. (1969). *Acoustic intra-aural reflexes in clinical diagnosis.* Dissertation, Department of Audiology, Karolinska Institute, Stockholm.

ANDERSON, H. and BARR, B. (1966). Conductive recruitment. *Acta Oto-Laryngologica* **62**, 171–184.

ANDERSON, H. and WEDENBERG, E. (1968). Audiometric identification of normal hearing carriers of genes for deafness. *Acta Oto-Laryngologica* **65**, 535–554.

ANDERSON, H. and WEDENBERG, E. (1970). Genetic aspects of hearing impairments in children. *Acta Oto-Laryngologia* **69**, 77–88.

ANDERSON, H., BARR, B. and WEDENBERG, E. (1969). Intraaural reflexes in retrocochlear lesions. In: *Nobel Symposium 10, Disorders of the Skull Base Region.* Stockholm: Almqvist & Wiksell.

ANDERSON, H., BARR, B. and WEDENBERG, E. (1970). The early detection of acoustic tumours by the stapedius reflex test. In: Wolstenholme, G.E.W. and Knight, J. (Eds.) *Ciba Foundation Symposium on Sensorineural Hearing Loss.* London: J & A Churchill.

BERGENIUS, J., BORG, E. and HIRSCH, A. (1983). Stapedius reflex test, brainstem audiometry and opto-vestibular tests in diagnosis of acoustic neurinomas. *Scandinavian Audiology* **12**, 3–9.

BLOM, S. and ZAKRISSON, J.E. (1974). The stapedius reflex in the diagnosis of myasthenia gravis. *Journal of Neurological Science* **21**, 71–76.

BLUESTONE, C.D. (1980). Assessment of Eustachian tube function. In: Jerger, J. and Northern, J.L. (Eds.) *Clinical Impedance Audiometry.* Stuttgart: Georg Thième Verlag.

BORG, E. (1973). On the neural organization of the acoustic middle ear reflex. A physiological and anatomical study. *Brain Research* **49**, 101–123.

BORG, E. (1982). Time course of the human acoustic stapedius reflex. *Scandinavian Audiology* **11**, 237–242.

BORG, E. and ZAKRISSON, J.E. (1974). Stapedius reflex and monaural masking. *Acta Oto-Laryngologica* **78**, 155–161.

BYLANDER, A. (1983). *Eustachian tube functioning in healthy children.* Dissertation, Department of Otorhinolaryngology, University of Lund.

CANTEKIN, E., BLUESTONE, C., SAEZ, C., DOYLE, W. and PHILLIPS, D. (1977). Normal and abnormal middle ear ventilation. *Annals of Otology, Rhinology and Laryngology* **86**, Suppl. 41.

CASSELBRANT, M. (1974) *Indirect determination of variations in the inner ear pressure in man.* Dissertation, Department of Otorhinolaryngology, University of Lund.

CHIVERALLS, K. (1977). A further examination of the use of the stapedius reflex in the diagnosis of acoustic neuroma. *Audiology* **16**, 331.

CHIVERALLS, K. and FITZSIMONS, R. (1973). Stapedial reflex action in normal subjects. *British Journal of Audiology* **7**, 105–110.

CLEMIS, J.D. and SARNO, C.N. (1980). The acoustic reflex latency test: clinical application. *The Laryngoscope* **90**, 601–611.

COLLETTI, V. (1974). Some stapedius reflex parameters in normal and pathological conditions. *Journal of Laryngology and Otology* **88**, 127–137.

COLLETTI, V. (1975). Stapedius reflex abnormalities in multiple sclerosis. *Audiology* **14**, 63–71.

DALLOS, P.J. (1964). Dynamics of the acoustic reflex: Phenomenological aspects. *Journal of the Acoustical Society of America* **36**, 2175–2183.

DECRAEMER, W.F., CRETEN, W.L. and VAN CAMP, K.J. (1984). Tympanometric middle-ear pressure determination with two-component admittance meters. *Scandinavian Audiology* **13**, 165–172.

DEUTSCH, L.J. (1972). The threshold of the stapedius reflex for pure tone and noise stimuli. *Acta Oto-Laryngologogica* **74**, 248–251.

DJUPESLAND, G. and KVERNVOLD, H. (1975). Acoustic impedance measured on ears with normal and diphasic impedance changes. *Scandinavian Audiology* **4**, 39–43.

DJUPESLAND, G. and ZWISLOCKI, J. (1973). On the critical band in the acoustic stapedius reflex. *Journal of the Acoustical Society of America* **54**, 1157–1159.

DJUPESLAND, G., FLOTTORP, G., SUNDBY, A. and SZALAY, M. (1973). A comparison between middle-ear muscle reflex thresholds for bone- and air-conducted pure tones. *Acta Oto-Laryngologica* **75**, 178–183.

ELNER, Å., INGELSTEDT, S. and IVARSSON, A. (1971). A method for studies of middle ear mechanics. *Acta Oto-Laryngologica* **72**, 191.

FISCH, U. and WEGMULLER, A. (1974). Early diagnosis of acoustic neuromas. *Oto-Rhino-Laryngology* **36**, 129.

FLISBERG, K. (1966). Ventilatory studies on the Eustachian tube. *Acta Oto-Laryngologica Supplementum* 219.

FLISBERG, K., INGELSTEDT, S. and ÖRTEGREN, U. (1963). Controlled 'ear aspiration' of air. A 'physiological' test of the tubal function. *Acta Oto-Laryngologica Supplementum* 182.

FLOTTORP, G. and DJUPESLAND, G. (1970). Diphosic impedance change and its applicability in clinical work. *Acta Oto-Laryngologica Supplementum* **263**, 200–204.

GREEN, K.W. and MARGOLIS, R.H. (1983). Detection of hearing loss with ipsilateral acoustic reflex thresholds. *Audiology* **22**, 471–479.

HALL, C.M. (1977). Stapedial reflex decay in retrocochlear and cochlear lesions. *Annals of Otology, Rhinology and Laryngology* **86**, 219–222.

HAYES, D. and JERGER, J. (1978). Impedance audiometry in otologic diagnosis. *Otolaryngologic Clinics of North America* **11**, 759–767.

HIRSCH, A. and ANDERSON, H. (1980a). Elevated stapedius reflex thresholds and pathologic reflex decay. *Acta Oto-Laryngologica Supplementum* 368, 11–28.

HIRSCH, A. and ANDERSON, H. (1980b). Audiological results in 96 patients with tumours affecting the eight nerve. A clinical study with emphasis on the early audiological diagnosis. *Acta Oto-Laryngologica Supplementum* 369, 1–26.

HOLBOROW, C.A. (1962). Deafness associated with cleft palate. *Journal of Laryngology* **76**, 762.

HOLMQUIST, J. (1969a). Eustachian tube function assessed with tympanometry. *Acta Oto-Laryngologica* **68**, 501–508.

HOLMQUIST, J. (1969b). Eustachian tube function in patients with ear drum perforations following chronic otitis media. *Acta Oto-Laryngologica* **68**, 391–401.

HOLMQUIST, J. and LINDEMAN, P. (1987). Eustachian tube function and healing after myringoplasty. *Otolaryngology Head and Neck Surgery* **96**, 80–82.

HOLMQUIST, J. and OLÉN, L. (1980). Evaluation of Eustachian tube function. *Journal of Laryngology and Otology* **94**, 15–23.

HOLMQUIST, J. and OLÉN, L. (1981). Measurement of Eustachian tube function using sonotubometry. *Scandinavian Audiology* **10**, 33–35.

HYDE, M.L., ALBERTI, P.W., MORGAN, P.P., SYMONS, F. and CUMMINGS, F. (1980). Pure tone threshold estimation from acoustic reflex thresholds – a myth? *Acta Oto-Laryngologica* **89**, 345–357.

IEC 118-10 (1986). *Guide to Hearing Aid Standards.* Geneva: International Electrotechnical Commission.

IEC 126 (1961). *IEC reference coupler for the measurement of hearing aids using earphones coupled to the ear by means of ear inserts.* Geneva: International Electrotechnical Commission.

IEC 1027 (1991). *Instruments for the Measurements of Aural Acoustic Impedance/Admittance.* Geneva: International Electrotechnical Commission.

INGELSTEDT, S. and ÖRTEGREN, U. (1963). Qualitative testing of the Eustachian tube function. *Acta Oto-Laryngologica Supplementum* **182**, 7–23.

ISO 389 (1985). *Acoustics – Standard Reference Zero for the Calibration of Pure Tone Audiometers.* Geneva: International Standards Organisation.

IVARSSON, A., TJERNSTRÖM, Ö, BYLANDER, A. and BENNRUP, S. (1983). High speed tympanometry and ipsilateral middle ear reflex measurements using a computerized impedance meter. *Scandinavian Audiology* **12**, 157–163.

JEPSEN, O. (1951). Threshold of the reflexes of the intertympanic muscles in a normal material examined by means of the impedance method. *Acta Oto-Laryngologica* **39**, 406–408.

JEPSEN, O. (1963). Middle ear muscle reflexes in man. In: Jerger, J. (Ed.) *Modern Developments in Audiology.* New York: Academic Press.

JERGER, J. (1970). Clinical experience and impedance audiometry. *Archives of Otolaryngology* **92**, 311–324.

JERGER, S. and JERGER, J. (1977). Diagnostic value of crossed vs. uncrossed acoustic reflexes. *Archives of Otolaryngology* **103**, 445–453.

JERGER, S. and JERGER, J. (1983). Evaluation of diagnostic audiometric tests. *Audiology* **22**, 144–161.

JERGER, J., JERGER, S. and MAULDIN, L. (1972). Studies in impedance audiometry. I. Normal and sensorineural ears. *Archives of Otolaryngology* **96**, 513–523.

JERGER, J., MAULDIN, L. and LEWIS, N. (1977). Temporal summation of the acoustic reflex. *Audiology* **16**, 177–200.

JERGER, J., OLIVER, T.A. and STACH, B. (1986). Problems in clinical measurement of acoustic reflex latency. *Scandinavian Audiology* **15**, 31–40.

JERGER, S., JERGER, J., MAULDIN, L. and SEGAL P. (1974a). Studies in impedance audiometry. II. Children less than 6 years old. *Archives of Otolaryngology* **99**, 1–9.

JERGER, J., ANTHONY, L., JERGER, S. and MAULDIN, L. (1974b). Studies in impedance audiometry. III. Middle ear disorders. *Archives of Otolaryngology* **99**, 165–171.

JERGER, J., BURNEY, P., MAULDIN, L. and CRUMP, B. (1974c). Predicting hearing loss from the acoustic reflex. *Journal of Speech and Hearing Disorders* **39**, 11–22.

JERGER, J., HARFORD, E., CLEMIS, J. and ALFORD, B. (1974d). The acoustic reflex in eighth nerve disorders. *Archives of Otolaryngology* **99**, 409–413.

JERGER, J., HAYES, D., ANTHONY, L. and MAULDIN, L. (1978). Factors influencing prediction of hearing levels from the acoustic reflex. *Monographs of Contemporary Audiology* **1**, 1–20.

JÖRGENSEN, F. and HOLMQUIST, J. (1987). Otitis media and the blocked nose. In: Lim, D. Bluestone, C.D., Klein, J.O. and Nelson, J.D. (Eds.) *Proceedings of the Fourth International Symposium on Recent Advances in Otitis Media*, pp. 80–82.

KANKKUNEN, A. and LIDÉN, G. (1984). Ipsilateral acoustic reflex thresholds in neonates and in normal-hearing and hearing-impaired pre-school children. *Scandinavian Audiology* **13**, 139–144.

KARLSSON, K. and HAGERMAN, B. (1984). A clinical comparison between a laboratory and a commercial impedance audiometer. *Scandinavian Audiology* **13**, 199–203.

KLOCKHOFF, I. (1961). Middle ear muscle reflexes in man. *Acta Oto-Laryngologica Supplementum* 164.

KLOCKHOFF, I. (1981). Impedance fluctuation and a 'tenor tympani syndrome.' In: *Proceedings of the Fourth International Symposium on Acoustic Impedance Measurements*, pp. 69–76 Lisbon: Universidade Nova de Lisboa.

KILLION, M.C. (1978). Revised estimate of minimum audible pressure: where is the missing 6 dB? *Journal of the Acoustical Society of America* **63**, 1501–1508.

KING, T.T., GIBSON, W.P.R. and MORRISON, A.W. (1976). Tumours of the eighth cranial nerve. *British Journal of Hospital Medicine* **16**, 259.

KOBRAK, H.G., LINDSAY, J.R. and PERLMAN, H.B. (1941). Experimental observations on the question of auditory fatigue. *The Laryngoscope* **51**, 1–12.

KUNOV, H. (1977). The 'eardrum artefact' in ipsilateral reflex measurements. *Scandinavian Audiology* **6**, 163–166.

LAUKLI, E. and MAIR, I.W.S. (1980). Ipsilateral and contralateral acoustic reflex thresholds. *Audiology* **19**, 469–494.

LIDÉN, G. (1970). The stapedius muscle reflex used as an objective recruitment test: a clinical and experimental study. In: Wolstenholme, G.E.W. and Knight, J. (Eds.) *Ciba Foundation Symposium on Sensorineural Hearing Loss*, pp. 295–211. London: J & A Churchill.

LIDÉN, G. and ROSENHALL, U. (1985). New dimensions in the assessment of auditory function. Special tests. In: Myers, E. (Ed.) *New Dimensions in Otorhinolaryngology – Head and Neck Surgery*, Vol. I, pp. 174–177. Amsterdam: Elsevier Science.

LIDÉN, G., PETERSON, J.L. and HARFORD, E.R. (1970). Simultaneous recording of changes in relative impedance and air pressure during acoustic and non-acoustic elicitation of the middle ear reflexes. *Acta Oto-Laryngologica* **263**, 208–217.

LINDEMAN, P. (1982). *The mastoid cell system – measurements in middle ear disease.* Dissertation, Department of Otorhinolaryngology and Audiology, University of Gothenburg.

LUSCHER, E. (1930). Function des Musculus Stapedius beim Menschen. *Zeitschrift für Hals- Nasen- und Ohren-Heilkunde* **25**, 462.

LUTMAN, M.E. (1984a). Phasor admittance measurements of the middle ear. I. Theoretical approach. *Scandinavian Audiology* **13**, 253–264.

LUTMAN, M.E. (1984b). Phasor admittance measurements of the middle ear. II. Normal phasor tympanograms and acoustic reflexes. *Scandinavian Audiology* **13**, 165–174.

LYON, M.J. (1978). The central location of the motor neurons to the stapedius muscle in cat. *Brain Research* **143**, 437–444.

McPHERSON, D.L. and THOMPSON, D. (1977). Quantification of the threshold and latency parameters of the acoustic reflex in humans. *Acta Oto-Laryngologica Supplementum* 353, 1–37.

MAGNUSON, B. (1980). *Middle ear disease of retractory type.* Dissertation, Department of Otorhinolaryngology, University of Linköping (in Swedish).

MARGOLIS, R.H. and SHANKS, J.E. (1985). Tympanometry. In: Katz, J. (Ed.) *Handbook of Clinical Audiology*, 3rd edn, pp. 438–475. Baltimore: Williams & Wilkins.

METZ, O. (1951). Studies on the contraction of the tympanic muscles as indicated by changes in the impedance of the ear. *Acta Oto-Larngologica* **39**, 397–405.

METZ, O. (1952). Threshold of reflex contractions of muscles of middle ear and recruitment of loudness. *Archives of Otolaryngology* **55**, 536–543.

MOLLER, A.R. (1961). Bilateral contraction of the tympanic muscles as indicated by changes in the impedance of the ear. *Annals of Otology, Rhinology and Laryngology* **70**, 735–745.

MOLLER, A.R. (1974). The acoustic middle ear muscle reflex. In: Keidel, W.D. and Neff, W.D. (Eds.) *Handbook of Sensory Physiology*, V/1, pp. 519–548. Berlin: Springer Verlag.

NIEMEYER, W. and SESTERHENN, G. (1974). Calculating the hearing threshold from the stapedius reflex threshold for different sound stimuli. *Audiology* **13**, 421–427.

NILSSON, R. (1983). *The role of the acoustic reflex in industrial noise exposure.* Dissertation, Department of Otolaryngology and Audiology, University of Gothenburg.

NORTHERN, J.L., GABBARD, S.A. and KINDER, D.L. (1985). The acoustic reflex. In: Katz, J. (Ed.) *Handbook of Clinical Audiology*, 3rd edn, pp. 476–495. Baltimore: Williams & Wilkins.

POPELKA, G.R., MARGOLIS, R.H. and WILEY, T.L. (1976). Effect of activating signal bandwidth on acoustic-reflex thresholds. *Journal of the Acoustical Society of America* **56**, 153–159.

REIMER, Å. (1987). Quantitative interpretation of audiological test battery. I. A comparison with ABR in 97 cases of unilateral sensorineural hearing loss. *Scandinavian Audiology* **16**, 101–108.

REKER, U. (1977). Methodological problems in the determination of homolateral stapedius reflex threshold. *Audiology* **16**, 487–498.

RIEDEL, C.L., WILEY, T.L. and BLOCK, M.C. (1987). Tympanometric measures of Eustachian tube function. *Journal of Speech and Hearing Research* **30**, 207–214.

ROSENHALL, U., LIDÉN, G. and NILSSON, R. (1979). Stapedius reflex decay in normal hearing subjects. *Journal of the American Auditory Society* **4**, 157–163.

SCHUKNECHT, H. (1974). *Pathology of the Ear.* Cambridge, MA: Harvard University Press.

SHAW, E.A.G. (1974). The external ear. In: Keidel, W.D. and Neff, W.D. (Eds.) *Handbook of Sensory Physiology*, V/1, pp. 455–490. Berlin: Springer Verlag.

STRUTZ, J., MUNKER, G. and ZÖLLNER, C. (1988). The motor innervation of the tympanic muscles in the guinea pig. *Archives of Otorhinolaryngology* **245**, 108–111.

THOMSEN, J. and TERKILDSEN, K. (1975). Audiological findings in 125 cases of acoustic neuromas. *Acta Oto-Laryngologica* **80**, 353–361.

THOMPSON, D.J. and ROBINETTE, L.N. (1988). Temporal characteristics of aural acoustic immittance instruments. *Ear and Hearing* 9, 290–295.

VANHUYSE, J.V., CRETEN, W.L. and VAN CAMP, K.J. (1975). On the W-notching of tympanograms. *Scandinavian Audiology* 4, 45–50.

VIRTANEN, H. (1977). *Eustachian tube sound conduction. Sonotubometry, an acoustical method for objective measurement of auditory tubal opening.* Dissertation, Department of Otorhinolaryngology, University of Helsinki.

WERSÄLL, R. (1958). The tympanic muscles and their reflexes. *Acta Oto-Laryngologica Supplementum* 139, 1–112.

WEVER, E.G. (1949). *Theory of Hearing.* New York: Wiley.

WILEY, T.L., OVIATT, D.L. and BLOCK, M.G. (1987). Acoustic immittance measures in normal ears. *Journal of Speech and Hearing Research* **30**, 161–170.

WILEY, T.L. and BLOCK, M.G. (1985). Overview and basic principles of acoustic immittance measurements. In: Katz, J. (Ed.) *Handbook of Clinical Audiology,* 3rd edn, pp. 423–437. Baltimore: Williams & Wilkins.

Chapter 9 Electrophysiological Methods

Electric Response Audiometry

'Electric response audiometry' (ERA) is the general term for a group of test methods based on the recording of the variations in electric potential difference, between two electrodes, due to the electric activity in neurons of the auditory pathways evoked by auditory stimulation (Jacobson and Hyde, 1985). The electrodes are usually placed on the skull, in the ear canal or in the middle ear; the choice of electrode positions depends on which part of the auditory system is to be evaluated.

The source of the electric activity which is recorded is normally not a concentrated point source, but rather many active neurons surrounded by conductive physiological tissues of various kinds with different electric conductive characteristics. This so-called volume conductor has a large influence on the electric potential pattern that can be recorded on the surface of the skull. The active sources are often described in electric terms as dipoles which are dynamic, i.e. vary in magnitude and direction with time during the stimulus cycle.

These facts explain the difficulty when trying to interpret the underlying neurophysiological processes from the electric activity recorded on the skull surface. However, in spite of this the methods have proved to be of great clinical importance. As is the case for many test methods, by learning from their results when used on test subjects with various known auditory disorders significant diagnostic conclusions can be drawn in a variety of clinical applications.

In a simplified scheme the auditory pathways from the inner ear to the primary auditory cortex can be considered as consisting of the following parts (Figure 9.1):

1. The inner ear or cochlea
2. The auditory nerve.

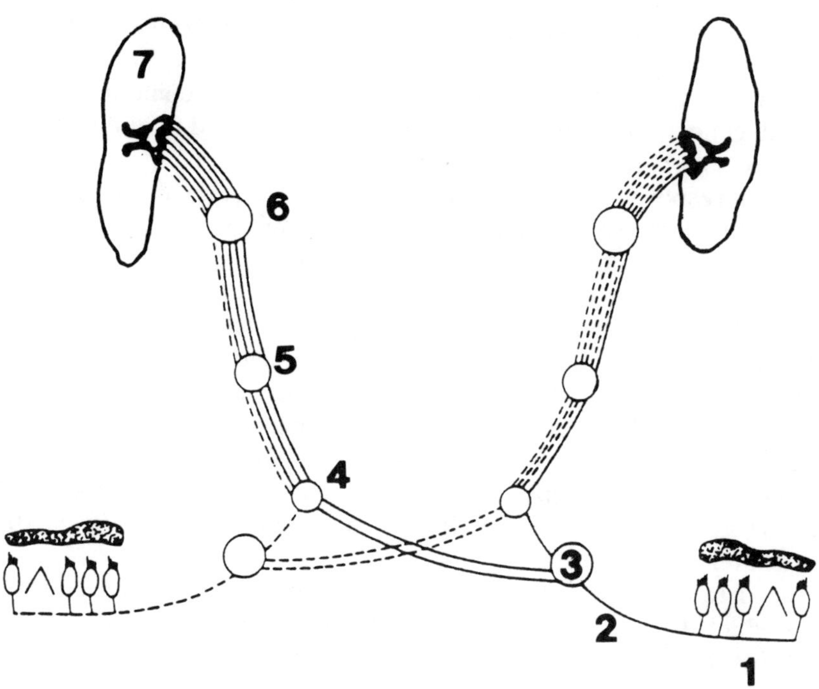

Figure 9.1 Simplified scheme of the afferent auditory pathways: 1=inner ear, 2=cochlear nerve, 3=cochlear nuclei, 4=superior olive, 5=inferior colliculus, 6=medial geniculate body, 7=primary auditory cortex.

3. The cochlear nuclei where the auditory nerve enters the brain stem.
4. The contralateral superior olive in the area called the trapezoid body.
5. The inferior colliculus which is reached via the lateral lemniscus.
6. The medial geniculate body.
7. The primary auditory projection area in the temporal lobe of the cortex. From here signals continue to secondary auditory areas.

This is the dominating pathway for the transmission of auditory information. About 90% of the neurons represent crossed pathways, i.e. transmit signals originating from the contralateral cochlea. Already at the level of the superior olive, a rich system of connections between ipsi- and contralateral pathways is present. These connections are of importance for many binaural listening tasks, e.g. directional hearing. Also, in addition to the afferent fibres which transmit information from the periphery to the cortex there are efferent fibres which are presumed to have mainly regulatory tasks.

A common system of defining the different types of auditory electric responses (AERs) is based on when the response occurs in relation to the stimulus. Common terms used are early responses, occurring in the time window 0–2 ms, fast (2–10 ms), middle latency (10–50 ms) and late or slow (50–300 ms).

The most important early response is the auditory compound action potential, generated by the auditory nerve and recorded by the technique called electrocochleography (ECoG).

The fast response refers to the auditory brain-stem response (ABR) dominated by five waves numbered by Roman numbers I–V according to Jewett (1970). The clinical technique for recording these responses is called brain-stem response audiometry (BRA).

Middle latency responses (MLR) (Galambos, Makeig and Talmachoff, 1981) have found some clinical use. By stimulating with a repetition frequency of 40 brief stimuli per second, response amplitude is enhanced and hearing threshold estimations can be made. In cortical response audiometry (CRA), late or slow responses with cortical origin are recorded. The main components are called P1, N1, P2 and N2, among which N1 and P2 dominate and typically occur in the latency range 100–200 ms after stimulus onset.

A very late response is the P300 wave (Michalewski, Prasher and Starr, 1986) which has been studied in relation to auditory discrimination in certain psychological and neurological experiments.

Equipment

The equipment which is needed for ERA is relatively complex and also rather costly as compared to most other audiometric equipment. Basically, it consists of three main functional parts as illustrated in Figure 9.2:

1. *Recording unit* consisting of electrodes, amplifier, filters and analogue-to-digital (A/D) converter.

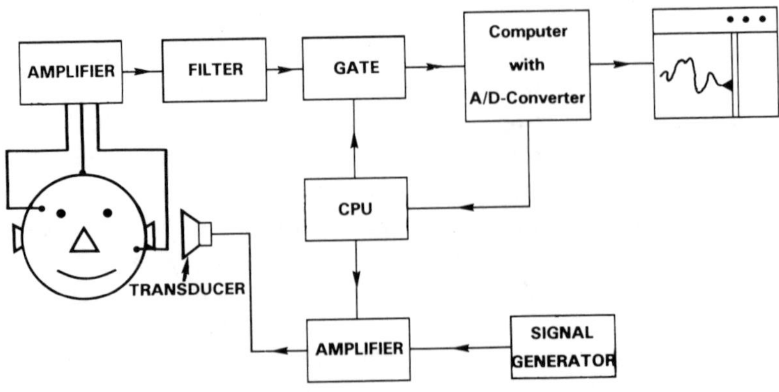

Figure 9.2 Principles of the equipment for ERA.

2. *Stimulus unit* consisting of signal generator, amplifier and transducer.
3. *Central processing and computing unit* which controls the stimulus and the recording units in order to coordinate stimulation and data collection. In its memory the summation of amplified records of the bioelectrical activity takes place. After the data collection is completed, the final results are presented as an averaged response on a visual display. A built-in or external recorder allows the printing of the response on paper for permanent storage.

Recording unit

Electrodes

Different types of electrodes may be used depending on what type of response is to be recorded. In ECoG needle electrodes are often used, e.g. the transtympanic needle electrode which penetrates the eardrum and is placed on the promontorial wall in the middle ear. For the recording of brain-stem and cortical responses, surface electrodes are usually the choice, either reusable or disposable. A double-sided adhesive tape collar keeps the electrode in place on the skin with a thin layer of electrode gel making the electrode contact between the electrode metal and the biological tissue.

Disposable electrodes of good quality are preferable; reusable types require careful cleaning and sometimes re-chloriding to retain stable electrical characteristics. The procedure of applying the electrodes is very important. An electrode impedance of less than about 5 kΩ should be reached to ensure good recording conditions. A higher contact impedance means more disturbing noise being generated at the electrode–tissue interface. This may be of the order of several hundred nanovolts and cause significant problems in ABR (Arlinger, 1981). High electrode impedance also increases the probability of interference from external disturbing sources through electrostatic and electromagnetic radiation.

An effective way of ensuring good electrode contact is first to clean the skin where the electrode is to be placed by rubbing with a piece of gauze soaked in alcohol. Then a small amount of electrode gel is applied and rubbed into the skin and the site is cleaned again with alcohol. Electrode gel is then applied to the electrode surface after which it is firmly pressed onto the skin.

In addition to low contact impedance, it is also essential to obtain approximately equal impedance with all electrodes applied. Imbalance between the positive and the negative recording electrodes will result in increased sensitivity to external interference. On most commercially available pieces of equipment, facilities are provided for the measurement of the contact impedance of individual electrodes. If the initial impedance measured is somewhat high, allowing a few minutes for stabilisation of the electrochemical conditions at the metal–electrolyte interface, often results in a decrease in contact impedance.

The combination of electrode metal and electrolyte provides a situation where polarisation can occur, corresponding to a galvanic battery with a direct current (d.c.) voltage difference between metal and tissue. If both batteries at the positive and the negative electrodes are equal, the two d.c. voltage differences balance each other to a net sum of zero. However, if they differ, the d.c. potential across the amplifier will be amplified and may cause overload of the amplifier. This situation occurs if the two electrodes contain different kinds of metal, e.g. in ECoG if one electrode is a stainless steel needle and the other is a silver/silver chloride surface electrode. Also, even a very small crack in the chloride layer of a silver/silver chloride electrode gives rise to a d.c. voltage which differs from that of an undamaged electrode of the same type and thus gives rise to the same potential problems. Therefore, it is of importance to handle such electrodes with great care.

Placement of electrodes

A practical way of placing electrodes is to use four electrodes: one on the vertex on the top of the skull, one on each mastoid and one in the forehead, the latter being used as ground electrode. This scheme allows the simultaneous recording of ipsi- and contralateral responses in ABR by equipment with two recording channels. The same electrode placement can be used for the recording of cortical potentials. From a practical point of view, the vertex placement may sometimes be difficult because of hair. Occasionally, the earphone headband can be used to help keep the electrode in place by pressing on it through, for example, a piece of foam plastic. As an alternative, the placement of this electrode at the very top of the forehead is possible with relatively little reduction in response amplitude.

Electrodes always have the capacity to pick up inductive interference from the earphone – a so-called stimulus artefact. In order to minimise this, it is essential to keep the earphone and its cable as far away from the electrode cables as possible and keep the electrode cables close together.

Amplifier

The amplifier has the task of amplifying the very small electric signals from the electrodes to a magnitude which is suitable for the A/D converter and the subsequent averaging. The electric potential to be amplified is of the order of tens or hundreds of nanovolts to 10 μv. Thus a gain in the range 100 000–1 000 000 is typically used to bring the input voltage to the A/D converter to the order of a few volts.

Low sensitivity to external interference is an important amplifier characteristic. This is accomplished by the use of a differential input amplifier. Such an amplifier requires three input connections: one non-inverting or positive, one inverting or negative and one common which constitutes a reference for the other two. The advantage with the differential input amplifier is that it amplifies only the difference in potential between positive and negative inputs. If the same voltage is applied to both input terminals, as is the case with many external interfering signals, this will have very little effect on the output voltage from the amplifier. The ability to suppress such in-phase signals is called the common mode rejection. A good differential amplifier often has a common mode rejection ratio of at least 100 dB, i.e. a voltage difference between the two input terminals is amplified 100 000 times more than a voltage applied in phase to the two input terminals.

Another important characteristic of an amplifier for bioelectrical activity is a high input impedance, of the order of mega-ohms (MΩ) or more. This is necessary to provide a low electric loading of the biological signal generator, otherwise the signal recorded will be distorted.

Four different types of interfering activity may disturb the recording of electric responses:

1. Electrostatic fields.
2. Electromagnetic fields.
3. Noise generated in resistive components.
4. Non-related bioelectrical activity.

Electrostatic fields are generated by electric charges. The transfer of such interference to the recording system of an ERA unit is through capacitative coupling. It can be effectively reduced by means of screening of cables with screens connected to the electrical 'earth' and by making cables as short as possible.

Magnetic fields are generated by electric currents and may become especially strong due to the presence of iron or other magnetic materials used in earphones, loudspeakers and transformers. Magnetic interference is much more difficult to shield. Special materials are required, e.g. μ metal with a special capacity to absorb magnetic energy. Again short cables are an advantage. It is also important to keep the electrode cables as close together as possible. In order to minimise electrostatic and electromagnetic interference, the amplifier is normally split into two parts: a preamplifier close to the patient and a main amplifier in the main unit.

Thermal or gaussian noise is generated in all resistive components with the noise voltage proportional to the square root of the resistance. This concerns the resistive part of the electrode impedance as well as resistances in connectors, cables and other electronic parts. At the electrodes, another kind of disturbance may arise caused by movements in the polarised layer between electrode metal and biological tissue if the patient moves or if muscles close to the electrodes contract. To avoid such movement artefacts a relaxed patient is very important.

Bioelectrical activity of various kinds is always generated in the living human body, e.g. EEG, the spontaneous activity of the central nervous system, responses to external stimuli other than the auditory stimuli under study, and the electrical activity of the heart and of all other muscles in the body. The degree of interference with ERA depends on both frequency spectrum of the activity and location of the generator in relation to the electrode positions used. EEG activity may cause significant interference when recording cortical responses to auditory stimuli, whereas electrical activity from the muscles may cause severe problems in brain-stem response audiometry.

Filter

The purpose of a filter is to accept signals in one frequency band and reject activity in others. Analogue filters are found in all types of ERA equipment and also, increasingly, digital filters in order to obtain optimum results (Svensson, Almqvist and Jönsson, 1987). Analogue filters are built by means of electronic components and circuits, whereas a digital filter is a mathematical calculation in a computer, resulting in a filtering effect.

Analogue filters occur basically in two types: low-pass and high-pass filters. A low-pass filter lets the low frequency range up to a certain cut-off frequency pass and rejects the high frequency range. A high-pass filter has the opposite characteristic. By combining low-pass and high-pass filters, band-pass and band-reject characteristics may be obtained. A notch-filter is a very narrow and sharp band-reject filter used to suppress one specific frequency, normally that of the mains system (50 or 60 Hz).

A disadvantage with the analogue filter is a distortion of the signal particularly in the frequency range around the cut-off frequency. Phase distortion is unavoidable, leading to changes in the shape of the signal recorded and thereby affecting the latencies of the response components. In order to minimise this effect, a relatively large bandwidth is often used which allows more undesired noise into the averaging procedure.

Digital filters can be made to perform their filtering function without phase distortion and can thus provide a smaller bandwidth and improved signal-to-noise ratio. However, the mathematical calculation in the computer usually takes too long to allow the filtering of each single sweep; the filtering is therefore made on the averaged response.

A/D conversion and averaging

In spite of the use of a differential amplifier and of filters, the auditory evoked response is still hidden in noise. Averaging is needed to increase the signal-to-noise ratio sufficiently to allow the identification of a response. The averaging is performed by a computer which requires the

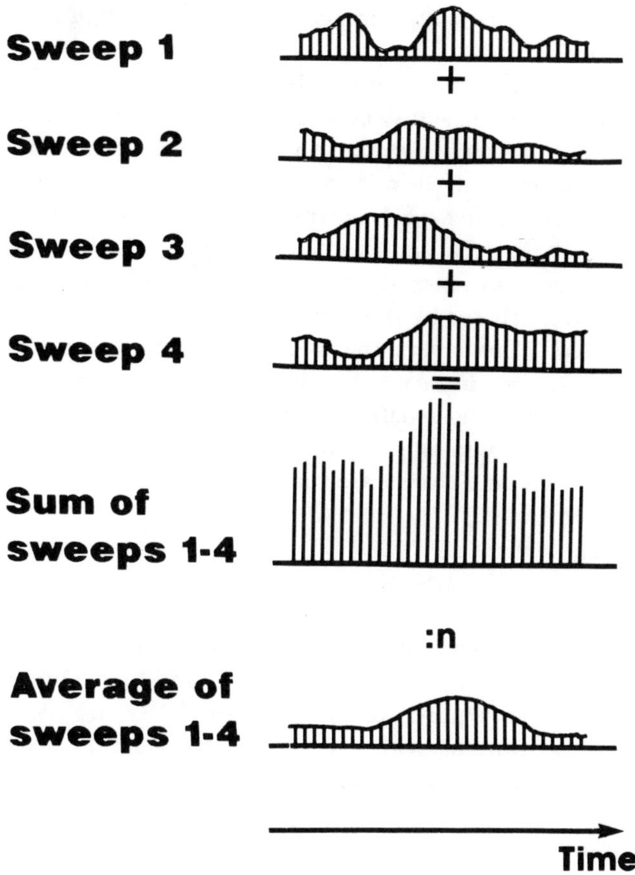

Figure 9.3 The principle of averaging in ERA.

conversion of the amplified signal from the analogue to the digital form. The A/D converter performs this procedure by sampling the analogue signal at fixed intervals. The amplitude in each sample is converted into a number to be stored in the computer memory. A sweep is a set of such samples that covers the desired time window of the signal, e.g. 10 ms in ECoG and BRA or 500 ms in CRA. Commonly, 200 samples are used for each sweep, i.e. sampling is performed each 50 μs in BRA and each 2.5 ms in CRA. Figure 9.3 illustrates the sampling and the summation of sweeps to obtain an averaged response.

The sampling procedure converts the instantaneous signal amplitude into a digital number. However, the A/D converter can use only a limited number of values – typically an 8-bit A/D converter is used allowing the quantisation of the signal amplitude into 256 different values. This procedure introduces a quantisation error, but the effect of this on the final average is negligible.

The use of the averaging procedure is based on the assumption that the small response hidden in each sweep has the same characteristic after each repeated stimulus, whereas the noise which covers the response part of the sweep varies randomly in relation to the auditory stimulation. By the summation procedure over a large number of sweeps, the sum of the responses grows with each sweep whilst the sum of the noise grows much more slowly because of its random character. Theoretically, the signal-to-noise (S/N) ratio increases by the square root of *n* where *n* is the number of sweeps added. Thus, averaging 100 sweeps increases S/N 10 times; averaging 1000 sweeps increases S/N approximately 31 times. In practice, the improvement in S/N is usually smaller due to the noise not being truly random but often containing periodic components, both from other bioelectrical activity and from external interference.

Stimulus unit

Stimulus types

Several types of auditory stimuli are used to evoke electric responses (Figure 9.4). A traditional requirement of auditory stimuli is to be frequency specific. A requirement specific for ECoG and BRA is transient stimulation, i.e. a stimulus with a very sudden onset, in order to excite synchronously as many neurons as possible to provide optimum conditions for recording and identifying the responses. These two requirements are inherently contradictory and thus compromises have to be made.

The most common stimulus when recording brain-stem responses is a broad-band click, generated by feeding a brief electric pulse to an earphone. The typical pulse duration is 0.1–0.2 ms. The acoustic click generated by the earphone consists of one or two half-waves followed by quickly decaying oscillations. The acoustic wave pattern is largely determined by the earphone's electromechanical characteristics and lasts considerably longer than the electric signal, typically a few milliseconds. Its frequency spectrum is broad with the maximum energy usually around 2–3 kHz (Figure 9.5).

A somewhat more frequency-specific click is the filtered click. This is generated by feeding a rectangular electric pulse through a band-pass filter. The resulting acoustic signal still has a fast onset, but its main energy is concentrated in the pass-band of the filter. Short tone bursts with rise and fall times of the order of 1 ms, or one or two periods and a very short plateau in between, also provide better frequency specificity (Davis and Hirsh, 1979). They have commonly been used in ECoG. When using such brief stimuli, it is important to remember that the acoustic stimulus actually obtained depends not only on the electric signal and the earphone

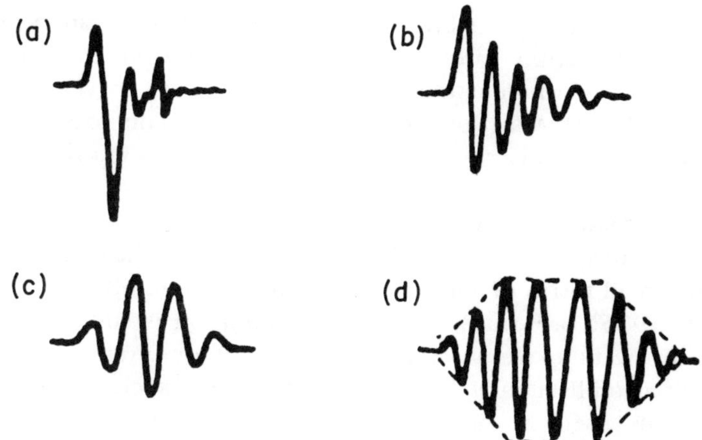

Figure 9.4 Typical brief sound stimuli used in ERA: (a) broad-band unfiltered click, (b) filtered click, (c) tone pip, (d) tone burst with well-defined rise and fall times and duration.

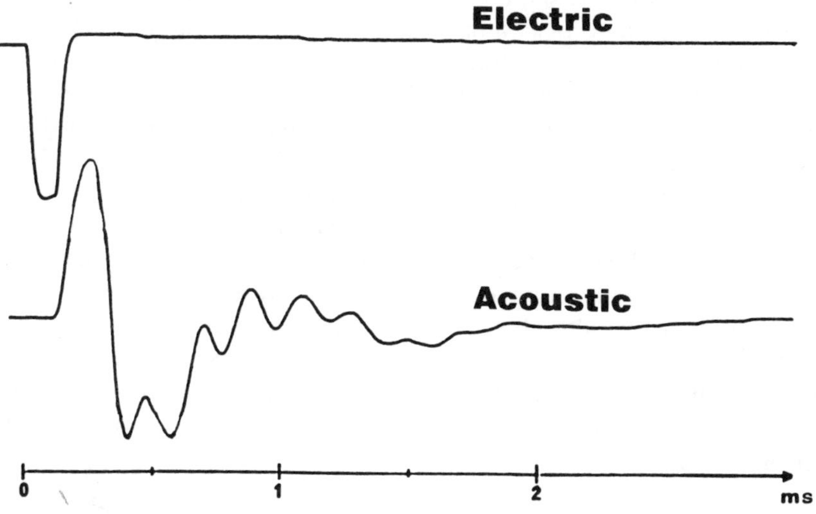

Figure 9.5 The electric square wave input delivered to the earphone (top) and the waveform of the resulting acoustic click (bottom).

characteristics but also on the coupling of the earphone to the ear (Laukli, 1983).

In CRA, longer rise times can be used, typically 20 ms, as well as longer durations of the tone burst. Therefore, the responses represent the response of a much more limited frequency range in the auditory system and have a high frequency specificity.

In most types of ERA stimulators, stimulus polarity can be selected between condensation, rarefaction or alternating. Condensation implies that the first and dominating acoustic wave is an increase in sound pressure, whilst in rarefaction mode the first wave is a decrease in pressure. In alternating mode every other stimulus is presented in opposite phase.

Calibration of stimulus level

A correct control of the stimulus level which reaches the eardrum is important in all forms of audiometry. A calibration in dB HL according to ISO 389 (1985) presumes that stimulus duration is sufficiently long in relation to the temporal integration of the auditory system, i.e. at least a few hundred milliseconds. In ERA, only CRA uses such stimuli. Thus the brief stimuli used in other types of ERA require other calibration principles.

Stimulus level can be calibrated either in an acoustic or a psychoacoustic scale. In the acoustic scale, the most commonly used principle is the peak equivalent sound pressure level (peSPL). Here the peak-to-peak amplitude of the brief stimulus is compared to a continuous pure tone adjusted to give the same peak-to-peak amplitude. This is most easily checked on an oscilloscope screen by evaluating the electric output signal from an acoustic coupler or artificial ear when the earphone is activated by the brief stimulus and a continuous tone, respectively. The peSPL of the brief stimulus is equal to the root mean square (RMS) sound pressure level of that continuous tone having the same peak-to-peak amplitude.

In the psychoacoustic calibration a hearing level scale is used. Zero dB HL is defined as the average hearing threshold of a reasonably large group (typically 20–50) of young, healthy, normally hearing listeners when the brief stimulus is presented by the particular transducer that is to be used for ERA. Naturally, the stimulus level can also be expressed in dB SL, i.e. relative to the test subject's threshold of hearing for the particular stimulus in use, provided that the subject can ccoperate in a threshold determination procedure.

Earphone or loudspeaker

The earphone or loudspeaker converts the electric signal from the stimulus generator into an acoustic signal. Usually conventional audiometer earphones are used, often provided with μ metal shielding to reduce the electromagnetic radiation.

Another way of reducing the electromagnetic stimulus artefact is to use earphone types with negligible magnetic fields, e.g. electrostatic or piezoelectric types, or insert earphones that may produce a smaller magnetic field.

A loudspeaker placed at some distance from the patient also provides a reduction of the magnetic stimulus artefact. A loudspeaker may also be indicated for some patients who refuse to wear earphones. However, calibration is less reliable than with earphones and latencies are influenced by the additional travelling time of the sound from the loudspeaker to the subject's ear. It is also worth noting that binaural stimulation usually occurs.

Central processing and computing units

The recording and the stimulus units are connected to a common control unit which handles the central process of initiating stimulation and collecting the amplified bioelectrical activity, including computation of the final average, digital filtering etc.

In some ERA equipment, the system is housed in a complete, self-contained unit and the test procedure is controlled by setting a limited number of switches and controls to the required positions. They are easy to use in clinical routine and are often portable. Typically, a small recorder is built into the system to provide a print-out on paper.

Other types of equipment are designed more like a small general computer with stimulus generator and amplifiers added as extension units. The setting of the various test parameters is handled by means of a keyboard, often based on a program menu. In general, such equipment provides greater flexibility, possibility for storing the results on disks and various kinds of off-line signal processing and analysis. Print-out is provided by means of a separate plotter.

Electrocochleography

Indication

Electrocochleography (ECoG) is a monaural electrophysiological hearing test and is used to assess the function of the inner ear. The main application has been the estimation of hearing thresholds in children and evaluation of binaural conductive or mixed hearing disorders with masking problems.

Physiological background

ECoG had its breakthrough at the end of the 1960s and early 1970s when efficient means of signal averaging had become available and made ERA clinically feasible. Pioneering studies were made by Aran and co-workers (Portmann, LeBert and Aran, 1967), Eggermont and co-workers (Eggermont and Odenthal, 1974) and Elberling (Salomon and Elberling, 1971; Elberling, 1973). A completely non-invasive technique was shown to be possible (Sohmer and Feinmesser, 1967). Two varieties of recording technique have developed. In one a transtympanic needle electrode is used with its tip placed on the promontory in the middle ear. This gives the

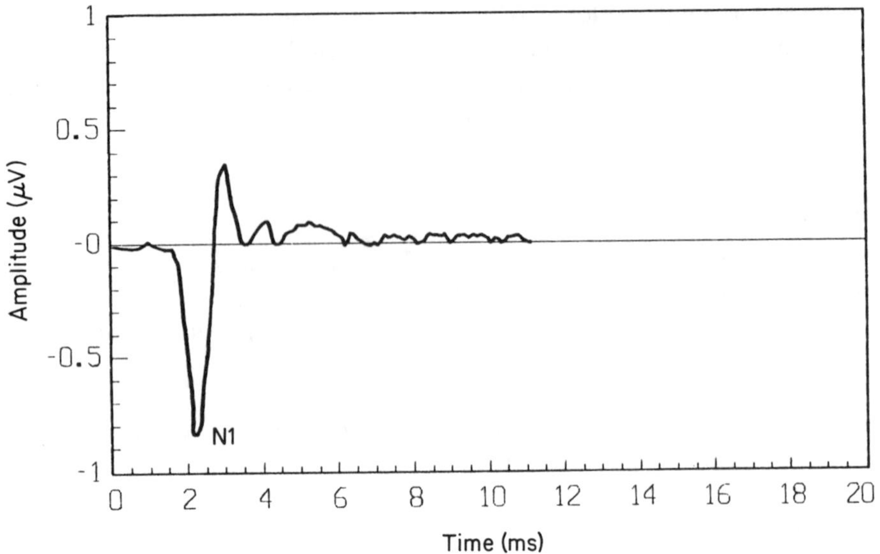

Figure 9.6 Example of a typical ECoG recording.

highest signal amplitude – up to 10–20 μV. The other utilises ear-canal electrodes placed either on the eardrum or the inner part of the ear-canal wall (Harder and Arlinger, 1981; Stypulkowski and Staller, 1987). With such electrodes response amplitudes may reach a few microvolts.

The response recorded in ECoG consists of several parts: the presynaptic activities cochlear microphonics (CM) and the summating potential (SP) from the cochlea, and the auditory compound action potential (ACAP) from the fibres of the auditory nerve. The latter part forms the dominating wave of the response, called N1, which typically occurs with a latency of 1.5–2 ms after stimulus onset at high stimulus levels (Figure 9.6).

Equipment

In ECoG needle electrodes are sometimes used, made from stainless steel, i.e. a different metal from that used in surface electrodes. If electrodes of different metals are connected to the two active amplifier input terminals, a difference in d.c. potential will occur. This requires the amplifier input stage to be a.c. coupled in order to prevent the amplifier becoming blocked by the d.c. potential difference.

Electrodes

A common electrode combination is a stainless steel needle electrode connected to the positive amplifier input and a silver/silver chloride surface electrode connected to the negative input. With this electrode polarity, the standard response type is obtained with the N1 component recorded downwards. The needle is inserted through the eardrum with its tip resting on the middle-ear promontory. The surface electrode is placed close to the ear to be tested, on the mastoid surface or the ear-lobe. The third common electrode is usually a silver/silver chloride surface electrode, where location is not very critical. Normally the forehead or cheek is used.

Several types of ear-canal electrodes have been devised to avoid the penetration of the eardrum (Stypulkowski and Staller, 1987). Their disadvantage is that they pick up the electrical activity further away from the cochlea than the transtympanic needle and thus provide lower response amplitude. The risk, although extremely small, of causing infection or mechanical damage with the promontory needle is, however, avoided (Crowley, Davis and Beagley, 1975).

Filter

The lower limiting frequency is selected to be typically in the range 20–300 Hz and the upper limit in the range 1000–3000 Hz.

Stimulus generator and transducer

Broad-band unfiltered clicks, filtered clicks or brief tone bursts are the most commonly used stimuli (Eggermont, Spoor and Odenthal, 1976) (see Figure 9.4). To allow the easy use of needle electrodes, an earphone construction with two parts has been used by many groups. A ring with a soft cushion is placed around the ear and held in place by means of a band around the head. Thin rubber bands provide support for the outer end of the needle electrode. The outer part contains the shielded earphone and is placed onto the ring and held in place by means of a thin circular permanent magnet.

Bone-conduction stimulation has also been used with some success for ECoG. Since the transtympanic needle electrode picks up electrical activity only from the ear in which it is placed, no contralateral masking is required. However, considerable problems with control of stimulus waveform may occur, in particular because of the limited ability of bone vibrators to transduce the transient stimuli used in ECoG (Arlinger and Kylén, 1977).

A stimulus repetition rate should be used which is not related to the mains frequency to reduce the effect of interfering hum picked up by the recording system. Examples of suitable repetition frequencies are 17 or 21 Hz.

Stimulus calibration

Click calibration should always be specified in dB peSPL. As a complement, a transfer to dB HL is often specified, typically of the order of 30–35 dB for broad-band clicks, i.e. a click level of 80 dB peSPL typically corresponds to 45–50 dB HL. The difference between the two scales depends mainly on the duration of the acoustic stimulation as a consequence of auditory temporal integration. The fact that temporal integration is level dependent (see Chapter 4) introduces an error in the transfer between sound pressure level and hearing level at levels significantly above 0 dB HL.

Sources of error and test reliability

The presence of a stimulus artefact will negatively influence the identification and analysis of a response. To reduce this problem, alternating stimulus polarity is often used. This technique also eliminates the cochlear microphonic part of the response which may or may not be desired.

The compound action potential has essentially the same decreasing waveform, dominated by the N1 component, independent of stimulus polarity (Figure 9.6). However, when analysed in more detail, some difference is often seen in N1 latency in response to rarefaction as compared to condensation stimuli (Elberling, 1973). This may result in some degradation of the final result when using alternating stimulus polarity.

For reliable clinical evaluation of ECoG recordings, normal material should be available showing mean latencies and standard deviations as a function of stimulus level. The data should be obtained with the particular equipment on a group of normally hearing subjects. In general, ECoG shows rather good reproducibility, in particular when using the transtympanic needle electrode. A standard deviation of 0.24 ms for the N1 latency at 75 dB HL broad-band click stimulation was reported by Bergholtz, Hooper and Mehta (1976). Lower stimulus levels typically result in larger standard deviations, but normally little effect is seen from sensorineural hearing loss. Eggermont and Odenthal (1974) report standard deviations of less than 0.2 ms for tone burst stimulation at 2, 4 and 8 kHz.

Clinical interpretation

An important clinical value of ECoG performed with transtympanic needle electrode is that it can be considered as a strictly monaural test which does not require contralateral masking. When other placement of the positive electrode is used, the relative risk of picking up activity from the contralateral ear increases but is still small for ear-canal placements. Another advantage is that ECoG is not influenced by sedation or general anaesthesia. A clear limitation is its low power in evaluating the auditory function at low frequencies – 1 kHz and below (Gibson, 1978). This is due to the inherent contradiction between a low frequency spectrum and a fast stimulus onset.

The most common clinical application is evaluation of the peripheral auditory function in children (Bergholtz et al., 1977), in particular the very

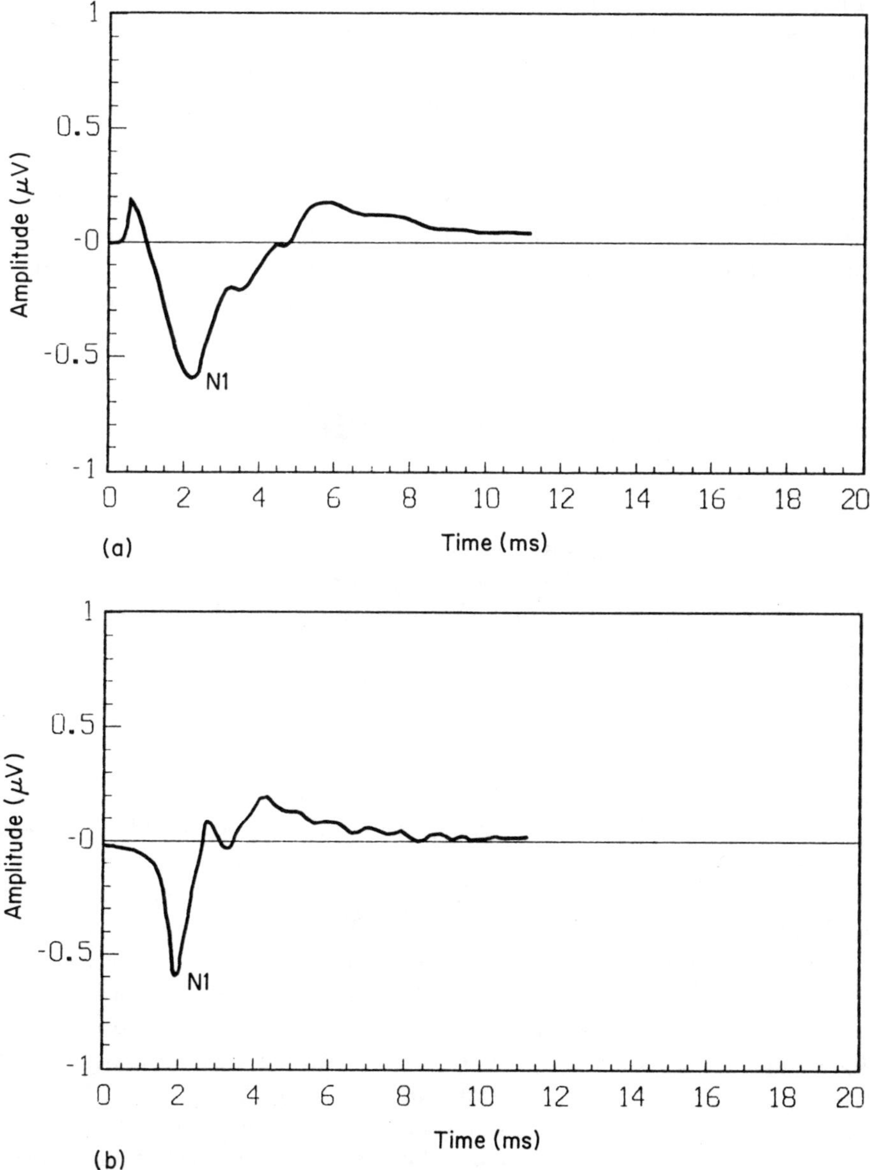

Figure 9.7 (a) The increased width of the N1 wave during an attack of Menière's disease. (b) Recording from the same patient when the hearing is normal again.

difficult-to-test children with multiple handicaps. The evaluation is normally based on determining the lowest stimulus levels for tone burst stimuli of various frequencies from 1 kHz that give rise to identifiable responses. ECoG has also been shown to give valuable clinical information on subjects having mixed hearing loss with large conductive components where conventional bone-conduction testing has limited success because of masking problems (Harder et al., 1980).

Patients with Menière's disease have been subject to several ECoG studies. The most common finding in this disease has been a widening of the response waveform, presumably due to an enlarged summating potential (Gibson, Moffat and Ramstad, 1977) (Figure 9.7).

The auditory compound action potential provides a good description of the cochlea since it is generated in the distal part of the auditory nerve. The cochlear microphonic component is generated by the hair cells and may thus provide a functional indicator for this specific part of the sense organ. One example is a report of abnormally large CM in ears with tinnitus in young subjects with normal pure-tone audiograms (Gibson, 1978).

Brain-stem Response Audiometry

Indication

Brain-stem response audiometry (BRA) is used for the clinical evaluation of sensorineural hearing disorders. The test provides a means of threshold estimation of difficult-to-test patients, e.g. children and multi-handicapped patients. The test has also become an important tool for the diagnosis of suspected brain-stem lesions with or without auditory symptoms.

Physiological background

BRA was developed as a clinically useful test method in the 1970s. A pioneering contribution was that of Jewett and Williston (1971) who used the same surface electrode locations as Sohmer and Feinmesser (1967). They showed that, following the compound action potential of the auditory nerve after auditory stimulation, a series of waves could be identified within a 10-ms time window. These waves are now known as the Jewett waves I to V (Figure 9.8). Normative data for latencies and amplitudes of these waves have been reported by several groups (e.g. Bergholtz, 1981). In addition to these waves, later waves denoted VI and VII may occur under certain conditions.

Considerable efforts have been devoted to the identification of the generators of the different waves in the auditory brain-stem response (ABR). A clear view is still lacking. An early interpretation given by Jewett (1970) was the following: wave I was generated by the cochlear nerve,

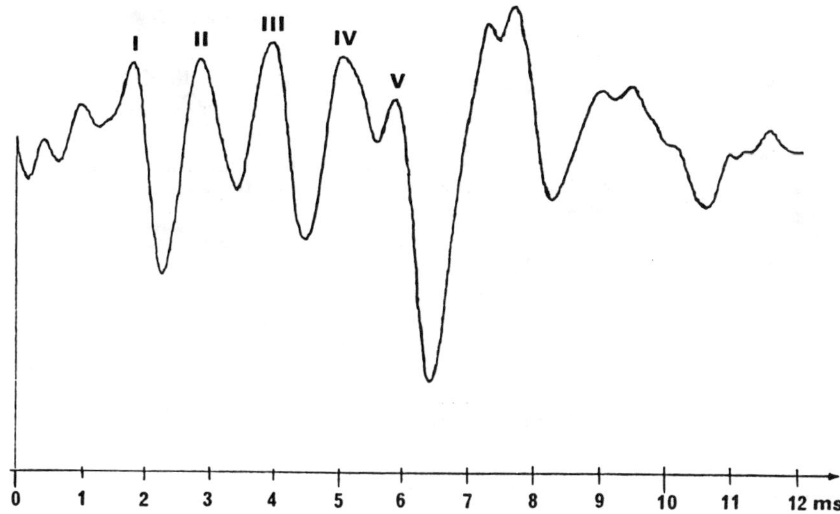

Figure 9.8 Example of a typical ABR recording.

wave II in the cochlear nuclei, wave III in the superior olive complex, wave IV in nuclei in the lateral lemniscus and wave V in the inferior colliculus. However, later studies have shown this interpretation to be too simple, e.g. Achor and Starr (1980) argue that only the first waves are derived from single neuroanatomical structures. Borg (1981) questions the role of the inferior colliculus as the sole generator of wave V and also assumes that wave III receives contributions from several sources. Moller (1983) has shown, in recordings made during skull surgery, that waves I and II have their origin in the auditory nerve. The following waves are probably generated by activity in brain-stem nuclei as well as tracts.

The absolute latency of the different waves is defined as the time from stimulus onset to the time corresponding to the amplitude maximum of the wave. Also interwave latencies are determined, in particular between waves I and V or III and V (Figure 9.9).

As with all types of electric responses, ABR latencies decrease and amplitudes increase when stimulus level is increased (Figure 9.10). Also, stimulus repetition frequency influences the response – increasing the repetition rate increases the wave latencies. Commonly used repetition rates are in the range 10–20 stimuli per second.

The distance between the stimulus transducer and the eardrum represents an acoustic delay determined by the velocity of sound. A distance between a loudspeaker and the test subject introduces a delay of approximately 3 ms. Also the transmission characteristics of the middle ear may affect response latencies due to phase distortion of the stimulus.

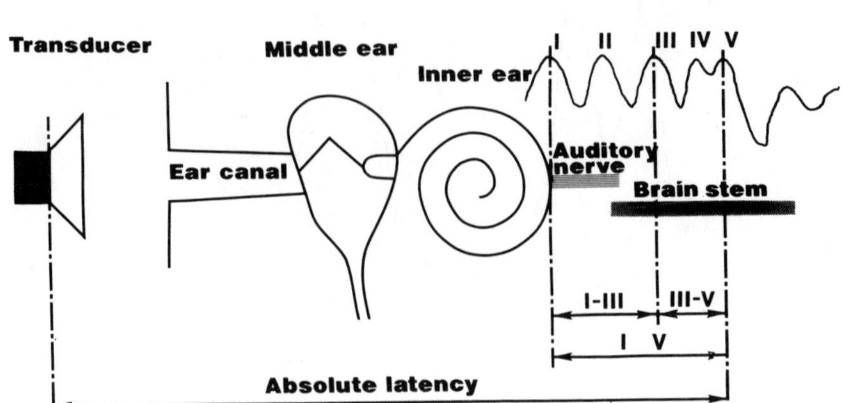

Figure 9.9 Illustration of different latencies in ABR.

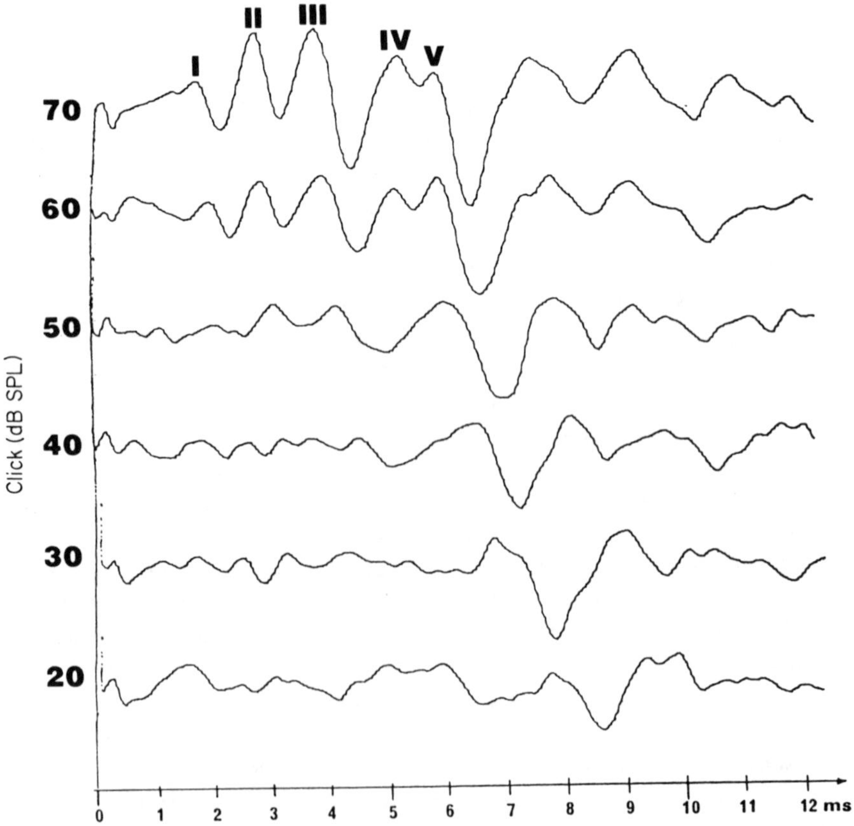

Figure 9.10 ABR recordings with decreasing stimulus level, showing increased latencies.

Biological factors which have been shown to influence ABR response are age, sex and body temperature. Wave latencies decrease significantly from birth to about 6 months of age (Hecox and Galambos, 1974; Starr et al., 1977; Harris et al., 1981). In elderly subjects they increase again. Rosenhall et al. (1985) found slightly increased latencies in the age group 55–75 as compared to 25–34 years. They also found men to have 0.1–0.2 ms longer wave III and V latencies than women in all age groups. Like most body functions, brain-stem activity is reduced by a decreased body temperature. A reduction of 1–2°C may increase latencies to pathological values in otherwise normal subjects.

Sleep or general anaesthesia as a rule has negligible effects on the ABR. Various sedatives have been used when testing children, e.g. chloral hydrate, barbiturates and benzodiazepines. The sedative effect of these drugs is often difficult to predict. Some clinics therefore prefer general anaesthesia as a reliable means of providing optimum testing conditions in children who cannot be tested in natural sleep.

Equipment

Since the auditory brain-stem response is of very low amplitude, typically a few hundred nanovolt at high stimulus levels, great care has to be taken to minimise noise and other interfering electrical activity (Arlinger, 1981).

Electrodes

Normally disposable silver/silver chloride surface electrodes are used. One recording electrode is placed either on the vertex or as high as possible in the forehead and the other close to the test ear, usually on the mastoid surface. Sometimes the latter is replaced by an ear-canal electrode in order to enhance wave I of the ABR. The common electrode is usually placed on the cheek. When the equipment allows two-channel recording, a third recording electrode is placed on the contralateral mastoid to provide simultaneous ipsi- and contralateral response recordings.

Depending on how the two recording electrodes are connected to the positive and negative inputs of the amplifier, the ABR waves I–V may be shown pointing upwards or downwards on the final recording of the averaged response. Connecting the vertex (forehead) electrode to the negative input normally results in the waves pointing downwards. This system shows wave I in the same direction as the N1 component in ECoG, which is logical because they represent the same activity – the compound action potential from the auditory nerve. A practical advantage is that this connection is the same as is used for the recording of cortical responses. Thus, when ABR and auditory cortical response (ACR) are to be recorded from the same patient in the same session, no change in electrode connections has to be made. However, the most commonly seen practice is the opposite, i.e. connecting the vertex (forehead) electrode to the positive amplifier input terminal and showing the ABR waves pointing upwards.

Filter

The lower limiting frequency of the analogue recording filter is normally set in the range 20–300 Hz and the upper in the range 1000–3000 Hz. The limits actually used affect the risk of phase distortion and consequent influence on the wave latencies of the ABR. Absolute latencies of the different waves obtained with recordings using different types of filters and settings of limiting frequencies are often not comparable therefore.

Stimulus generator and transducer

The most common stimulus used to evoke the ABR is the broad-band click, generated by either a rectangular or half-sinusoid electric pulse with duration in the range 0.1–0.2 ms. Most earphones used are magnetically shielded to reduce the risk of stimulus artefacts. The experience using short tone bursts shows that the increase in frequency specificity is obtained at the expense of the response amplitude. A stimulus repetition rate in the range 10–20/s that is not simply related to the mains frequency is recommended.

Stimulus calibration

Click calibration should always be specified in dB peSPL. As a complement, a transfer to dB HL is often used. The HL scale is typically 30–35 dB less than the peSPL scale for broad-band clicks. The fact that temporal integration is dependent on sound level makes threshold estimations at higher sound levels less reliable when expressed in dB HL. In some applications of BRA, the scale of sensation level, i.e. decibels relative to the test subject's detection threshold for the click train, is used.

Sources of error and test reliability

A number of factors may influence the response latencies. The analogue filter characteristics are important technical factors – both the type of filter and cut-off frequencies. Because of phase distortion, which occurs in particular in the frequency range close to the cut-off frequencies, the response waveform is affected. This in turn implies a shift in time when the various peaks occur, i.e. wave latencies. Ideally, a very wide frequency band should be used in the recording system. However, since the reduction of noise is of great importance, the band limits have to be kept relatively narrow (Osterhammel, 1981). Because of the risk of phase distortion, the normal material with which clinical test results are

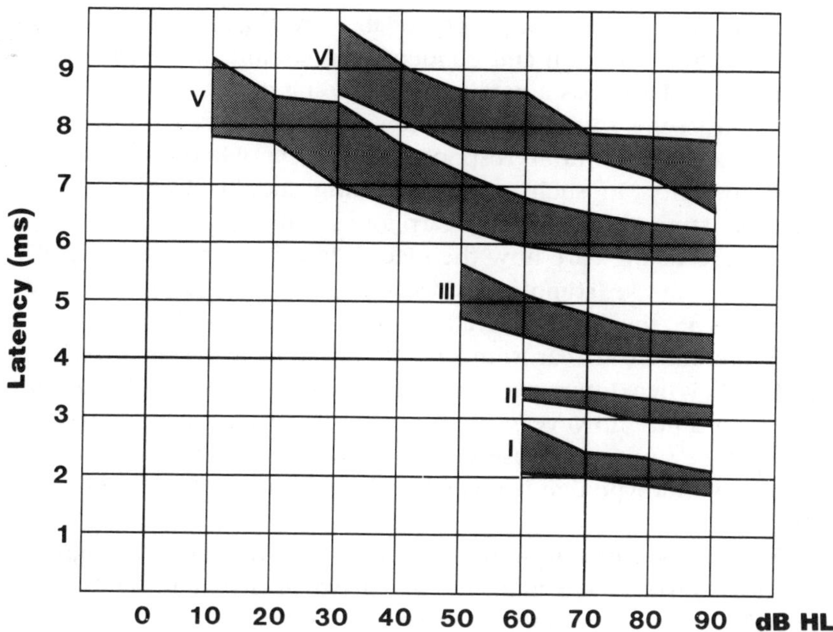

Figure 9.11 Examples of ABR latencies of a normal material, shown as mean value ± 2 standard deviations at different stimulus levels.

compared has to be obtained on the same equipment and with the same filter settings as used in the clinical practice.

The most practical way of presenting the normal material is as a latency range defined by the mean plus/minus two standard deviations for different stimulus levels. Such data reported from different laboratories (Thornton, 1975; Rosenhamer, Lindström and Lundborg, 1978; Chiappa, 1983) show good agreement with regard to reliability. The standard deviations are found in the range 0.1–0.3 ms, typically being larger for the later waves and at lower stimulus levels. An example of a normal material presented graphically is shown in Figure 9.11.

Contralateral masking is rarely needed in the recording of ABR, particularly in the otoneurological application of the test where stimulus levels are relatively high above the hearing threshold. Since the stimuli normally used have their main energy in the high frequency range, the effective transcranial attenuation is typically of the order of 60 dB. Thus, when the test is used for the estimation of hearing thresholds, contralateral masking has to be used only seldomly.

A stimulus artefact sometimes occurs due to magnetic radiation from the earphone. Alternating stimulus polarity is a means of reducing this, because the artefacts from every stimulus pair cancel each other in the summation process. Normally, very small or negligible differences occur in response to rarefaction and condensation stimuli, and thus alternating the stimulus polarity has a negligible degrading effect on the response in comparison to the advantage of eliminating the artefact (Gibson, 1978). In rare cases, a very poor response may occur when using alternating stimulus polarity. In such cases, recording should also be made with rarefaction stimuli only. Using earphones with good quality magnetic shielding and taking care how the electrode cables are placed relative to the earphone in use, stimulus artefacts are normally no problem.

Variations in the acoustic transmission time from earphone or loudspeaker membrane to eardrum due to variation in distance have to be considered. When interwave latencies are evaluated this factor has no effect. Sometimes, however, the presence of a wave I may be difficult to establish. One way to increase wave I amplitude is to replace the mastoid electrode with a type that is placed in the ear canal (Harder and Arlinger, 1981).

Different types of earphone reproduce a brief electric signal with different acoustic wave patterns, in particular when using broad-band clicks. This may also affect ABR wave latencies.

Clinical interpretation

The clinical evaluation of ABR is normally based on wave I–V latencies whilst the amplitudes of the waves have relatively little quantitative significance. Waves II and IV are often very small or non-existent. At low stimulus levels, usually only wave V and/or the wave of opposite polarity following wave V (FFP7, the 7-ms far field potential according to Terkildsen, Osterhammel and Huis in't Veld (1974)) are identifiable.

Reliable identification of an ABR requires that two repeated tests have been made with the same stimulus and recording parameters. If a conductive component is known to exist in the ear tested, this is important to consider. Basically, its effect on the ABR corresponds to a reduction of the stimulus level by the same amount as the magnitude of the conductive loss (Borg, Löfqvist and Rosén, 1981).

Sensorineural hearing loss

Brain-stem response audiometry has been shown to be the most sensitive audiological test for differentiating between cochlear and retrocochlear hearing disorders. The most important characteristic is the prolongation of wave V latency in retrocochlear cases (e.g. Rosenhamer, 1980). Commonly, wave V latencies for left and right ears are compared and the interaural latency difference determined. A value exceeding 0.3 ms when stimulating the two ears at the same sensation level is typically considered as an indication for retrocochlear disorder (Brackmann, 1978). An example is shown in Figure 9.12.

In subjects with cerebellopontine angle tumours and particularly acoustic neuromas the sensitivity of ABR is very close to 100%. Thus, ABR has become extremely important as a diagnostic tool for the early detection of such tumours (Rosenhamer, 1980; Rosenhall, 1981; Josey, 1985).

The absence of a reproducible ABR pattern may also indicate a retrocochlear pathology and is often seen in cases with large tumours or brain-stem lesions. Sudden transitory hearing loss with reversible ABR pathology may indicate a haemorrhage in a cerebellopontine angle tumour.

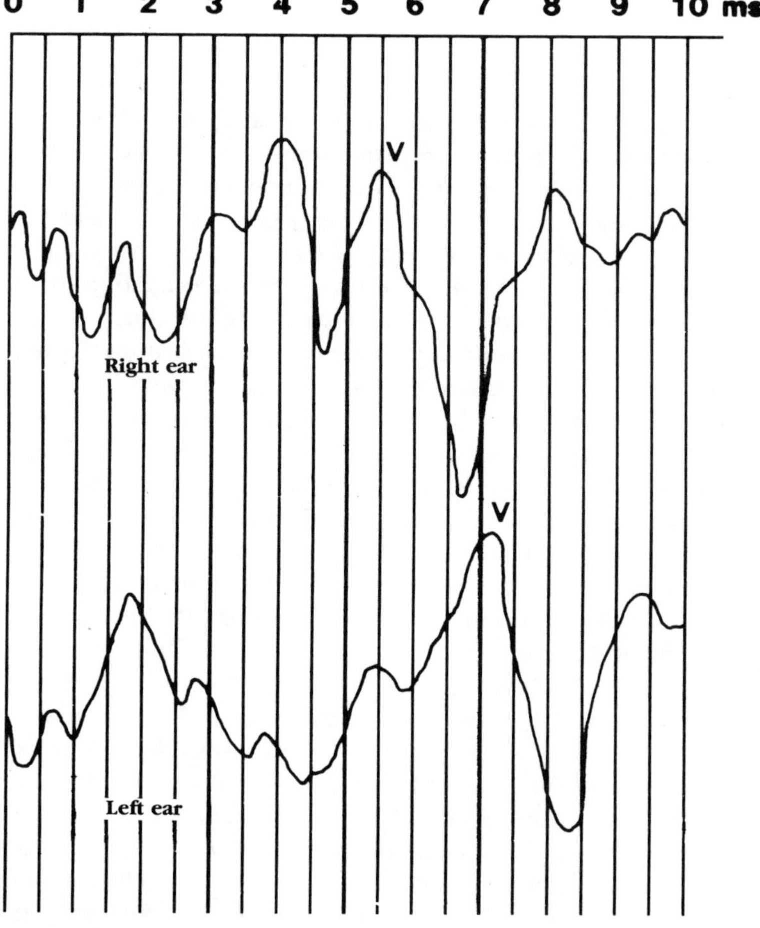

Figure 9.12 Pathological prolongation of wave V latency in patient with left-sided cerebellopontine angle tumour.

In patients with severe hearing loss in the mid- and high frequency range, the probability of obtaining an ABR is low (Borg and Löfqvist, 1982; Bauch and Olsen, 1988). No exact limit can be defined but in cases where the average hearing threshold (0.5/1/2 kHz) is of the order of 70 dB or more, a recordable ABR cannot be expected (Harris and Almqvist, 1981; Rosenhall, 1981).

ABR indicating a retrocochlear lesion but with negative findings on subsequent radiological testing may occur, i.e. false negative findings with regard to the tumour diagnosis. Other retrocochlear disease may be the reason in some cases. To exclude the possibility of a conductive component being the cause, an evaluation of interwave latencies is often helpful. In a typical retrocochlear case the I–V and III–V interwave latencies are longer than normal whilst they remain unaffected by a conductive disorder.

Estimation of hearing thresholds

ABR is also important for the estimation of hearing thresholds in subjects where conventional audiometric methods have failed (Fria, 1985). Compared to cortical responses, the brain-stem responses have the advantage of being virtually unaffected by degree of wakefulness or sleep. The test can be performed therefore in general anaesthesia if deemed necessary. This also allows a detailed otoscopic investigation by means of microscope on subjects who otherwise would refuse this.

The neonatal period allows a period of a number of weeks where the child will easily fall asleep after feeding and permit testing without sedation. Broad-band click stimuli will give an estimate of hearing thresholds in the high frequency range. Filtered clicks will make the test somewhat more frequency specific, but it will still not be possible to determine hearing thresholds at discrete frequencies. The basic principle in the testing is to determine the lowest stimulus level that evokes a reproducible response. The recording of cortical responses permits the use of frequency-specific tone bursts, but requires that the test subject is tested relaxed and awake. Typically, this is very difficult at an age below 10–12 years.

A negative ABR test cannot be interpreted as an indication of total deafness because the efficiency of the method to evaluate low frequency hearing is very low. Thus, the negative outcome should not be interpreted as indicating that a hearing aid will be of no benefit.

In patients with a psychomotor handicap, hearing loss may be a component in the total situation which is often very difficult to evaluate with conventional psychoacoustic methods. BRA has been shown to be a valuable tool in obtaining an estimate of the auditory function and of considerable value for the continued care of the patient and information to parents and staff (Harris, Broms and Möllerström, 1981; Stein et al., 1987). This applies also to geriatric patients in whom sometimes disturbed communication may be due to either senile dementia or hearing loss or both. Also in this population BRA has been applied with some success (Soucek, Michaels and Frohlich, 1986).

Neurological diagnosis

BRA is becoming an increasingly important tool for the diagnosis of brain-stem lesions which do not primarily or only concern the auditory pathways. The evaluation of suspected multiple sclerosis is an example of this where often abnormal ABR is recorded as a consequence of the demyelinising disease. The most common finding is the absence of the later waves in the ABR complex whilst earlier waves appear within limits. Jerger et al. (1986) found ABR abnormalities in 52% of a group with verified multiple sclerosis.

In intensive care, ABR has been used to test patients with reduced degrees of consciousness, e.g. after intoxication, haemorrhage or skull trauma (Hall, 1988). Also, in such cases the common effect on ABR is increased wave latency or absence of later waves.

Intraoperative monitoring during tumour or vascular surgery in the skull is also an area in which ABR is being used. The aim is to reduce the risk of causing damage to the auditory pathways during surgery (Kileny et al., 1988).

Brain-stem response audiometry has evolved as the most widely used test in the ERA 'family' with important clinical applications since its start in the mid-1970s. Because the equipment has become easier to use, it is frequently found in smaller clinics. However, the clinical reliability of the test assumes that the staff who perform the test and evaluate the recordings use it often enough to obtain continuous and broad experience.

Cortical Response Audiometry

Indication

Cortical response audiometry (CRA) is mainly used for the estimation of hearing thresholds on adult subjects and children from the age of about 10 years. Indications for the test may be a suspected non-organic hearing loss or to obtain confirmation of hearing threshold levels in cases of insurance compensation. CRA has also proved to be of value as a diagnostic tool in otoneurological evaluations.

Physiological background

The basic studies of CRA as a clinical test method were published in the 1960s (e.g. Davis and Yoshie, 1963). The cortical response is a wave

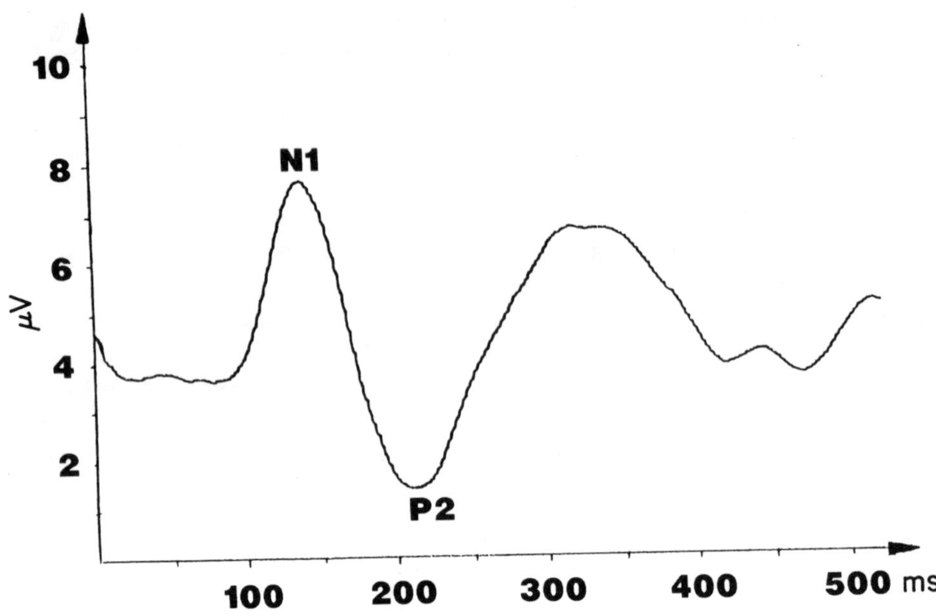

Figure 9.13 Example of a typical CRA recording.

pattern that occurs in the latency range 100–300 ms after stimulus onset. The main energy of the response is in the frequency range 4–6 Hz and its amplitude may reach 20 μV. The dominating components are called N1 or N100 and P2 or P200 (Figure 9.13), occurring with approximate latencies of 100 and 200 ms, respectively.

The source of the auditory cortical response has not been uniquely defined as the auditory projection areas in the temporal lobes. Vaughan (1969) published isopotential maps showing how the response amplitude varied as a function of recording site on the skull surface. His results showed amplitude maximum on the vertex, and Vaughan interpreted this as evidence for the primary auditory projection areas being the generator site. Other studies, e.g. Picton et al. (1974), argue that the slow auditory cortical response was generated in a diffuse area related to the frontal lobes of the brain. Later studies using recordings of magnetic fields from the brain evoked by auditory stimulation clearly indicate that the major parts of the evoked cortical potentials and the evoked magnetic fields are generated in the same areas in the temporal lobes (Elberling et al., 1981).

The wave pattern obtained in response to auditory stimulation is very similar to that obtained in visual or tactile stimulation. This fact may be used to make sure that the recording equipment functions correctly, for example, in cases where no identifiable auditory responses can be recorded.

Amplitude and latency of the cortical responses are influenced by a number of factors. As is the case with all electric responses to auditory stimulation, latency increases and amplitude decreases when the stimulus level is reduced. These relations may be used to estimate the hearing threshold by extrapolation (Skinner, Antinoro and Shimota, 1974; Arlinger, 1976a).

Wave amplitudes are also influenced by the interval between successive stimuli. Maximum amplitude is obtained with intervals of 10 s or longer. Also irregular variation of interstimulus intervals increases the amplitude (Tyberghein and Forrez, 1969). This is probably due both to reducing the risk of phase locking to periodic activity in the EEG and to increased attention effects in the test subject (Mast and Watson, 1968; Picton and Hillyard, 1974).

In clinical testing, a compromise between maximum amplitude and short testing time is usually made leading to interstimulus intervals in the range 1–3 s being most common. Summation of 30–50 stimuli typically provides a sufficient improvement of the signal-to-noise ratio to allow the identification of a response.

Sleep and wakefulness have been shown to influence the cortical responses. Therefore, reliable testing presumes that the subject is tested awake. Closing the eyes tends to produce a clear alpha-activity in the EEG which may give rise to severe interference in the averaged response. The response pattern changes with age over a much larger range than the more peripherally generated electric responses. Normal adult response latencies cannot be expected until the age of 12–15 years (McCandless, 1967).

Binaural stimulation influences the response pattern. Contralateral masking is therefore recommended assuming a transcranial sound attenuation of 40 dB. The risk of over-masking must be considered.

Equipment

The main technical difference between CRA and other ERA methods is the use of frequency-specific stimuli with lower repetition rates and the recording bandwidth being in the very low frequency range. The number of sweeps added to obtain an averaged response is smaller, primarily because of the initial signal-to-noise ratio being more favourable than, for instance, in ABR.

Electrodes

Disposable silver/silver chloride surface electrodes are used. A vertex electrode is connected to the negative amplifier input terminal and a mastoid electrode is connected to the positive input. The common electrode is usually placed on the cheek or forehead. This scheme gives the conventional recordings with vertex negativity shown upwards.

Filter

The frequency range set by the analogue filter is typically from about 1 Hz to 15–30 Hz. Due to the phase characteristics of analogue filters, the use of low-pass filters with very steep slope and low cut-off frequency may significantly influence the wave latencies measured.

Stimulus generator and transducer

The most common stimulus is a tone burst with a duration of 20–200 ms and rise and fall times of the order of 20 ms. Increasing the duration above 30–50 ms has little effect on the response recorded (Skinner and Jones, 1968). As is the case with more peripherally generated responses, the onset is the most important part of the stimulus – the response represents the reaction of the sensory system to a change in the acoustic environment. A rise time of 20 ms has been found to be a good compromise between the wish for frequency specificity and for a distinct onset. Stimulus repetition rate is normally set in the range 0.3–1/second. If available, irregularly varying interstimulus intervals should be used.

Stimulus calibration

Stimulus levels are calibrated in dB HL according to the ISO 389 (1985) standard as for conventional pure-tone audiometers.

Sources of error and test reliability

In the evaluation of wave latency both technical and biological factors have to be considered. Technical factors of importance are stimulus rise time and repetition rate, and settings of the filters in the recording system.

The background electrical activity may vary during the recording and reduce the signal-to-noise ratio significantly. Movement artefacts caused by mechanical movement in the polarised layer between the metal electrode and the biological tissue may cause large potential variations. An electronic artefact rejection system is of considerable help in reducing the influence of such disturbing activity.

Biological factors which may influence the reliability of a CRA recording concern the state of the test subject. Wakefulness is important because sleep significantly alters the cortical activity, presumably both that evoked by the stimulation and the non-related background EEG activity. The subject closing his eyes usually gives rise to a clear increase in the alpha-activity of the EEG. Drugs which affect the function of the central nervous system may also influence the CRA recording. It is therefore important to check such factors when relevant.

The subject's attention towards the stimulus has been shown to have some influence on cortical responses. Letting the subject read a book or magazine during testing, avoiding excessive movements, may be used as a means of reducing the risk for changes in attention.

The N1 latency is normally around 100 ms and the P2 between 150 and 200 ms at high stimulus levels. In a group of normal adults standard deviation for the N1 latency was found at about 9 ms and for the P2 latency around 20 ms (Kileny and Kripal, 1987).

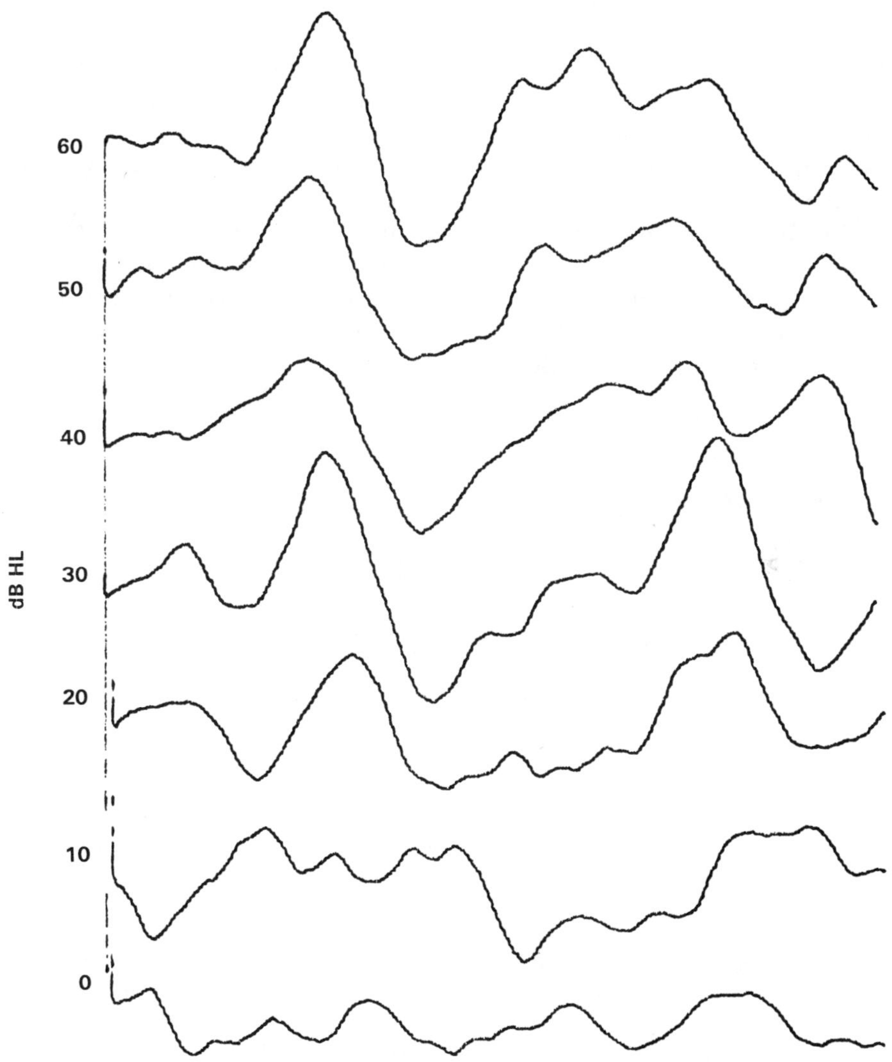

Figure 9.14 Example of the relation between wave latency and stimulus level in CRA recordings.

Clinical interpretation

The interpretation of the auditory cortical response (ACR) presumes the identification of the N1 and P2 components. Threshold estimation is based on the presentation of a series of stimuli at various levels (Figure 9.14) to allow for the determination of the lowest level that gives a reproducible response.

This level can usually be assumed to be 10–20 dB above the psychoacoustic hearing threshold on adults (Beagley and Kellogg, 1968). Responses to suprathreshold levels show the general pattern of shorter latencies and larger amplitudes at higher levels.

Responses recorded on subjects who may be using drugs which influence the conditions for reliable CRA must be interpreted with caution. Also test subjects below 12–15 years of age introduce extra difficulty because of the risk of insufficient maturation of response latencies.

CRA has also been used in otoneurological evaluations. Using a special stimulus, frequency glides of a continuous pure tone, Arlinger (1976b, 1983) showed significant differences in ACR response latencies on subjects with cochlear and with retrocochlear lesions. Using the same type of stimulus, Ödkvist et al. (1987) found pathological wave latencies in the cortical responses recorded on a group of test subjects with significant occupational exposure to industrial solvents.

References

ACHOR, L.J. and STARR, A. (1980). Auditory brain stem recordings in cat. I. Intracranial and extracranial recordings. *Electroencephalography and Clinical Neurophysiology* **48**, 154–173.

ARLINGER, S.D. (1976a). N1 latencies of the slow auditory evoked potential. *Audiology* **15**, 370–375.

ARLINGER, S.D. (1976b). *Auditory responses to frequency ramps – a psychoacoustic and electrophysiological study.* Dissertation, University of Linköping.

ARLINGER, S.D. (1981). Technical aspects on stimulation, recording and signal processing. *Scandinavian Audiology* Suppl. 13, 41–53.

ARLINGER, S.D. (1983). Auditory evoked cortical responses to frequency glides in subjects with retrocochlear hearing impairment. *Journal of Neurology, Neurosurgery and Psychiatry* **46**, 917–923.

ARLINGER, S.D. and KYLÉN, P. (1977). Bone conducted stimulation in electrocochleography. *Acta Oto-Laryngologica* **84**, 377–384.

BAUCH, C.D. and OLSEN, W.O. (1988). Auditory brainstem responses as a function of average hearing sensitivity for 2000–4000 Hz. *Audiology* **27**, 156–163.

BEAGLEY, H.A. and KELLOGG, S.E. (1968). A comparison of evoked response and subjective auditory thresholds. *International Audiology* **7**, 420–421.

BERGHOLTZ, L.M. (1981). Normative data in clinical ABR. *Scandinavian Audiology Supplement* 13, 75–81.

BERGHOLTZ, L.M., HOOPER, R.E. and MEHTA, D.C. (1976). Test–retest reliability in clinical electrocochleography. *Annals of Otology, Rhinology and Laryngology* **86**, 679–685.

BERGHOLTZ, L.M., ARLINGER, S.D., KYLÉN, P. and JERLVALL, L.B. (1977). Electrocochleography used as a clinical hearing test in difficult-to-test children. *Acta Oto-Laryngologica* **84**, 385–392.

BORG, E. (1981). Physiological mechanisms in auditory brainstem evoked potentials. *Scandinavian Audiology Supplement* 13, 11–22.

BORG, E. and LÖFQVIST, L. (1982). A lower audiometric limit for auditory brainstem response (ABR). *Scandinavian Audiology* **11**, 277–278.

BORG, E., LÖFQVIST, L. and ROSÉN, S. (1981). Brainstem response (ABR) in conductive hearing loss. *Scandinavian Audiology Supplement* 13, 95–97.

BRACKMANN, D.E. (1978). Electric response audiometry: clinical applications. *Otolaryngologic Clinics of North America* **11**, 7–18.

CHIAPPA, K.H. (1983). Brainstem auditory evoked potentials. In: Stålberg, E. and Young, R.R. (Eds.) *Clinical Neurophysiology*, pp. 259–277. London: Butterworths.

CROWLEY, D.E., DAVIS, H. and BEAGLEY, H.A. (1975). Survey of clinical use of electrocochleography. *Annals of Otology, Rhinology and Laryngology* **84**, 1–11.

DAVIS, H. and HIRSH, S. (1979). A slow brainstem response for low-frequency audiometry. *Audiology* **18**, 445–461.

DAVIS, H. and YOSHIE, N. (1963). Human evoked cortical responses to auditory stimuli. *The Physiologist* **6**, 164.

EGGERMONT, J.J. and ODENTHAL, D.W. (1974). Action potentials and summating potentials in the normal human cochlea. *Acta Oto-Laryngologica Supplementum* **317**, 39–61.

EGGERMONT, J.J., SPOOR, A. and ODENTHAL, D.W. (1976). Frequency specificity of tone-burst electrocochleography. In: Elberling, C. and Salomon, G. (Eds) *Electrocochleography* pp. 215–246. Baltimore: University Park Press.

ELBERLING, C. (1973). Transitions in cochlear action potentials recorded from the ear canal in man. *Scandinavian Audiology* **2**, 151–159.

ELBERLING, C., BAK, C., KOFOED, B., LEBECH, J. and SAERMARK, K. (1981). Auditory magnetic fields from the human cortex: influence of stimulus intensity. *Scandinavian Audiology* **10**, 203–207.

FRIA, J.F. (1985). Threshold estimation with early latency potentials. In: Katz, J. (Ed.) *Handbook of Clinical Audiology*, 3rd edn, pp. 549–564. Baltimore: Williams & Wilkins.

GALAMBOS, R., MAKEIG, S. and TALMACHOFF, P.J. (1981). A 40 Hz auditory potential recorded from the human scalp. *Proceedings of the National Academy of Science of the USA* **78**(4), 2643–2647.

GIBSON, W.P.R. (1978). *Essentials of Clinical Electric Response Audiometry.* London: Churchill Livingstone.

GIBSON, W.P.R., MOFFAT, D.A. and RAMSTAD, R.T. (1977). Clinical electrocochleography in the diagnosis and management of Menière's disorders. *Audiology* **16**, 389–401.

HALL, J.W. III (1988). Auditory evoked responses in the management of acutely brain-injured children and adults. *American Journal of Otology* **9**, 36–46.

HARDER, H. and ARLINGER, S. (1981). Ear-canal compared to mastoid electrode placement in BRA. *Scandinavian Audiology Supplement* 13, 55–57.

HARDER, H., KYLÉN, P., ARLINGER, S.D. and EKVALL, L. (1980). Preoperative bone-conducted electrocochleography in otosclerosis. *Archives of Otolaryngology* **106**, 757–762.

HARRIS, S. and ALMQVIST, B. (1981). ABR in operatively verified cerebello-pontine angle tumours. *Scandinavian Audiology Supplement* 13, 113–114.

HARRIS, S., BROMS, P. and MÖLLERSTRÖM, B. (1981). ABR in the mentally retarded child. *Scandinavian Audiology Supplement* 13, 149–150.

HARRIS, S., MÖLLERSTRÖM, B., REIMER, Å. and GRENNERT, L.G. (1981). Auditory brainstem response and gestational age in the newborn. *Scandinavian Audiology Supplement* 13, 147–148.

HECOX, K. and GALAMBOS, R. (1974). Brainstem auditory evoked responses in human infants and adults. *Archives of Otolaryngology* **99**, 30–39.

ISO 389 (1985). *Acoustics – standard reference zero for the calibration of pure tone air conduction audiometers.* Geneva: International Standards Organisation.

JACOBSON, J.T. and HYDE, M.L. (1985). An introduction to auditory evoked potentials. In: Katz, J. (Ed.) *Handbook of Clinical Audiology*, 3rd edn, pp. 496–533. Baltimore: Williams & Wilkins.

JERGER, J.F., OLIVER, T.A., CHMIEL, R.A. and RIVERA, V.M. (1986). Patterns of auditory abnormality in multiple sclerosis. *Audiology* **25**, 193–209.

JEWETT, D.L. (1970). Human auditory evoked potentials: possible brainstem components detected on the scalp. *Science* **167**, 1517–1518.

JEWETT, D.L. and WILLISTON, J.S. (1971). Auditory-evoked far fields averaged from the scalp of humans. *Brain* **94**, 681–696.

JOSEY, A.F. (1985). Auditory brainstem response in site of lesion testing. In: Katz, J. (Ed.) *Handbook of Clinical Audiology*, 3rd edn, pp. 534–548. Baltimore: Williams & Wilkins.

KILENY, P.R. and KRIPAL, J.P. (1987). Test–retest variability of auditory event-related potentials. *Ear and Hearing* **8**, 110–114.

KILENY, P.R., NIPARKO, J.K., SHEPARD, N.T. and KEMINK, J.L. (1988). Neurophysiologic intraoperative monitoring: I. Auditory function. *American Journal of Otology* **9** (Suppl.), 17–24.

LAUKLI, E. (1983). Stimulus waveforms used in brainstem audiometry. *Scandinavian Audiology* **12**, 83–89.

McCANDLESS, G.A. (1967). Clinical application of evoked response audiometry. *Journal of Speech and Hearing Research* **10**, 468–478.

MAST, T.E. and WATSON, C. (1968). Attention and auditory evoked responses to low detectability signals. *Perception and Psychophysics* **4**, 237–240.

MICHALEWSKI, H.J., PRASHER, D.K. and STARR, A. (1986). Latency variability and temporal interrelationships of the auditory event-related potentials (N1, P2 and P3) in normal subjects. *Electroencephalography and Clinical Neurophysiology* **65**, 59–71.

MOLLER, A.R. (1983). Interpretation of brainstem auditory evoked potentials: results from intracranial recordings in humans. *Scandinavian Audiology* **12**, 125–133.

ÖDKVIST, L.M., ARLINGER, S.D., EDLING, C., LARSBY, B. and BERGHOLTZ, L.M. (1987). Audiological and vestibulo-oculomotor findings in workers exposed to solvents and jet fuel. *Scandinavian Audiology* **16**, 75–81.

OSTERHAMMEL, P. (1981). The unsolved problems in analog filtering of the auditory brain stem responses. *Scandinavian Audiology Supplement* 13, 69–74.

PICTON, T.W. and HILLYARD, S.A. (1974). Human auditory evoked potentials II: Effects of attention. *Electroencephalography and Clinical Neurophysiology* **36**, 191–199.

PICTON, T.W., HILLYARD, S.A., KRAUSZ, H.I. and GALAMBOS, R. (1974). Human auditory evoked potentials I: Evaluation of components. *Electroencephalography and Clinical Neurophysiology* **36**, 179–190.

PORTMANN, M., LEBERT, G. and ARAN, J.M. (1967). Potentiels cochleares obtenus chez l'homme en dehors de toute intervention chirurgicale. *Revue de Laryngologie* **88**, 157–164.

ROSENHALL, U. (1981). ABR in cerebello-pontine angle tumours. *Scandinavian Audiology Supplement* 13, 115.

ROSENHALL, U., BJÖRKMAN, G., PEDERSEN, K. and KALL, A. (1985). Brainstem auditory evoked potentials in different age groups. *Electroencephalography and Clinical Neurophysiology* **62**, 426–430.

ROSENHAMER, H.J. (1980). *On brainstem electric responses in audiological diagnosis.* Doctoral thesis, Karolinska Institute, Stockholm.

ROSENHAMER, H.J., LINDSTRÖM, B. and LUNDBORG, T. (1978). On the use of click-evoked electric brainstem responses in audiological diagnosis. *Scandinavian Audiology* **7**, 193–205.

SALOMON, G. and ELBERLING, C. (1971). Cochlear nerve potentials recorded from the ear canal in man. *Acta Oto-Laryngologica* **71**, 319–325.

SKINNER, P.H. and JONES, H.C. (1968). Effects of signal duration and rise time on the auditory evoked potential. *Journal of Speech and Hearing Research* **11**, 301–306.

SKINNER, P.H., ANTINORO, F. and SHIMOTA, J. (1974). An evaluation of linear extrapolation to threshold in electroencephalic response audiometry. *Journal of Auditory Research* **12**, 26–31.

SOHMER, H. and FEINMESSER, M. (1967). Cochlear action potentials recorded from the external ear in man. *Annals of Otology, Rhinology and Laryngology* **76**, 427–435.

SOUCEK, S., MICHAELS, L. and FROHLICH, A. (1986). Evidence for hair cell degeneration as the primary lesion in hearing loss of the elderly. *Journal of Otolaryngology* **15**, 175–183.

STARR, A., AMLIE, R.N., MARTIN, W.H. and SANDERS, S. (1977). Development of auditory function in newborn infants revealed by auditory brainstem potentials. *Pediatrics* **60**, 831–839.

STEIN, L.K., KRAUS, N., ÖZDAMAR, Ö., CARTEE, C., JABALEY, T., JEANTET, C. and REED, N. (1987). Hearing loss in an institutionalized mentally retarded population. *Archives of Otolaryngology, Head and Neck Surgery* **113**, 32–35.

STYPULKOWSKI, P.H. and STALLER, S.J. (1987). Clinical evaluation of a new ECoG recording electrode. *Ear and Hearing* **8**, 304–310.

SVENSSON, O., ALMQVIST, B. and JÖNSSON, K.E. (1987). Effects of low-frequency components and analog filtering on auditory brainstem responses. *Scandinavian Audiology* **16**, 43–47.

TERKILDSEN, K., OSTERHAMMEL, P. and HUIS IN'T VELD, F. (1974). Far field electrocochleography – electrode postions. *Scandinavian Audiology* **3**, 123–129.

THORNTON, A.R.D. (1975). Statistical properties of surface-recorded electrocochleographic responses. *Scandinavian Audiology* **4**, 91–102.

TYBERGHEIN, J. and FORREZ, G. (1969). Cortical audiometry in normal hearing subjects. *Acta Oto-Laryngologica* **67**, 24–32.

VAUGHAN, H.G. (1969). The relationship of brain activity to scalp recordings of event related potentials. In: *Averaged Evoked Potentials.* Washington DC: NASA.

Chapter 10
Test Battery for Clinical Evaluation

Introduction

An early medical evaluation is important in the management of a person with hearing loss, because diagnosis at an early stage generally provides better conditions for any kind of required intervention. The history of the impairment is essential and to be complete it has to include information on the following:

1. The duration of the symptoms and if the onset was slow and gradual or sudden.
2. Possible hereditary factors.
3. Past ear diseases.
4. Infectious diseases, e.g. meningitis, certain viral diseases and Lyme disease (borreliosis).
5. Neurological diseases.
6. Head trauma.
7. Use of potentially ototoxic drugs.
8. Exposure to high noise levels.
9. Tinnitus.
10. Vertigo or other problems related to balance.

The medical examination should include otoscopy, preferably otomicroscopy, and relevant parts of an otoneurological evaluation with regard to the function of the cranial nerves which are anatomically close to the cochlear nerve (the vestibular, facial and trigeminal nerves).

The course of the audiological evaluation of the patient with hearing loss depends on a number of factors. Initially, pure-tone audiometry, and sometimes routine speech audiometry, are used to provide information on whether a conductive or a sensorineural loss is at hand. Normally, the comparison of air- and bone-conduction thresholds gives a reliable answer to this question. Sometimes, however, the pure-tone audiogram is unreliable in this respect. This may occur in cases of otosclerosis where the audiogram may show a more or less pronounced bone-conduction loss (see Figure 8.11). Menière's disease, which is a cochlear disorder, may sometimes give rise to an air–bone gap in the low frequency range. In such cases, additional information from impedance audiometry using stapedius reflex thresholds should be obtained (Klockhoff, 1961). Since this test requires very little time, it has been suggested that tympanometry and the determination of stapedius reflex thresholds may well be part of the initial standard test battery.

Evaluation of Conductive Disorders

A detailed otomicroscopic examination is of great value in the evaluation of patients with suspected conductive disorders. Not only must the presence of chronic otitis media be determined but also of scarred or calcified parts of the eardrum or the presence of atticus retraction etc.

A patient with a conductive hearing loss usually shows good agreement between average pure-tone hearing thresholds (500, 1000 and 2000 Hz) and the speech recognition threshold, and the maximum speech recognition score is typically within the normal range. In particular, the comparisons between pure-tone and speech audiometric data are of importance for patients with otosclerosis, where the presence of poorer than normal bone-conduction hearing thresholds may be due to either Carhart's notch or cochlear otosclerosis. In the former case, speech recognition will be normal but typically reduced in the latter.

The Weber test and impedance audiometry will, in most cases, provide valuable information in the initial audiological evaluation.

Bilateral severe hearing impairments often give rise to special test problems due to the so-called masking dilemma: the contralateral masking level required may become so high that it gives rise to masking of the test ear – over-masking. The shape of the pure-tone audiogram provides important clinical information. A conductive component in the low frequency range is most commonly seen in cases with ossicular fixation. A conductive component in the high frequency range indicates a partial ossicular discontinuity (see Figure 8.12) or a collapsed ear canal. Theoretically, an air–bone gap could attain any value, but in practice it rarely exceeds 60 dB due to the transmission of sound as vibrations from the earphone through the skull to the inner ear. Thus, hearing thresholds which exceed 60 dB HL are caused by either sensorineural or combined lesions (both conductive and sensorineural components). Large conductive components, e.g. as caused by total ossicular discontinuity, typically have a flat character, i.e. are of equal magnitude over the whole frequency range. If the eardrum is whole, the evaluation will always include tympanometry and stapedius reflex testing (Figure 10.1). It is worth noting

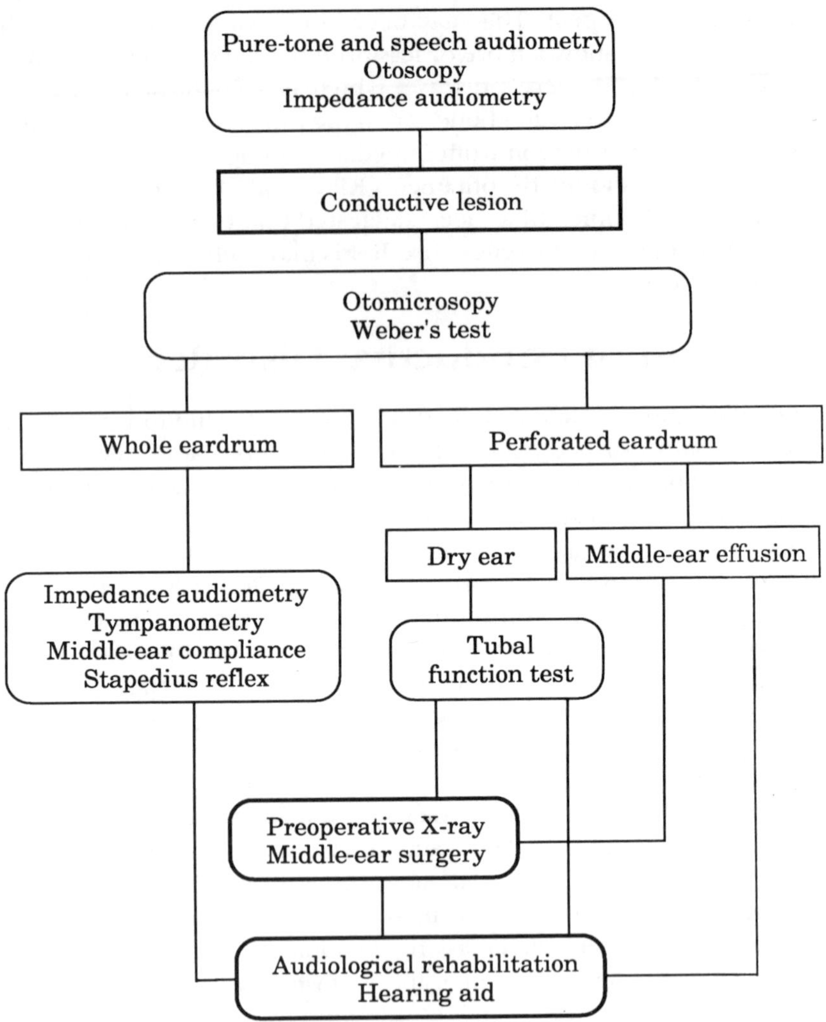

Figure 10.1 Evaluation of and suitable action for cases with conductive hearing loss.

that a moderate scarring of the eardrum may make the interpretation of impedance audiometric test results more difficult. With a normal eardrum as seen by otomicroscopy, tympanometry may show a middle-ear compliance that is higher than normal in ears with ossicular discontinuity and lower than normal in ears with otosclerosis or other type of ossicular fixation. Tympanometry using a higher probe tone frequency may be of value in indicating an ossicular discontinuity (Lidén, Peterson and Björkman, 1970).

After tympanometry, stapedius reflex thresholds are determined. A conductive component causes the absence of a reflex response in the impaired ear for both ipsi- and contralateral stimulation. Exceptions from this rule are partial discontinuities and a discontinuity caused by fracture of the crura of the stapes. In such cases, reflex responses with abnormally large amplitude can often be seen (see Figure 8.12), and the pure-tone audiogram often shows a conductive loss in the high frequency range (Anderson and Barr, 1971). In patients with early otosclerosis, low-amplitude reflex responses may often be seen, sometimes inverted or diphasic (see Figure 8.11) (Flottorp and Djupesland, 1970; Djupesland and Kvernbold, 1975). In unilateral otosclerosis, conductive recruitment (see Figure 8.10) is often present when the diseased ear is stimulated and the response is recorded in the normal ear (Anderson and Barr, 1966; Terkildsen, Osterhammel and Bretlau, 1973). In cases with epitympanic fixation conductive recruitment does not occur.

In ears with a dry eardrum, perforation tubal function tests may be performed. Although the value of such tests is questioned by some, it may give some prognostic information with regard to the further treatment of the case.

In general, the audiological evaluation preceding middle-ear surgery is of great importance. A commonly followed rule in bilateral cases is to operate on the poorer ear, since there is always a certain probability of inner-ear damage, or even deafness, after middle-ear surgery even when performed by the most experienced middle-ear surgeon. In addition to the results from pure-tone and speech audiometry, other factors important to everyday hearing should be regarded when decisions on middle-ear surgery are to be made, e.g. which ear the patient uses for telephoning or for a hearing aid. A patient with a bilateral hearing loss should be recommended to obtain experience with a properly fitted hearing aid. If the patient functions well with a hearing aid fitted to one ear, as a rule the other ear should be chosen if middle-ear surgery is decided upon.

Evaluation of Sensorineural Hearing Loss

A sensorineural hearing loss may be either cochlear, retrocochlear or central. In *cochlear* hearing loss which is much more common than the other two types, the lesion is localised to the receptor organ in the inner ear. The most common types of cochlear lesion are presbyacusis (hearing loss due to old age) and noise-induced hearing loss. Menière's disease is another example of a cochlear disorder. Hereditary hearing loss is usually of the cochlear type and this is also the case for impairments caused by infectious diseases, ototoxic drugs and skull trauma. A typical characteristic of cochlear hearing loss is recruitment of loudness. Maximum speech recognition scores usually deteriorate with increasing cochlear hearing loss.

In *retrocochlear* hearing loss, the lesion is localised in the cochlear nerve. This type is relatively uncommon; examples are acoustic neuromas and other types of cerebellopontine angle tumours as well as a consequence of some types of infectious diseases, vascular malformations and hereditary degenerative disorders. A retrocochlear lesion typically gives rise to a significant qualitative deterioration of hearing, which leads to speech recognition that is significantly poorer than could be expected from the pure-tone audiogram. Speech audiometry is therefore an important part of the evaluation of cases suspected of having a retrocochlear lesion (Figure 10.2). However, a considerable number of patients with acoustic neuromas still have good speech recognition. Speech audiometry thus has low sensitivity in this diagnostic application and its specificity is also relatively low. An example of this is seen with patients suffering from Menière's disease who often show quite poor speech recognition scores.

In *central* hearing disorders, the lesion is localised to the pathways in the brain stem or higher in the central nervous system (CNS), including

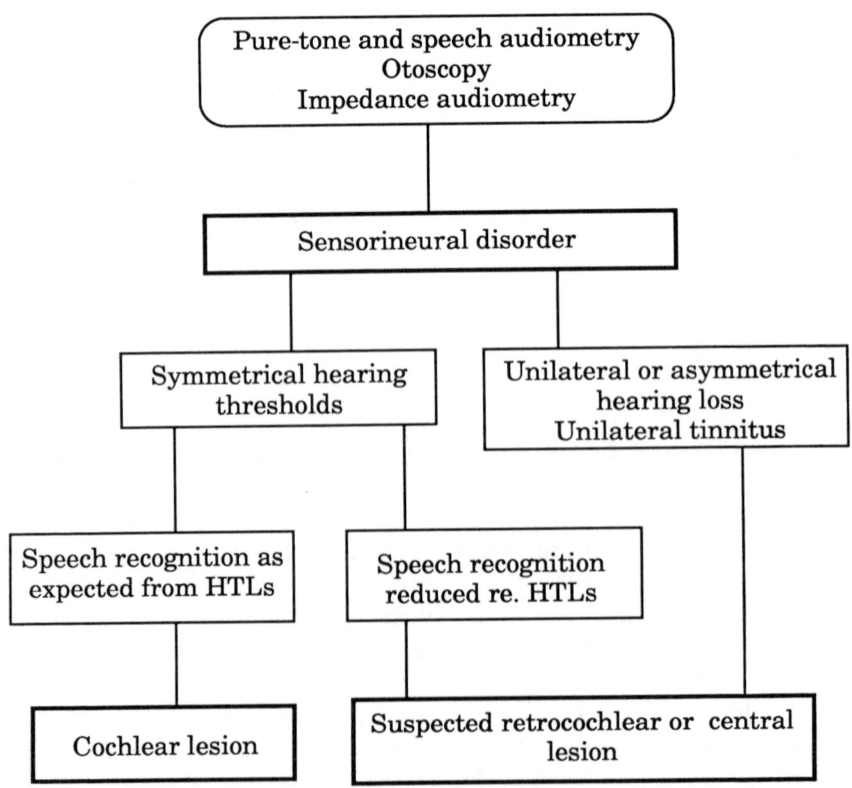

Figure 10.2 Initial evaluation of sensorineural hearing loss. Cases with suspected retrocochlear hearing loss must be examined further as illustrated in Figures 10.3–10.5.

the primary auditory projection areas in the temporal lobes of the cortex. Examples of diseases which can give rise to central auditory lesions are circulatory disturbances in the brain, CNS infections, brain tumours and multiple sclerosis. As a rule, such diseases do not cause hearing impairment with conventional symptoms. The pure-tone audiogram is typically within normal limits and this is often true for the results from normal speech audiometry. However, distorted speech audiometry often identifies central lesions. The borderline between central auditory lesions and perceptive disorders such as impressive aphasia is often not clear, and the borderline between central and retrocochlear lesions is also often unclear. The reason for this is that a lesion situated laterally in the brain stem may give rise to retrocochlear symptoms; however, the pure-tone audiogram is still typically within normal limits. The proximal part of the cochlear nerve contains glia cells and is histologically part of the central nervous system. Multiple sclerosis, which is a CNS disease, may engage the root of the cochlear nerve and then cause a typical retrocochlear hearing disorder.

In order to be able to diagnose lesions on various levels in the auditory pathways, a test battery which extends beyond pure-tone and speech audiometry is needed. A variety of special test methods has been devised to make a more detailed analysis of sensorineural lesions possible.

Such special test methods fall into the three main categories: psychoacoustic tests, impedance audiometric tests and electrophysiological tests (ERA). Psychoacoustic tests require active cooperation by the patient and thus contain an evidently subjective component. From the patient's point of view, the other two categories can be considered objective because they require no active cooperation on the part of the patient. However, significant subjective components exist in the interpretation of the results produced by such tests.

Psychoacoustic special tests can be divided into the main groups of recruitment tests (loudness balance tests): threshold tone decay tests and sound localisation tests. A schematic view of the ability of a number of test methods to differentiate between different types of auditory lesions is shown in Table 10.1.

Sensitivity and specificity are important characteristics of a diagnostic method with regard to its ability to identify a certain disease (compare Chapter 3). The balance between a high sensitivity and a high specificity may be difficult. A very common diagnostic question is whether a unilateral sensorineural hearing loss is caused by an acoustic neuroma or not (Figure 10.2). Such a tumour is a serious condition for which surgery is the recommended form of treatment. Therefore, as high a sensitivity as possible is required of the test methods used, whereas the requirement on specificity may be set lower. It is important not to miss a patient with a tumour, but a few cases being referred for further examinations without having a tumour can be tolerated. However, a test method with too low a

Table 10.1 Audiometric test profiles: schematic view of the ability of a number of test methods to differentiate between different types of sensorineural auditory lesions

Test method	Localisation of lesion			
	Cochlea	Auditory nerve	Brain stem	Cortex
Stapedius reflex threshold	(+)	+	+	−
Stapedius reflex decay	−	+	+	−
BRA	(+)	+	+	−
ECoG	(+)	+	−	−
CRA	(+)	(+)	(+)	(+)
Pure-tone audiometry	+	+	(+)	−
Speech audiometry	(+)	+	(+)	−
Distorted speech audiometry	−	+	+	+
Phase audiometry	−	+	+	−
Threshold tone decay	−	+	+	−
Loudness balance test	R	NR	NR	NR
Békésy audiometry	II	III,IV	III,IV	I

A plus sign indicates that an abnormal test result is typical for the kind of lesion and a minus sign that a result within the normal limits chosen is typical. A plus within brackets indicates that the test may be sensitive for the type of lesion, but that results are often difficult to interpret or that the sensitivity is low. Results of loudness balance tests are shown as indicating recruitment (R) or no recruitment (NR). For Békésy audiometry, curve-type numbers are shown. For further details see text and also Chapters 5–9.

specificity will be costly because too many patients are then sent for unnecessary X-ray examinations and time is spent with the stressful suspicion of having a brain tumour.

A factor of importance in diagnostic evaluations is the degree of hearing loss. The more severe the loss, the more difficult the differentiation between cochlear and retrocochlear lesions. Brain-stem audiometry (BRA) is a method which is affected by a severe high frequency hearing loss. As a rule of thumb, the test is usually meaningful if the hearing threshold for at least one of the frequencies (3, 4 or 6 kHz) does not exceed 70 dB HL (Figure 10.3). If this condition is not fulfilled, an ABR may still be recorded if the hearing threshold at 2 kHz is at most 40 dB HL. If reproducible ABR responses are found which indicate a cochlear lesion, this is a very important finding. However, the absence of reproducible ABR responses in a case with poor high-frequency hearing thresholds does not provide any reliable diagnostic information.

Stapedius reflex tests are also influenced by severe hearing loss. However, as a rule reflex responses can be recorded in cases with more severe hearing loss than limits the usefulness of ABR recordings. This is

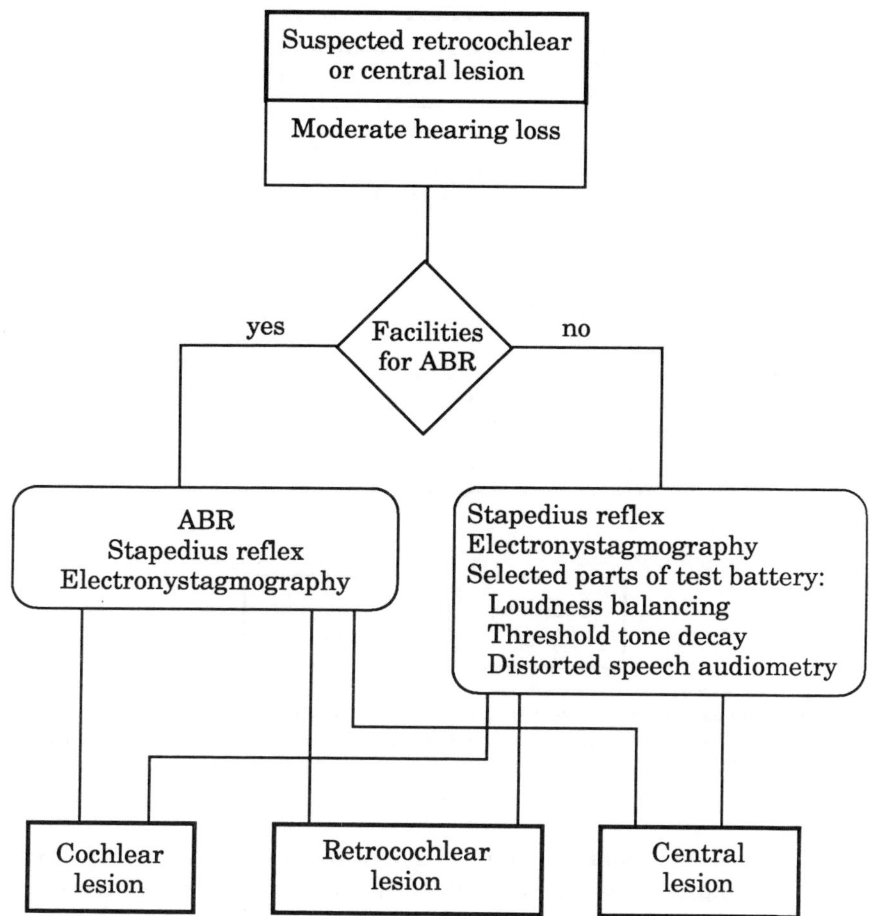

Figure 10.3 Evaluation of suspected retrocochlear hearing loss with moderate pure-tone audiometric hearing loss.

partly due to the fact that the stapedius reflex is determined using stimuli in the mid- and low frequency range.

Earlier, extensive audiological test batteries were used in the diagnosis of sensorineural hearing loss (Lidén and Korsan-Bengtsen, 1973; Jerger and Jerger, 1974; Clemis and Mastricola, 1976; Johnson, 1977; Palva et al., 1978). Various single psychoacoustic test methods as a rule have a rather low sensitivity in the diagnosis of retrocochlear lesions. The idea with the large test battery is that the limited sensitivity of each test separately is counterbalanced by using several tests, increasing the probability that at least some of the tests will have a correct outcome. However, the drawbacks due to long testing time are considerable and, in addition,

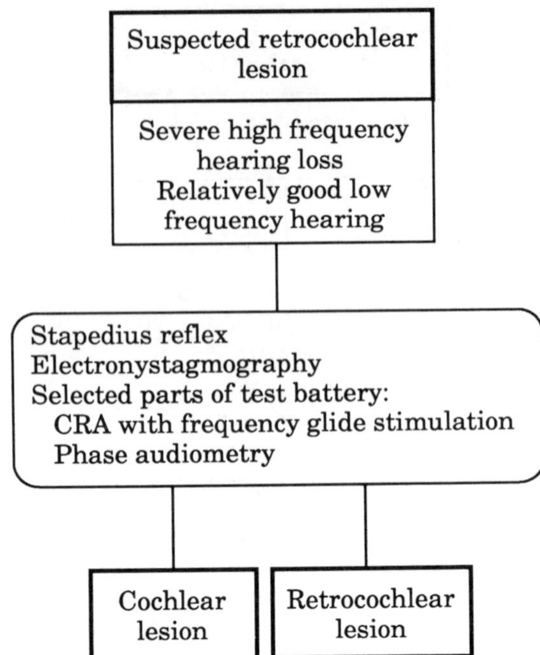

Figure 10.4 Evaluation of suspected retrocochlear hearing loss with pure-tone hearing thresholds showing severe loss for high frequencies but relatively well-preserved hearing for low frequencies.

better sensitivity is obtained at the cost of lower specificity. A very obvious trend over the last few years has been the smaller number of tests being used in diagnostic evaluations. This development is partly due to the increased use of ABR and stapedius reflex testing, both having high sensitivity in the diagnosis of retrocochlear lesions (Rosenhamer, 1977; Selters and Brackmann, 1977; Eggermont, Don and Brackmann, 1980; Hirsch and Anderson, 1980; Thomsen et al., 1981; Bergenius, Borg and Hirsch, 1983; Cohn et al., 1986; Kanzaki, 1986; Abramovich, 1987; Reimer, 1987; Zöllner, Weigel and Friedburg, 1987).

An important factor in the choice of test methods for the otoneurological evaluation is what equipment and other investigative resources are available. The single most important factor is whether facilities for ABR recording are present or not. Not only is the equipment necessary, but also experience in using it and in interpreting the recordings.

In Figures 10.3–10.6 are shown proposals for test strategies in cases with suspected retrocochlear or central hearing loss. It should be noted that the diagnosis of retrocochlear hearing loss does not refer only to cerebellopontine angle tumours. Whether a tumour is present or not can be evaluated only by means of neuroradiological methods (Figure 10.6).

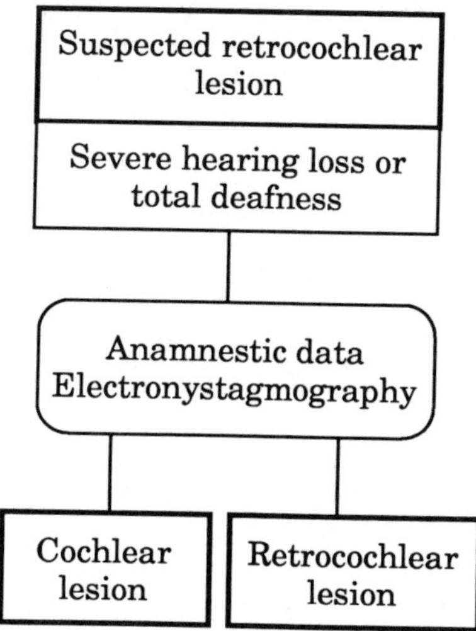

Figure 10.5 Evaluation of suspected retrocochlear hearing loss in cases with severe hearing loss or total deafness.

At present, computed tomography (CT) scanning is the most common method by means of which both the cerebellopontine angle region and the internal auditory meatus can be examined. However, small tumours often go undetected in a CT scan, except intracanalicular tumours that have caused a widening of the internal auditory meatus. Special methods using air-contrast may increase the chance of detecting a small tumour. A new technique based on magnetic resonance imaging (MRI) may in the future replace the CT scan in radiographic evaluation of the cerebellopontine region.

The two basic tests suggested – ABR and stapedius reflex recordings – both have high sensitivity in differentiating between cochlear and retrocochlear disorders. The third otoneurological test method suggested is electronystagmography (ENG). If one or both of the audiological tests indicate a retrocochlear lesion, and/or if ENG shows a significantly reduced vestibular response to caloric stimulation, clear indication for CT or MRI examination is present. Loss of other cranial nerve functions, e.g. reduced corneal reflex, should also be taken as an indication for detailed radiographic examinations. If the results of radiographic studies are negative, the patient should be followed by an audiometric check-up at suitable intervals.

The brain-stem response audiometry is not available, stapedius reflex testing and ENG should be performed and, in addition, suitable parts of a psychoacoustic test battery (loudness balance testing, threshold tone decay, phase audiometry, distorted speech audiometry).

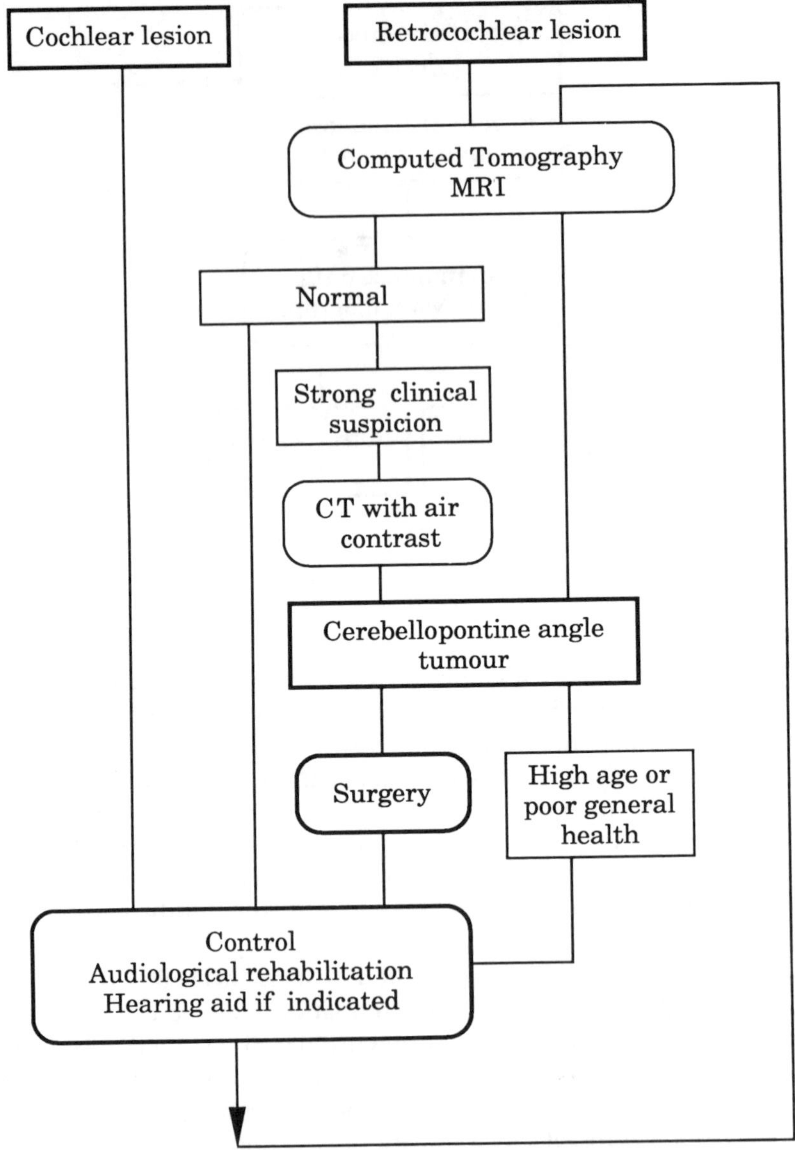

Figure 10.6 General scheme for the audiological care of cases with sensorineural hearing loss.

As mentioned previously, a severe hearing loss is more difficult to evaluate diagnostically than a moderate one. If ABR cannot meaningfully be performed because of severe high-frequency loss, the recording of cortical responses to frequency glides (Arlinger, 1983) or phase audiometry may be performed, provided that hearing thresholds are reasonably good in the low and mid-frequency range. Cortical evoked responses to frequency glides may also be affected by central disorders (Ödkvist et al., 1987).

In cases with severe loss over the complete frequency range or total deafness, the medical history of the patient, clinical observations and electronystagmography will provide the basis for a diagnostic decision. Naturally, the indications for advanced radiographic techniques become wider in such cases.

Evaluation of Suspected Non-organic Hearing Loss

A non-organic hearing loss may be an unconscious functional disorder or a conscious simulation or aggravation of a smaller organic hearing loss. Anamnestic data usually provide important information in this type of diagnosis. The patient's reactions to various sounds are also important to consider. When comparing the pure-tone audiogram and the speech recognition threshold, agreement within 10 dB is to be expected in organic hearing loss, with the possible exception of very steeply sloping audiograms and retrocochlear lesions. Non-organic hearing loss should be suspected if the speech recognition threshold is significantly better than the average loss for pure tones. Other indicators of non-organic hearing loss may be unreliable hearing thresholds for pure tones with poor reproducibility, and high speech discrimination scores at speech levels close to the measured hearing thresholds for pure tones.

Békésy audiometry or repeated pure-tone audiometry on different occasions are other means of obtaining further information on suspected non-organic hearing loss, as is of course electric response audiometry (ERA). Determination of stapedius reflex thresholds may also be of value, in particular in cases with poor pure-tone audiograms. If the stapedius reflex thresholds obtained are less than 20 dB above the hearing thresholds, this supports a diagnosis of non-organic hearing loss.

Several psychoacoustic tests have been developed specially for the detection of simulated hearing loss. In unilateral cases, Stenger's test may be used. In bilateral cases the Doerfler–Stewart test is available. Still other tests are the diversion test and the delayed feedback speech test.

ERA testing for the purpose of estimating hearing thresholds are often of great help. However, such methods permit no exact determination of hearing thresholds, and a small degree of aggravation is usually difficult to detect. CRA using tone pulse stimulation is the recommended method.

References

ABRAMOVICH, S.J. (1987). Auditory brain stem response and computed tomography in acoustic tumour investigations. *Journal of Laryngology and Otology* **101**, 334–345.

ANDERSON, H. and BARR, B. (1966). Conductive recruitment. *Acta Oto-Laryngologica* **62**, 171–184.

ANDERSON, H. and BARR, B. (1971). Conductive high-tone hearing loss. *Archives of Otolaryngology* **93**, 599–605.

ARLINGER, S. (1983). Auditory evoked cortical responses to frequency glides in subjects with retrocochlear hearing impairment. *Journal of Neurology, Neurosurgery and Psychiatry* **46**, 917–923.

BERGENIUS, J., BORG, E. and HIRSCH, A. (1983). Stapedius reflex test, brainstem audiometry and opto-vestibular tests in diagnosis of acoustic neuromas. *Scandinavian Audiology* **12**, 3–9.

CLEMIS, J.D. and MASTRICOLA, P.G. (1976). Special audiometric test battery in 121 proved acoustic tumours. *Archives of Otolaryngology* **102**, 654–656.

COHN, A.I., LeLIEVER, W.C., HOKANSON, J.A. and QUINN, F.B. (1986). Acoustic neurinoma diagnostic model evaluation using decision support systems. *Archives of Otolaryngology, Head and Neck Surgery* **112**, 830–835.

DJUPESLAND, G. and KVERNBOLD, H. (1975). Acoustic impedance measured on ears with normal and diphasic impedance changes. *Scandinavian Audiology* **4**, 39–43.

EGGERMONT, J.J., DON, M. and BRACKMANN, D.E. (1980). Electrocochleography and auditory brainstem electric responses in patients with pontine angle tumours. *Annals of Otology, Rhinology and Laryngology* **89** (Suppl.75), 1–19.

FLOTTORP, G. and DJUPESLAND, G. (1970). Diphasic impedance change and its applicability in clinical work. *Acta Oto-Laryngologica Supplementum* 263, 200–204.

HIRSCH, A. and ANDERSON, H. (1980). Audiological test results in 96 patients with tumours affecting the eighth nerve. A clinical study with emphasis on the early audiological diagnosis. *Acta Oto-Laryngologica Supplementum* 369.

JERGER, J. and JERGER, S. (1974). Audiological comparison of cochlear and eighth nerve disorders. *Annals of Otology, Rhinology and Laryngology* **83**, 275–285.

JOHNSON, E.W. (1977). Auditory test results in 500 cases of acoustic neuroma. *Archives of Otolaryngology* **103**, 152–158.

KANZAKI, J. (1986). Present state of early neuro-otological diagnosis of acoustic neuroma. *Oto-Rhino-Laryngology* **48**, 193–198.

KLOCKHOFF, I. (1961). Middle ear muscle reflexes in man. *Acta Oto-Laryngologica Supplementum* 164.

LIDÉN, G. and KORSAN-BENGTSEN, M. (1973). Audiometric manifestations of retrocochlear lesions. *Advances of Oto-Rhino-Laryngology* **20**, 271–287.

LIDÉN, G., PETERSON, J.C. AND BJÖRKMAN, G. (1970). Tympanometry. *Acta Oto-Laryngologica Supplementum* 263, 218–224.

ÖDKVIST, L.M., ARLINGER, S.D., EDLING, C., LARSBY, B. and BERGHOLTZ, L.M. (1987). Audiological and vestibulo-oculomotor findings in workers exposed to solvents and jet fuel. *Scandinavian Audiology* **16**, 75–81.

PALVA, T., JAUHIAINEN, T., SJÖBLOM, C.-J. and YLIKOSKI, J. (1978). Diagnosis and surgery of acoustic tumours. *Acta Oto-Laryngologica* **86**, 233–240.

REIMER, Å. (1987). Quantitative interpretation of audiological test battery. *Scandinavian Audiology* **16**, 101–108.

ROSENHAMER, H.J. (1977). Observations on the electric brain-stem responses in retrocochlear hearing loss. *Scandinavian Audiology* **6**, 205–210.

SELTERS, W.A. and BRACKMANN, D.E. (1977). Acoustic tumor detection with brain stem electric response audiometry. *Archives of Otolaryngology* **103**, 181–187.

TERKILDSEN, K., OSTERHAMMEL, P. and BRETLAU, P. (1973). Acoustic middle ear muscle reflex in patients with otosclerosis. *Archives of Otolaryngology* **98**, 152–155.

THOMSEN, J., NYBOE, J., BORUM, P., TOS, M. and BARFOED, C. (1981). Acoustic neuromas. Diagnostic efficiency of various test combinations. *Archives of Otolaryngology* **107**, 601–607.

ZÖLLNER, C., WEIGEL, K. and FRIEDBURG, H. (1987). Sensitivity and specificity of brain stem potentials as a means of differentiating cochlear and retrocochlear disorders (acoustic neuromas). *Oto-Rhino-Laryngology* **49**, 123–132.

Chapter 11 Audiometry in Schoolchildren

Screening audiometry in schoolchildren is an audiological activity that is routinely undertaken in some countries and in Sweden since the 1960s. The organisation of screening may vary, and also the classes of children tested and the criteria for referral for further medical evaluation.

For such a programme to be meaningful, it has to have a defined purpose and goal, adapted to the local resources and other conditions. Big cities and rural areas naturally pose different problems in the organisation of the programme. However, the test method used should be the same and the criteria for referral should, as far as possible, be identical.

Goal of School Screening Programme

During the first year in school, one purpose of the programme is to detect children with hearing loss of a degree that may affect the child's ability to follow the lessons. The most common findings are hearing loss caused by blocked eustachian tubes (otosalpingitis) and mild sensorineural hearing loss. Children with otosalpingitis of long duration should be referred for medical follow-up and treatment in order both to provide as good a hearing as possible for the child at school and to diagnose those cases which develop into chronic otitis media. Occasionally, cases of undetected unilateral hearing loss are discovered. This discovery is important with regard to how the child is located in the classroom, i.e. with his or her good ear towards the rest of the class.

Since parotitis is a known risk factor with regard to unilateral deafness, a special audiometric test on children who are known to have had this disease is recommended.

In older age, the prevalence of mild, high-frequency sensorineural hearing loss tends to increase. These cases are probably most often caused by noise exposure. Although small and of little practical significance at an early age, they are important indicators of sensitivity to noise exposure.

They should be considered with regard to future noise exposure and the risk for significant further deterioration.

In Sweden the most common grades where audiometric screening is performed are the first and eighth, corresponding to ages 7 and 15 years. These are often complemented by tests in trade training schools which eventually will lead the students to professional areas where occupational noise exposure is a common auditory hazard.

Staff

Commonly, school screening programmes are run by the school health authorities with a school nurse responsible for the actual testing. It is of great importance that they have received proper training in the audiometric procedures to be used. Cooperation with a local audiological/otological unit is of advantage in order to establish a continuous system for taking care of children with hearing loss.

Test Methods

The outcome of a school screening programme is highly dependent on the test methods used, the test conditions, and the skill and experience of the person who performs the testing. The basic test method to be used is screening audiometry with threshold determination as described in Volume 1 of this manual.

Sometimes screening audiometry is complemented by tympanometry (Lidén and Renvall, 1980; Gimsing and Bergholtz, 1983). Tympanometry is a very sensitive method for indicating abnormal middle-ear pressure or fluid in the middle ear. Screening audiometry with a screening level of 20 dB HL, a common choice in school programmes, is considerably less sensitive in detecting mild-to-moderate, middle-ear disorders. A flat tympanogram curve or a middle-ear pressure below −150 daPa is usually considered as an indicator of significant middle-ear pathology. However, there is no general agreement as to whether such findings should automatically be followed by medical treatment. Otosalpingitis often heals spontaneously. A safe procedure is to retest with tympanometry after 4–6 weeks. If pathology is still present, the child should be referred for medical treatment and control.

Test Site

When choosing a suitable screening level for audiometry, ambient sound levels at the test site are of utmost importance. Since most school programmes have to manage with a normal room for testing, without access to a special, sound-insulated, audiometric test booth, a screening level of better than 20 dB HL is rarely possible. This is usually considered acceptable in the lower grades where middle-ear disorders dominate the problems found, because a lower screening level increases the sensitivity for detecting such disorders at the expense of a marked reduction in specificity. However, in higher grades where the detection of noise-induced, high-frequency hearing loss is perhaps the most important goal, a screening level of 10 dB is clearly preferable.

The test site should always be chosen so as to avoid sounds from other children awaiting their turn, telephone sounds etc. Tympanometry is a test method that accepts much higher ambient sound levels and thus can be performed in basically any normal room.

Criteria for Referral

The following criteria are suggested as a standard scheme, naturally open to modification according to local conditions.

1. Children with uni- or bilateral hearing loss of 25 dB HL or more for at least two of the frequencies 500, 1000, 2000 and 3000 Hz should be retested at the school programme after a period in the range 2 weeks to 3 months. If the criterion is fulfilled also at retest, the child should be referred for medical examination. The retest procedure reduces significantly the number of false positives caused by occasional temporary otosalpingitis.
2. Average bilateral hearing loss exceeding 30 dB HL (average of 500, 1000, 2000 and 3000 Hz) should be referred directly for medical diagnosis and possibly treatment.
3. A uni- or bilateral hearing loss exceeding 25 dB HL, averaged over the frequencies 4000, 6000 and 8000 Hz, should result in written information for the child and his or her parents regarding the probable cause as noise exposure and the need to protect the child from further exposure to loud sounds.
4. A uni- or bilateral hearing loss exceeding 30 dB HL on average should lead to a referral to a clinic for a serious evaluation of the cause and risks for progression.

These criteria assume a screening level of 20 dB HL. For other screening levels, the limits may have to be changed.

Care of Hearing-impaired Students

Students who have such a hearing loss as to warrant use of a hearing aid and other technical devices in order to be able to follow the lessons have to be followed up and receive audiometric evaluation at regular intervals. The importance of a good acoustic environment in their classroom(s) cannot be overrated. Acoustic absorption material covering a considerable part of the ceiling gives a short reverberation time which is particularly important for the hearing-impaired listener. Suitable floor covering which reduces the disturbing sounds produced by steps, falling objects, chairs etc. is very important in providing as low a background noise level as possible. This is of great importance in order to obtain the maximum benefit of the aids in use.

References

GIMSING, S and BERGHOLTZ, L.M. (1983). Audiological screening of seven- and ten-year-old children. *Scandinavian Audiology* **12**, 171–177.

LIDÉN, G. and RENVALL, U. (1980). Impedance and tone screening of school-children. *Scandinavian Audiology* **9**, 121–126.

Chapter 12 Audiometry in Occupational Health

Introduction

A complete occupational hearing health care programme should contain both medical and technical programmes and therefore have qualified staff in both areas. Considering the wide range of knowledge that must be covered by a high quality occupational health service, it is desirable to create formal means of cooperation with other departments and institutions which may complement the existing resources. In such cases, it is of course important to define the limits within which the occupational health services operate on their own resources and what external cooperation will take place. These limits will be determined by the conditions present with regard to economy, knowledge and experience.

Goals

Occupational hearing health care or occupational audiology has first the goal of preventing hearing loss caused by occupational noise exposure. To achieve this, as early a detection as possible of an initial hearing loss is essential in order to provide preventive measures before the hearing loss has become significant. For people with an already established hearing loss, it is important to keep this under control to prevent further deterioration.

If a hearing loss is of such magnitude that it fulfils the requirements for insurance compensation, the occupational audiology programme should be able to assist in such cases. Furthermore, the occupational audiology programme should complement regular audiological services in the discovery of hearing loss that affects the social function of the impaired or threatens important aspects of his or her well-being. In such cases, well-organised routine procedures should be available for referral for the fitting of hearing aids when such are indicated, or to an otological or audiological clinic when a diagnostic evaluation needs to be undertaken.

Staff

The occupational nurses are the type of staff who usually have the most knowledge in audiometry, assuming that they are the ones who perform the audiometry and have most of the direct contact with the employees examined. However, an occupational health physician, with medical responsibility for the occupational health services provided, also needs a thorough knowledge about audiometry, its possibilities and limitations, and how to interpret test results.

The main responsibility of the safety engineers regarding audiometry is to assist in the evaluation of ambient sound levels in the room where audiometry is to be performed. Indirectly, their concern with evaluation of occupational noise exposure of single individuals is also of importance, in addition to their role in suggesting and implementing improvements in the acoustic conditions at the work sites.

The consequences of hearing loss, independent of its origin, mainly affect communication between the impaired person and other people. This may give rise to isolation with regard to fellow workers and sometimes also to problems in handling the work tasks. Knowledge about the risk for such problems is also of importance for the occupational health team.

Test Methods and Test Site

The types of audiometry performed are usually limited to hearing threshold determinations by means of pure-tone air-conduction audiometry or Békésy audiometry using fixed frequencies.

Since the most important goal is to detect small hearing losses as early as possible, it is important to choose the method and practical test conditions for audiometry so as to obtain both test validity and reliability that are as good as possible. The overwhelming experience supports the conclusion that manual pure-tone audiometry and Békésy audiometry have comparable test reliability (Burns, 1968; Cluff, 1980; Jerlvall and Arlinger, 1986), although some arguments have been put forward about the advantage of Békésy audiometry (Erlandsson et al., 1979). By evaluating a mean value of hearing thresholds from several test frequencies in the high range, a reduction of the effects of some sources of error can be obtained and thereby an improved sensitivity for early detection (Erlandsson et al., 1980).

The single most important factor for reliable early detection of hearing loss is to secure a very silent test environment in order to allow for the measurement of hearing threshold levels as low as possible. In order to be able to evaluate reliably the results of audiometry, and in particular to detect changes in subjects with good hearing threshold levels, it is necessary to know the ambient sound levels of the test room and the lowest measurable hearing threshold levels. On the basis of test reliability in the determination of hearing threshold levels and the biological variation of hearing thresholds in young normally hearing subjects, hearing threshold levels of about 15 dB HL are considered significantly different from zero, i.e. from the normal average. Therefore, it is desirable to be able to measure hearing threshold levels at least down to 10 dB HL and preferably down to 0 dB HL.

The most logical approach is first to decide which is the lowest hearing threshold level that should be measurable. Then the ambient sound levels are measured in the room selected. If required, sound attenuation measures are then undertaken to reach the maximum permissible ambient sound levels.

In Békésy audiometry, the audiometer has a certain lowest test level, which is either 0 or −10 dB HL. If the ambient sound levels of the test site are not sufficiently low in relation to this lowest test level of the equipment, recordings of relatively good hearing threshold levels may be unreliable. This is because of the uncertainty about whether the result shows a true hearing threshold or merely reflects a hearing threshold that is masked by the ambient sound in the room.

Sometimes the situation arises where a room is available for audiometry but no measures have been undertaken for reducing the ambient sound in the room. The first thing to do is to have the ambient sound levels measured. The results of those measurements must then be evaluated to see if the specific goal chosen with regard to lowest measurable, hearing threshold levels can be reached. If that is not the case, the source(s) of noise have to be attenuated or a sound-attenuating test booth has to be aquired or, as a last resort, the audiometric goal has to be adjusted.

Some audiometers are equipped with earphones mounted in large sound-attenuating ear muffs to reduce the requirements on ambient sound levels. Unfortunately, such ear muffs have the drawback of sometimes preventing the earphone from being in close contact with the outer ear of the listener, which is the intention of a supra-aural earphone. This provides some sound leakage between the earphone and the outer ear into the larger cavity of the ear muff, giving rise to a reduction in the sound level reaching the eardrum and thus falsely to poor hearing threshold values. The additional attenuation of ambient sounds, provided by the ear muff, is quite small at the relatively low frequencies where it is needed most. Therefore, the value of such ear muffs is very limited and their use in general not recommended.

Screening audiometry combined with hearing threshold determination is the logical choice of method on the basis of a certain defined goal of lowest hearing threshold level to be measured and/or of the limitations set by the ambient sound levels of the test site. As a screening level, the lowest measurable hearing threshold level at the test site should be chosen. If Békésy audiometry is to be used, it is important to remember the limitations set by the ambient sound levels at the test site. Variations in hearing threshold levels at or close to that limit may be due to variations in ambient sound levels just as much as to variations in auditory function of the test subject.

Equipment

The audiometric equipment used in occupational audiology is a pure-tone audiometer for air-conduction testing, i.e. with earphone output, either of manual or of Békésy type. The market offers models of both types which may be connected to a computer. The computer can be used both for control of the testing and for storing and analysing the test results.

As for all audiometric test equipment, the need for regular electroacoustic calibration procedures is important. A suitable interval is in the range 3–12 months depending on degree and type of use. An audiometer which is in use every day and often in mobile use, where mechanical risk factors are more imminent than in stationary use, needs to be controlled more often than an audiometer which is used only occasionally and is never moved. The electroacoustic control and calibration should be performed by a competent laboratory, which may be available at an audiology department of a large hospital, university or other official institution, or with the manufacturer. When transporting the audiometer, it is necessary to have it packed very carefully to avoid mechanical shock and other hazards, both on its way to the calibration and in particular on its return to the user.

Intervals between Repeated Audiometric Testing

An important question in occupational audiology concerns the choice of suitable intervals between repeated audiometric testing. An interval which is too long increases the risk of significant hearing deterioration in noise-exposed people going undetected and therefore of no measures being taken to improve the situation. Intervals which are too short mean inefficient use of the resources of the occupational health services, because the probability of significant change is too low. Since exposure to noise of higher levels increases the risk of damage, it is logical to adapt the interval to the exposure conditions present.

The following scheme is based on the current occupational noise exposure regulations in Sweden, which permit a maximum equivalent noise level of 85 dB(A) per 8-hour working shift, a time-intensity trading of 3 dB for halving of daily exposure and a maximum peak level of 140 dB(C, peak). It assumes that ear protectors of different suitable types are easily available and generally being used when needed:

Equivalent noise level:	80–89 dB(A)	Interval:	≤ 5 years
	90–94 dB(A)		2 years
	≥ 95 dB(A)		1 year
Peak sound level	≥ 140 dB(C)		1 year

Every employee is tested at the beginning of employment.

This programme is based on the primary goal of detection of noise-induced hearing loss. From a general hearing health care view, shorter intervals may sometimes be indicated. One group for which this may be particularly valid is the age group 55–65 years, where the age-related hearing loss often begins to show up and causes a growing number of problems, both at work and in spare time.

Selection Criteria for Referrals

Occupational audiometry has no merit of its own, but it is performed to provide data on which the necessary action can be taken. Thus, there is a need to know when action should be undertaken, and some basic criteria for that purpose may be specified as guidance. The following rules have been applied over a period of more than a decade by a large number of occupational health centres in a Swedish county. They were formulated by the Department of Audiology at the University Hospital in Linköping, Sweden, and are implemented in a detailed form with clear quantitative limits on a computer program for the evaluation of audiograms from occupational health services (Arlinger and Ivarsson, 1985).

1. Test subjects whose audiograms fulfil current requirements with regard to insurance compensation.
2. Subjects who need to be referred for medical diagnostic evaluation because of:
   (a) significant asymmetry; usually, occupational noise exposure gives rise to relatively symmetrical hearing loss. Although exceptions occur, the probability of pronounced asymmetry having a cause other than noise exposure is so high that these subjects are referred for further testing;
   (b) type of hearing loss other than noise-induced as indicated by an audiogram which is atypical for that impairment, i.e. either audiograms of relatively flat form or showing low-frequency loss on one or both ears.
3. Subjects who need to be referred for hearing aid fitting or regarding other assistive devices.

4. Subjects who have significant deterioration of hearing in relation to a previous audiogram. These cases should be handled by the occupational health staff and evaluated with regard to noise exposure, the use of hearing protection, need and possibilities for noise reduction measures at work site etc.

References

ARLINGER, S. and IVARSSON, U. (1985). A data bank on hearing and use of hearing protection among 45 000 workers in small industries. *Proceedings of Internoise*, Volume II. Bremerhaven: Wirtschaftsverlag NW.

BURNS, W. (1968). *Noise and Man.* London: J. Murray.

CLUFF, G.L. (1980). Audiometry reliability with a noise exposed population. *Sound and Vibration*, January 1980, 18–20.

ERLANDSSON, B., HÅKANSON, H., IVARSSON, A. and NILSSON, P. (1979). Comparison of the hearing threshold measured by manual pure-tone and by self-recording (Békésy) audiometry. *Audiology* **18**, 414–429.

ERLANDSSON, B., HÅKANSON, H., IVARSSON, A. and NILSSON, P. (1980). The accuracy of hearing measurements for detection of hearing impairment caused by noise. In: Ivarsson, A. and Nilsson, P. (Eds.) *Advances in Measurements of Noise and Hearing.* Lund: Department of Otolaryngology, University of Lund.

JERLVALL, L. and ARLINGER, S. (1986). A comparison of 2 dB and 5 dB step size in pure-tone audiometry. *Scandinavian Audiology* **15**, 51–56.

Chapter 13 Audiometry in Hearing Aid Fitting

Introduction

The term 'hearing aid fitting' is used here to refer to the complete procedure of selecting an aid for a particular patient, adjusting the aid for optimum performance and evaluation of hearing aid function on the patient, as well as the patient's benefit from the aid.

The first step in the procedure is to decide whether a patient who presents with some hearing problem really is a hearing aid candidate. This is the hearing aid indication stage. If an aid is indicated, the next question is what degree of acoustic amplification is the likely target, considering the type and degree of hearing loss, and which hearing aid(s) available might provide that gain. This is the prescription stage.

When a certain hearing aid has been selected for trial, it is desirable to know what acoustic gain this aid will provide the ear of a particular patient with its individual ear mould. The technical specifications for a particular model of a hearing aid presented by the manufacturer are determined by the use of an acoustic coupler or ear simulator. The actual performance of the aid on a specific human ear may differ considerably from such technical data. Therefore, the actual measurement on the patient is of great importance, in order to know both how far from the prescribed target the performance is and the performance itself, in order to understand the user's reactions to it.

Finally, it is often desirable to be able to quantify the user's performance with the aid in different listening situations. These measurements on and with the user may be termed 'the verification stage'.

Hearing Aid Indication and Prescription

The pure-tone audiogram is the most common description of auditory function and also the most commonly used basis for the evaluation of a person's need for a hearing aid. The audiogram basically shows the ability of the listener to detect pure tones of various frequencies. The auditory reactions to barely audible pure tones are of course quite different from the reactions to complex sounds at higher levels, which happen in most everyday listening situations. In spite of this, experience has shown that the pure-tone audiogram, on average, is a surprisingly good basis for the evaluation of hearing aid indication. This is probably due to the fact that a large number of more complex auditory characteristics regarding signal analysis are correlated with pure-tone hearing thresholds. The poorer the hearing threshold, as a rule the poorer the auditory frequency analysis, the ability to detect fast changes in amplitude etc. However, in single cases, which cannot easily be predicted, the pure-tone audiogram is a poor basis for the prediction of the benefit from a hearing aid.

In spite of considerable development and improvement in electroacoustic characteristics, the hearing aid still provides an imperfect compensation for the effects of a sensorineural hearing loss. This sometimes has the consequence that for a small hearing loss a hearing aid may be of little benefit. Traditionally, the limit where the possible benefit of a hearing aid is to be evaluated has been based on the average hearing loss at the frequencies 500, 1000 and 2000 Hz. However, experience with modern well-fitted hearing aids has shown that benefit may be possible for users with smaller losses. This is particularly the case for those with pronounced high-frequency losses where the hearing thresholds may be close to normal at 500 and 1000 Hz, and occasionally at 2000 Hz.

Thus, it is not possible to identify a single absolute limit in terms of pure-tone audiometric hearing thresholds as an indication for the benefit of a hearing aid. A general evaluation has to be made where, in addition to the pure-tone audiogram, the patient's expressed degree of difficulty and the need for the aid are of significant importance. The pure-tone audiogram is still the single, most important, quantitative measure to evaluate the degree of acoustic gain the patient needs and forms the basis for the preliminary selection of suitable type(s) of hearing aid.

The speech audiogram is usually considered to be of limited importance in the evaluation of the possible benefit of a hearing aid. Cases with extremely poor speech recognition ability may be interpreted as a poor prognosis for a successful fitting. However, an ear which has not been in active use for a considerable time may show a relatively poor speech recognition performance and this can be improved considerably by training through the help of acoustic amplification.

Over the last few years our knowledge about changes in auditory signal analysis caused by sensorineural hearing impairment has increased considerably. Various methods have been applied to illustrate this, e.g. the measurement of spectral resolution by means of psychoacoustic tuning curves and of temporal resolution by means of gap detection. Statistical correlations have been shown in several studies between such characteristics and the ability to recognise speech in noise (Dreschler and Plomp, 1980, 1985; Lyregaard, 1982; Patterson et al., 1982; Lutman and Clark, 1986). However, this knowledge is still not at a level that allows any simple application to evaluating indications for a hearing aid.

An important basis for the need of a hearing aid is, naturally, the evaluation by patients themselves of their various difficulties caused by the hearing loss in various situations. For a systematic evaluation of such factors several different handicap scales have been developed to quantify a hearing handicap index. The Danish system Social Hearing Handicap Index (SHHI) (Ewertsen and Birk Nielsen, 1973; Birk Nielsen and Ewertsen, 1974) is based on the answers to 21 questions regarding difficulties in recognising speech and voices in various everyday listening situations. Giolas et al. (1979) have proposed a more complex formula – the Hearing Performance Inventory – which also includes listening situations other than those concerning the recognition of human speech.

Hearing aid gain

To an increasing extent, rules are being used in order to calculate and predict the gain curve (the acoustic gain as a function of frequency) of the hearing aid that may best fit a prospective user with a certain degree of hearing loss. Several methods have been suggested. In general they may be described in one of the following two categories:

1. Methods based on the pure-tone audiogram.
2. Methods based on the most comfortable loudness level as a function of frequency.

Often the loudness discomfort levels of the patient are also considered in the selection of the type of aid, because it is of importance that the maximum output level of the hearing aid does not cause discomfort.

Table 13.1 Predicted values for hearing aid gain at different frequencies according to POGO

Frequency (Hz)	Gain (dB)
250	½ HTL – 10
500	½ HTL – 5
1000	½ HTL
2000	½ HTL
3000	½ HTL
4000	½ HTL

HTL = hearing threshold level at that frequency.

The half gain rule is the oldest method for estimating hearing aid gain (Lybarger, 1944). It implies that the hearing aid should provide a gain equal to half the hearing loss as measured by an audiogram. A further development of the same idea is the POGO method (prescription of gain and output) proposed by McCandless and Lyregaard (1983). It is aimed at cases of cochlear hearing loss with recruitment. The predicted gain value at a certain frequency is shown in Table 13.1.

The gain values represent the real ear gain on the patient. In the frequency range up to 2000 Hz, deviations of up to 5 dB may be acceptable, and possibly 10 dB at a single frequency. In addition, the maximum output level of the hearing aid in dB SPL as measured on a 2 cm^3 coupler should not exceed the average loudness discomfort levels of the patient at 500, 1000 and 2000 Hz, expressed in dB HL, by more than 4 dB.

A further calculation rule for the prediction of hearing aid gain on the basis of the pure-tone audiogram is the NAL method, proposed by Byrne and Dillon (1986) of the National Acoustic Laboratories in Australia. The gain at various frequencies is obtained according to Table 13.2. Here, x represents 0.05 times the sum of the hearing threshold levels at 500, 1000 and 2000 Hz or 0.15 times the average at these frequencies.

The calculated insertion gain, according to the NAL formula, can be read from Table 13.3 as a sum of two terms: basic gain and additional gain. The additional gain is equivalent to x in Table 13.2 and is added to the basic gain to give the calculated insertion gain. When a significant conductive component is present, one-fourth of the air–bone gap has to be added as a third term for each frequency.

In a simplified form, the difference obtained in results from applying the POGO and the NAL rules is quite small for flat audiograms, but is larger

Table 13.2 Formulae for the prediction of hearing aid gain at different frequencies according to NAL

Frequency (Hz)	Gain (dB)
250	$0.31 \times \text{HTL} + x - 17$
500	$0.31 \times \text{HTL} + x - 8$
750	$0.31 \times \text{HTL} + x - 3$
1000	$0.31 \times \text{HTL} + x + 1$
1500	$0.31 \times \text{HTL} + x + 1$
2000	$0.31 \times \text{HTL} + x - 1$
3000	$0.31 \times \text{HTL} + x - 2$
4000	$0.31 \times \text{HTL} + x - 2$
6000	$0.31 \times \text{HTL} + x - 2$

Table 13.3 Predicted gain values, according to NAL, as sum of basic gain (left) and additional gain (right) for different levels of hearing loss and pure-tone frequencies

HTL (dB HL)	Basic gain in dB at frequency (Hz) of								Average HTL (dB HL)	Additional gain in dB
	250	500	1000	1500	2000	3000	4000	6000		
0	–17	–8	1	1	–1	–2	–2	–2	0	0
5	–15	–6	3	3	1	0	0	0	5	1
10	–14	–5	4	4	2	1	1	1	10	2
15	–12	–3	6	6	4	3	3	3	15	2
20	–11	–2	7	7	5	4	4	4	20	3
25	–9	0	9	9	7	6	6	6	25	4
30	–8	1	10	10	8	7	7	7	30	4
35	–6	3	12	12	10	9	9	9	35	5
40	–5	4	13	13	11	10	10	10	40	6
45	–3	6	15	15	13	12	12	12	45	7
50	–1	8	17	17	15	14	14	14	50	8
55	0	9	18	18	16	15	15	15	55	8
60	2	11	20	20	18	17	17	17	60	9
65	3	12	21	21	19	18	18	18	65	10
70	5	14	23	23	21	20	20	20	70	10
75	6	15	24	24	22	21	21	21	75	11
80	8	17	26	26	24	23	23	23	80	12
85	9	18	27	27	25	24	24	24	85	13
90	11	20	29	29	27	26	26	26	90	14

for sloping audiograms. In general the NAL rule predicts lower gain values than the POGO rule, particularly at frequencies of 2 kHz and above (Byrne, 1987). Figures 13.1 and 13.2 illustrate four simple examples of audiograms with calculated gain curves.

Libby (1985) is of the opinion that the POGO method often overestimates the gain needed by the hearing aid user and that the factor 1/3 often agrees better than 1/2, particularly at small and moderate degrees of hearing loss. However, Lyregaard (1986) found good agreement with the factor 1/2 in a group of elderly users fitted with behind-the-ear aids. In general, the experience available with these methods is still too limited to allow the general conclusion that one is superior to the other. The individual variation between different users is also large, making it important to consider any such procedure as a preliminary starting point for the fitting, but with no guarantee of the ideal gain curve being fitted in every single case.

The most comfortable level as a target curve for the amplified average speech level was suggested in 1940 by Watson and Knudsen. Pascoe (1975, 1978) has applied the same principle in his work. Skinner et al. (1982) makes use of three quantities – hearing threshold levels, most comfortable levels and loudness discomfort levels – in order to adjust the

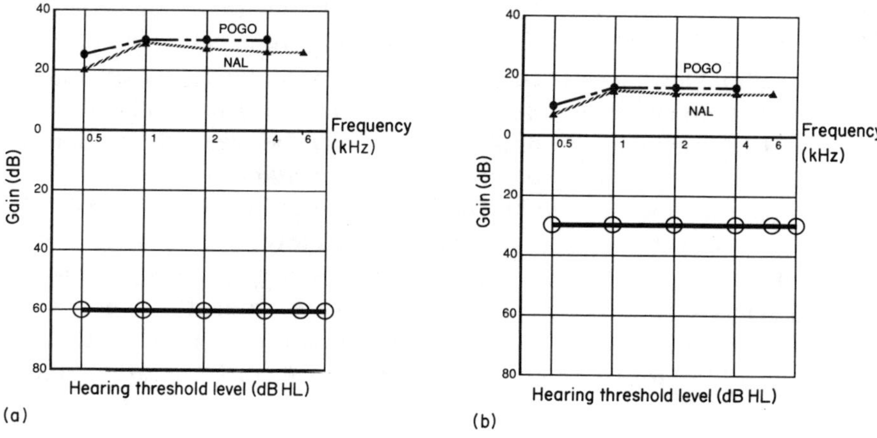

Figure 13.1 Two flat audiograms at (a) 30 and (b) 80 dB HL and the corresponding estimated hearing aid gain values according to POGO and NAL, respectively.

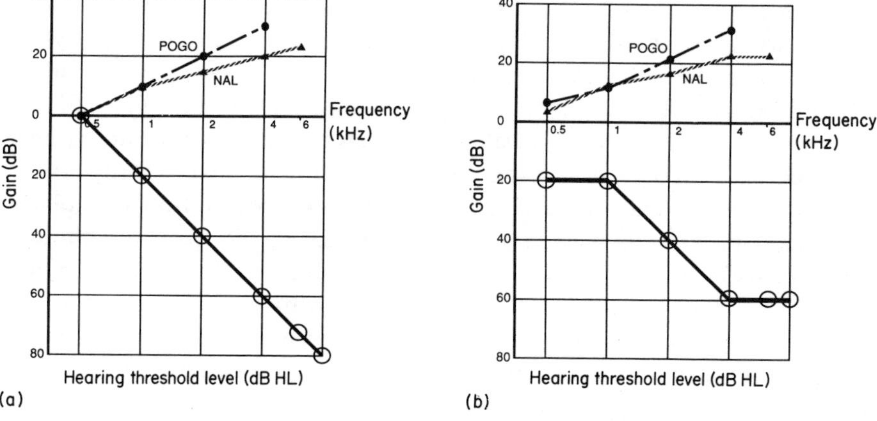

Figure 13.2 Two examples of sloping audiogram curves with the corresponding estimated hearing aid gain values according to POGO and NAL, respectively.

hearing aid gain curve to provide an amplified speech spectrum that fits optimally between the threshold and the loudness discomfort curves.

Still another model for hearing aid fitting makes use of the patient's masked hearing thresholds as determined against a background noise, the spectrum of which corresponds to that of average speech, presented at an overall level of 65 dB SPL (Lindström et al., 1983). The patient's masked hearing thresholds are compared with the average threshold curve for a group with normal hearing. The difference between these two curves is considered to represent the expected need of acoustic gain for the patient.

If the patient's hearing threshold at a certain frequency is significantly worse than the noise level in the corresponding third octave band, the hearing threshold level measured is not affected by masking since the noise is below threshold and inaudible in that critical band. The estimated gain needed at that frequency is thus the difference between the patient's hearing threshold level and the average normal masked threshold at that frequency (in the range 40–50 dB HL). If the unmasked hearing threshold level is better than the masked normal threshold level, the masking noise in this critical band will be audible and the result may reflect reduced frequency selectively caused by the impairment. At frequencies where the patient has normal frequency selectivity and unmasked hearing thresholds in the range 40–50 dB HL or better, this model will consequently predict a needed gain of 0 dB.

Evaluation of Hearing Aid Function on a User

When it has been decided that a hearing-impaired person is to be fitted with a hearing aid, the common procedure is to select one or more types of aid that may be suitable according to one of the prescription models discussed above. Then the actual gain curve has to be verified by measurement of the hearing aid gain on the patient's ear. Experience shows that the actual gain obtained in the higher frequency range is usually rather limited, where the gain needed according to the prescription formula is usually the largest. This may also occur for a hearing aid, whose technical specifications indicate a high gain at high frequencies. The reason for this discrepancy is the influence of the ear mould and the acoustic characteristics of the user's ear. Unless a real-ear gain measurement is performed, such a case may go unnoticed, leaving a high risk that the patient will receive a poor fitting (Ringdahl, Leijon and Lidén, 1984).

Two different methods, one acoustic and one psychoacoustic, are used to measure real-ear hearing aid gain. The acoustic method is based on the recording of the sound pressure in the external ear canal close to the eardrum without and with the hearing aid in its place. The difference between these two measurements is the *insertion gain* (IG) of the hearing aid. The psychoacoustic method is based on the measurement of hearing thresholds in a sound field with and without the hearing aid in use. The difference between these unaided and aided threshold levels is the *functional gain* of the hearing aid.

Insertion gain (IG)

In the earlier application of IG, a miniature microphone was used, placed in the ear canal (Harford, 1980). However, the probe microphone is now the most commonly used transducer. Here the actual microphone is placed outside but close to the ear and connected to the ear canal by means of a small probe tube, a flexible silicone tube with diameter of the order of 0.5 mm internally and 1 mm external.

The loudspeaker producing the acoustic test signal is usually placed in front of the test subject at a relatively short distance (0.5–1 m) to reduce the influence of the room acoustics as much as possible. For the same reason, a frequency-modulated (warble) tone is most commonly used or, as an alternative, a narrow-band noise, rather than a pure tone. The test signal frequency is swept or stepped in small steps from 100–200 Hz to 8–10 kHz. In some types of commercially available equipment a broad-band noise signal is used and, by means of advanced signal analysis technology, the IG curve can be calculated from the noise spectrum.

The IG test systems available on the market may differ with regard to the technique by which the test signal level is regulated as it sweeps or steps across its frequency range (Madsen, 1986; Preves and Sullivan, 1987). For this purpose a reference microphone is usually included in addition to the actual probe microphone. This may be used for the purpose of measuring the sound pressure at a certain reference point during the recording or be connected to regulate the sound pressure from the loudspeaker actively. Figure 13.3 illustrates the three main principles in use.

The simplest way to determine the IG curve is to place the reference microphone in the ear canal of the unaided ear and the probe microphone in that of the aided ear. Provided that the ears are quite symmetrical and that the subject sits straight in front of a loudspeaker that produces a

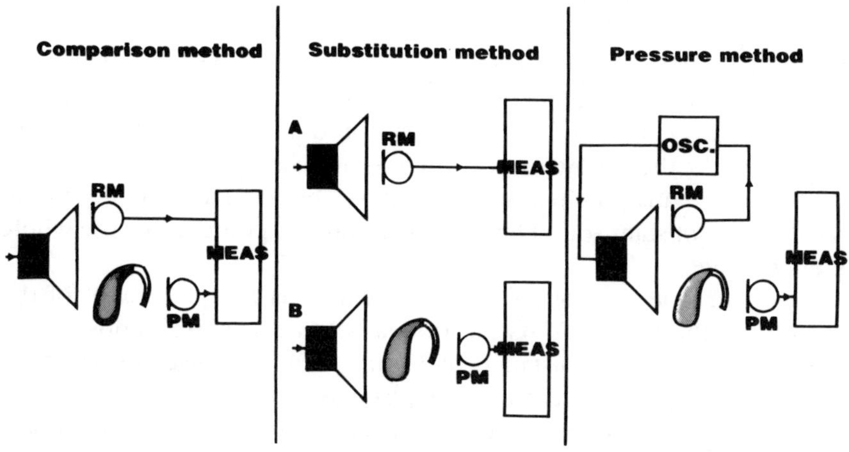

Figure 13.3 Illustration of the three different principles for measurement and regulation of the test sound level in insertion gain measurement systems. PM = probe microphone, RM = reference microphone.

symmetrical sound field, the difference in sound pressure reaching the two microphones represents directly the insertion gain of the hearing aid. Thus, the use of this method does not require computerised equipment with memory and provisions for subtractions between successive recordings. However, it is more sensitive than others to deviations from the assumptions given regarding symmetrical conditions. This method using the simultaneous measurement with two microphones is called the comparison method.

A variation of the comparison method – the modified comparison method – places the reference microphone just behind or below the ear to be fitted. The probe microphone is placed in the ear canal and an initial recording of probe sound pressure without the hearing aid represents the acoustic amplification of the external ear, sometimes called the external ear effect. After careful placement of the hearing aid in the ear, a new recording is made. A subtraction of the first recording from the second in the computer of the test system produces the IG curve.

Another method is the pressure method, where the reference microphone is placed very close to the position of the hearing aid microphone. The reference microphone records the sound pressure level at this point continuously during the test and, if this deviates from the level set for the test, the electric signal level to the loudspeaker will be adjusted automatically to keep this reference sound pressure constant. The probe microphone in the ear canal is used for the unaided and the aided ear canal responses, and the difference curve is calculated in the computer. The placement of the reference microphone in close proximity to the hearing aid may be a source of error in the aided measurement because of sound leaking out from the hearing aid to the reference microphone. This can be of particular importance when using ear moulds with large vents or open-mould fittings.

In the substitution method the test sound level is recorded in that point of the room where the subject's head will be located but in its absence. The result of this calibration recording is stored in the computer memory of the system. At the following recording of the aided and unaided sound levels in the ear canal, the test signal level will be regulated by the system so as to keep a constant sound level at the reference point across the whole frequency range.

The most critical part of an IG measurement is the placement of the probe tube in the ear canal. Its location should be as close as possible to the eardrum – within a distance of 5 mm – to minimise the effect of changes in probe position. Further, the placement of the hearing aid or ear mould in the ear canal has to be undertaken very carefully to avoid any change in probe position, along the length of the ear canal as well as across it. In addition, the subject must remain in an unchanged position during the testing. This is of particular importance if the distance between subject and loudspeaker is small and when the test is performed in a small room without acoustic treatment.

Functional gain

In order to measure the functional gain of a hearing aid, aided and unaided hearing threshold levels are determined in a sound field. The test is usually performed in a normal audiometric booth, which should have a floor area of at least 3–4 m^2 to permit a distance between the listener and loudspeaker of at least 1 m. Pure tones should be avoided because of the uncertainty due to standing waves in the room. Instead, frequency-modulated (FM) tones or narrow band-filtered noise should be used. Sound-absorbing screens should be placed across windows in the audiometric room during testing. This, of course, has the disadvantage that the patient cannot be seen by the tester outside the room but is essential to avoid sound reflections from the glass surface(s). A small head-rest attached to the back of the subject's chair makes it easier for him or her to keep the head at a fixed position. This head-rest may be equipped with a small electric switch to indicate to the tester that the subject's head is in contact with the head-rest.

FM tones are commonly available in clinical audiometers. The only additional equipment required is a power amplifier and a relatively small loudspeaker of reasonable quality. As a rule, it is desirable to be able to reach sound levels up to about 100 dB HL. The variation of the sound level across different positions in the test room is usually minimised if modulation frequencies in the range 10–20 Hz are used together with frequency deviations in the range 10–25% (Walker and Dillon, 1983). However, these factors seem to have negligible influence on test reliability (Arlinger and Jerlvall, 1987). A frequency deviation of 25% (±12.5%), in combination with centre frequencies in steps of one-third octave in the range from 1 or 2 kHz to 8 kHz, in addition to 500 Hz, is a practical compromise between the wish for a detailed description of the functional gain curve and a limited test time.

To make sure that the test subject perceives the test signals in the intended ear, a soft ear-canal plug with good fit should be placed in the non-test ear. When testing subjects with relatively good hearing thresholds, it is important to remember the requirements on low ambient sound levels in the test room. This is a possible source of error, of particular relevance in the low frequency region, where hearing thresholds often are near normal whilst ambient sounds are most likely to be audible (Macrae, 1982). If the internal noise of the hearing aid is audible to the test subject, this may also cause measurement errors. The actual test method used to determine hearing threshold levels should be the standardised method for pure-tone audiometry with earphones. However,

Békésy audiometry with frequency sweep can also be used. The test–retest reliability of sound-field audiometry using FM tones has been shown to be somewhat superior to conventional pure-tone testing with earphones (Arlinger and Jerlvall, 1987).

Comparison of methods, sources of error and test reliability

A comparison of the acoustic and the psychoacoustic methods of determining real-ear gain shows that both methods have their advantages and limitations. A general rule is that the average result of the two methods is the same, i.e. the validity of the two methods is the same (Mason and Popelka, 1986; Tecca and Woodford, 1987). However, in individual cases differences of up to 10–15 dB may arise, caused by the fact that the two methods have different sources of error.

The main source of error in IG testing is the placement of the probe tube in the ear canal and the risk for change of position when the hearing aid or ear mould is placed in the ear canal. In addition, the way the sound field is regulated and the placement of the loudspeaker in relation to the test subject and sound reflecting surfaces in the test room may also cause errors.

In the determination of functional gain, errors may be caused by the usual uncertainties involved in psychoacoustic hearing threshold testing, i.e. the ability and willingness of the listener to concentrate on the test and the ambient sounds in the test room. In addition, variations in the test sound field may influence the test result.

Test–retest experiments usually show the IG method to be superior in the frequency range below about 2 kHz with a standard deviation for single gain values of the order of 1.5–2 dB (Ringdahl and Leijon, 1984; Mueller and Sweetow, 1987; Tecca, Woodford and Kee, 1987). In the frequency range 2.5–6 kHz, the standard deviation typically increases to 3–4.5 dB. This implies that a statistically significant ($P<0.05$) difference in gain between two test results, e.g. when comparing two types of hearing aid being tested on the same subject, is at least in the range 3–4 dB for frequencies up to 2 kHz and 6–9 dB for frequencies above 2 kHz.

Therefore, in the frequency range above 2 kHz, the two methods have about the same test–retest reliability (Arlinger and Jerlvall, 1987). In the range below 2 kHz, the standard deviation for the difference in sound-field hearing threshold for repeated tests, which corresponds to a functional gain value, was found to be 3–3.5 dB. Thus a difference between two gain values of 6–7 dB is required to indicate a significant difference or change in gain. In the range 2.5–6 kHz, the standard deviation was found to be 3–4 dB, implying a significant difference of at least 6–8 dB.

In the hands of an experienced tester, the IG measurement requires considerably less test time than the functional gain test, which is of

Table 13.4 Comparison of different aspects on real-ear hearing aid gain measurements

Characteristic	Insertion gain	Functional gain
Test reliability	Better in low and mid-frequency range	Somewhat better at high frequencies
Speed	Fast	Rather slow
Equipment cost	Relatively high	Low (5–10% of IG)
Test room requirements	Modest	High – as for pure-tone bone-conduction testing
Test procedure	Technically rather advanced	Simple and well known
Frequency resolution	Almost continuous	Continuous possible (Békésy), but half or one-third octave usual

importance when several types of hearing aid or settings of the controls of one aid are to be tested. An advantage with functional gain testing is the considerably less expensive equipment required if an audiometer with FM tones and a usable audiometric test room are already available. The actual testing is performed by means of a technique which is well known to any tester and thus provides a good control of the test situation. For those who lack experience with computers, the more sophisticated IG equipment will require significant training until acceptable reliability is achieved.

Small portable IG units are now available on the market. Considering the very modest requirements on the test room, it is very easy to take such a unit to various places for testing, e.g. homes for the elderly, clinical out-stations etc.

The results of a comparison between the two methods may be tabulated as in Table 13.4.

Evaluation of the User's Function with Hearing Aid

The measurement of functional gain as described above includes the determination of aided hearing thresholds. The results of this measurement may be considered as a description of one characteristic concerning the user's function with a hearing aid, namely his or her sensitivity in detecting narrow-band sounds.

Speech audiometric test results without and with a hearing aid are functionally more important in providing a quantitative measure of the improvement in speech communication provided by the hearing aid.

However, conventional speech audiometry, i.e. speech recognition threshold and maximum speech recognition score in quiet, has shown a relatively too poor sensitivity to be of any value in this respect (Libby, 1985).

Speech audiometric tests using sentences rather than single words, and presented in a sound field at a normal speech level against a background of broad-band noise, provide better conditions for useful results (Hagerman, 1982, 1984). To make full use of the sound-field situation, the speech signal may be presented from a frontally located loudspeaker and background noise sounds from loudspeakers at 45–90° on both sides of the listener. The purpose of the actual test is usually to determine the signal-to-noise ratio which provides 50% correct speech recognition by varying the noise level while the speech level is kept constant.

If test lists made up of complete sentences are not available, phonetically balanced monosyllabic test words may be used. However, the lower slope of the psychometric function of monosyllabic words, as compared to sentences, makes this version less sensitive.

Computer-aided speech audiometry may eventually be developed into a valuable tool with improved sensitivity in hearing aid fitting (Miltich, 1987). The computer may be used to perform a fast analysis of speech recognition errors made by the listener and then to produce a detailed confusion matrix. This matrix can provide improved insight into the listener's particular problems in speech recognition and into possible improvement by changing the electroacoustic characteristics of the hearing aid.

When considering the indication for hearing aid use, the patient's own evaluation of his or her hearing problems in various everyday situations with the hearing aid on, and the problems of handling the wearing of the hearing aid and manipulation of its controls are important aspects of the value of a hearing aid fitting. The social hearing handicap index and the hearing performance inventory, as previously mentioned, are examples of methods for systematic evaluation of such aspects. The difference in index obtained before and after the fitting is an important measure of the benefit experienced by the user.

In binaural hearing aid fitting, each hearing aid should first be evaluated separately. In addition, it is an advantage to evaluate the user's binaural function with both aids on by using test methods adapted for that purpose. Speech recognition scores in a sound field with background noise from source(s) other than the loudspeaker used for the speech, and comparison of monaural and binaural results, are examples of such testing.

Another suitable test method could use the loudness balance between the two aided ears. FM tones in a sound field from a frontally placed loudspeaker are recommended. The test subject is asked to tell in which ear the test sound is heard loudest (left, right or equal). The following centre frequencies and sound levels are recommended:

1000 Hz: 50, 60, 70 dB HL
1500 Hz: 45, 55, 65 dB HL
2000 Hz: 40, 50, 60 dB HL
3000 Hz: 35, 45, 55 dB HL
4000 Hz: 30, 40, 50 dB HL

By analysing the test results the hearing aids and ear moulds may be adjusted to obtain the best possible loudness balance.

References

ARLINGER, S.D. and JERLVALL, L.B. (1987). Reliability in warble-tone sound field audiometry. *Scandinavian Audiology* **16**, 21–27.

BIRK NIELSEN, H. and EWERTSEN, H.W. (1974). Effect of hearing aid treatment. *Scandinavian Audiology* **3**, 35–38.

BYRNE, D. (1987). Hearing aid selection formulae: same or different? *Hearing Instruments* **38** (1), 5–11.

BYRNE, D. and DILLON, H. (1986). The National Acoustic Laboratories (NAL) new procedure for selecting the gain and frequency response of a hearing aid. *Ear and Hearing* **7**, 257–265.

DRESCHLER, W.A. and PLOMP, R. (1980). Relation between psychophysical data and speech perception for hearing-impaired subjects. I. *Journal of the Acoustical Society of America* **68**, 1608–1615.

DRESCHLER, W.A. and PLOMP, R. (1985). Relations between psychophysical data and speech perception for hearing-impaired subjects. II. *Journal of the Acoustical Society of America* **78**, 1261–1270.

EWERTSEN, H.W. and BIRK NIELSEN, H. (1973). Social Hearing Handicap Index. *Audiology* **12**, 180–187.

GIOLAS, T.G., OWENS, E., LAMB, S.H. and SCHUBERT, E.D. (1979). Hearing Performance Inventory. *Journal of Speech and Hearing Disorders* **44**, 169–195.

HAGERMAN, B. (1982). Sentences for testing speech intelligibility in noise. *Scandinavian Audiology* **11**, 79–87.

HAGERMAN, B. (1984). Clinical measurements of speech reception threshold in noise. *Scandinavian Audiology* **13**, 57–63.

HARFORD, E.R. (1980). The use of a miniature microphone in the ear canal for the verification of hearing aid performance. *Ear and Hearing* **1**, 329–337.

LIBBY, E.R. (1985). State-of-the-art of hearing aid selection procedures. *Hearing Instruments* **36**(1), 30–38, 62.

LINDSTRÖM, B., SVÄRD, I, BREDBERG, G. and LUNDBORG, T. (1983). A method to establish the effect of the hearing aid in noise using Victoreen signal threshold and speech discrimination. *Scandinavian Audiology Supplementum* **18**, 45–55.

LUTMAN, ME. and CLARK, J. (1986). Speech identification under simulated hearing-aid frequency response characteristics in relation to sensitivity, frequency resolution, and temporal resolution. *Journal of the Acoustical Society of America* **80**, 1030–1040.

LYBARGER, S.F. (1944). US Patent Application, SN 543-278.

LYREGAARD, P.E. (1982). Frequency selectivity and speech intelligibility in noise. *Scandinavian Audiology Supplementum* **15**, 113–122.

LYREGAARD, P.E. (1986). On the practical validity of POGO. *Hearing Instruments.* **37**(5), 13–16.

McCANDLESS, G.A. and LYREGAARD, P.E. (1983). Prescription of gain/output (POGO) for hearing aids. *Hearing Instruments* **34**(1), 16–21.

MACRAE, J. (1982). Invalid aided thresholds. *Hearing Instruments* **33**(9), 20–22.

MADSEN, P.B. (1986). Insertion gain optimization. *Hearing Instruments* **37**(1), 28–32.

MASON, D. and POPELKA, G.R. (1986). Comparison of hearing aid gain using functional, coupler and probe-tube measurements. *Journal of Speech and Hearing Research* **29**, 218–226.

MILTICH, A.J. (1987). A clinical comparison of probe microphone systems. *Hearing Instruments* **37**(1), 33.

MUELLER, H.G. and SWEETOW, R.W. (1987). A clinical comparison of probe microphone systems. *Hearing Instruments* **38**(6), 20–21, 57.

PASCOE, D.P. (1975). Frequency responses of hearing aids and their effects on the speech perception of hearing-impaired subjects. *Annals of Otology, Rhinology and Laryngology* **84**, Supplement 32.

PASCOE, D.P. (1978). An approach to hearing aid selection. *Hearing Instruments* **29**, 12–16, 36.

PATTERSON, R.D., NIMMO-SMITH, I., WEBER, D.L. and MILROY, R. (1982). The deterioration of hearing with age: frequency selectivity, the critical ratio, the audiogram, and speech threshold. *Journal of the Acoustical Society of America* **72**, 1788–1803.

PREVES, D.A. and SULLIVAN, R.F. (1987). Sound field equalization for real ear measurements with probe microphones. *Hearing Instruments* **38**(1), 20–26, 64.

RINGDAHL, A. and LEIJON, A. (1984). The reliability of insertion gain measurements using probe microphones in the ear canal. *Scandinavian Audiology* **13**, 173–178.

RINGDAHL, A., LEIJON, A. and LIDÉN, G. (1984). Analysis of hearing aid fittings using insertion gain measurements. *Scandinavian Audiology* **13**, 179–185.

SKINNER, M., PASCOE, D.P., MILLER, J.D. and POPELKA, G.R. (1982). Measurements to determine the optimal placement of speech energy within the listener's auditory area: a basis for selecting amplification characteristics. In: Studebaker, G.A. and Bess, F.H. (Eds.). *The Vanderbilt Hearing-Aid Report.* Upper Darby, PA: Monographs in Contemporary Audiology.

TECCA, J.E. and WOODFORD, C.M. (1987). A comparison of functional gain and insertion gain in clinical practice. *Hearing Journal* **40**(6), 23–27.

TECCA, J.E., WOODFORD, C.M. and KEE, D.K. (1987). Variability of insertion-gain measurements. *Hearing Journal* **40**(2), 18–20.

WALKER, G. and DILLON, H. (1983). The selection of modulation rates for frequency modulated sound field stimuli. *Scandinavian Audiology* **12**, 151–156.

WATSON, N.A. and KNUDSEN, V.O. (1940). Selective amplification in hearing aids. *Journal of the Acoustical Society of America* **11**, 406–419.

Chapter 14 Measurements in Tinnitus Evaluation

Tinnitus evaluation is performed in order to define the character of the perceived sound, its level and the possibility of masking it. Measurements may also be indicated for recording the sounds generated by muscular, vascular or respiratory sources in the region of the ear.

Indication

The measurements to be performed are part of the general evaluation and care of patients who complain of tinnitus.

Physiology and Psychoacoustics

Tinnitus is defined as a perception of sound without any external sound source. The word tinnitus stems from the Latin word *tinnire* which means to ring or to sound. The character of the perceived sound may vary considerably from a continuous tone or noise to pulsating sounds or clicks. Tinnitus is not a disease in itself, but a symptom which may have a variety of causes. Tinnitus of short duration – of the order of a few seconds – is a very common phenomenon which most people notice occasionally. Annoying, long-duration tinnitus is commonly but not always found together with a hearing loss.

Two basic types are distinguished, based on the underlying cause: objective and subjective tinnitus. In objective tinnitus, the sound usually has its source in vascular, muscular or respiratory processes and can be recorded objectively. Subjective tinnitus is caused in the auditory sense organ or pathways and the term has its basis in the fact that usually the sound can only be perceived by the subject but not by anybody else and it cannot be recorded. When it is possible to localise its presumed site of origin, a subdivision is sometimes made into cochlear, retrocochlear or central tinnitus.

Recent studies have shown the existence of spontaneous acoustic emissions from the cochlea, probably generated by the hair cells through their contractile properties (Zurek, 1985). It has been suggested that some cases of tinnitus generated in the cochlea might be objective in the sense that it could be recorded as an acoustic signal in the ear canal. However, the results so far seem to indicate that spontaneous cochlear acoustic emissions only rarely can explain a tinnitus generated in the auditory sense organ or pathways.

Objective Tinnitus

Vascular tinnitus

This typically presents as a pulse-synchronous sound of relatively low pitch. The most common causes are arteriovenous fistula, vascular stenosis or glomus tumour (Harris, Brismar and Cronqvist, 1979). A lack in the bone cover of the bulbus of the jugular vein or carotid artery in the middle ear may also cause this symptom, in addition to diseases with increased pulse amplitude, e.g. aortic insufficiency.

Muscular tinnitus

This may be due to tonic–clonic twitches or tics in muscles in the middle ear or around the eustachian tube. Sometimes simultaneous twitches may be seen in the soft palate (Boeck, 1967). A low-pitched sound is heard, often described as nails flicking against each other. One or more of the following muscles may be involved:

1. The stapedius muscle (innervated by the facial nerve).
2. The tensor tympani muscle (trigeminal nerve).
3. The tensor veli palatini muscle (trigeminal nerve).
4. The levator veli palatini muscle (trigeminal, facial or glossopharyngeal nerve).
5. The palatopharyngeal muscle (glossopharyngeal nerve).

Lesions in the brain stem and particularly in the area around the olives may be the cause of such muscular tinnitus. Patients with pseudobulbar paresis can show this symptom. Usually no other neurological abnormalities are found. Psychosomatic factors can often be found with the symptoms increasing in periods of stress. The tensor tympani syndrome (Klockhoff, 1981) may be considered as part of this group. Recording of the acoustic impedance of the middle ear may indicate increased tonus of the tensor tympani muscle.

Respiratory tinnitus

This is perceived by patients with an open eustachian tube – tuba aperta. The patient's own voice is heard abnormally loud (autophony) and also breathing sounds are annoying. This problem often is preceded by significant loss of weight or hormonal changes, e.g. pregnancy or the use of contraceptive pills.

Subjective Tinnitus

Cochlear tinnitus

This is the dominating subgroup. Typically, a cochlear lesion causes both a hearing loss and tinnitus, the pitch of which is mostly found to correspond to the frequency range where the hearing loss is largest. However, it is not uncommon that the degree of hearing loss is very small. The tinnitus can usually be masked (Feldmann, 1971). In some patients, exposure to a masking sound for some minutes or more may give rise to a release from tinnitus for some time after exposure. This is called residual inhibition, and it may be total or partial, depending on whether the tinnitus disappears completely or is only reduced but still present. Vernon (1977) has suggested a standardised method of measuring residual inhibition.

The majority of tinnitus sufferers are found among patients with the most common types of cochlear lesions: presbyacusis, noise-induced hearing loss and Menière's disease. Several explanations have been proposed for the direct mechanism behind the tinnitus (Hazell, 1987; Coles, 1988). Results from animal experiments indicate an increased neural activity from the area corresponding to the lesion (Jastreboff and Sasaki, 1986). Similarly to phantom pain, the patient may perceive a phantom sound due to the increased spontaneous activity from the damaged area.

Retrocochlear tinnitus

This is caused mostly by cerebellopontine angle tumours. An early study of patients with acoustic neuroma found an incidence of tinnitus of more than 50% and, in 10–15%, the tinnitus was the primary reason for seeking medical help (Lundborg, 1952). For retrocochlear as well as for cochlear tinnitus, the dominating pitch usually corresponds to the frequency range with the largest hearing loss. Masking is often effective and residual inhibition is also often found.

Central tinnitus

This is due to central lesions and often gives rise to more unspecific sound perception with a broad-band noise character diffusely localised in or around the head. It is usually not possible to mask central tinnitus. Its cause may be a tumour, infection or trauma. After encephalitis and meningitis, a severe tinnitus may appear, prolonging the duration of convalescence. A high incidence of tinnitus has been reported after skull trauma causing damage to the temporal bone and temporal lobe of the cortex (Schucart and Tenner, 1981).

In addition to classification based on the anatomical location of the lesion and its relation to a disease, tinnitus may also be classified according to severity. Klockhoff and Lindblom (1967) have proposed a classification of three groups for patients with Menière's disease, which is generally applicable:

1. Type 1: intermittent tinnitus.
2. Type 2: continuous but distractable.
3. Type 3: continuous and not distractable.

The word 'distractable' means that, in many situations, the patient is distracted by external sounds and other events and is not aware of the tinnitus although it is continuous. This classification, however, is not always simply related to degree of annoyance caused by the tinnitus. Intermittent tinnitus may be just as annoying when it is present as continuous tinnitus. For most patients, difficulties in going to sleep are the main complaint. The reporting of sleep disturbance and use of sleep-inducing drugs is therefore of importance when trying to determine the degree of annoyance by tinnitus.

Methods and Equipment

Various types of methods and equipment may be used for the evaluation of tinnitus. In objective tinnitus, the main purpose is to record pathological sounds. Sometimes a stethoscope, preferably an electronic type to obtain better sensitivity, and careful auscultation in and at the ear and neck area of the side to which the patient localises the sound is recommended. For permanent recording and analysis, a miniature microphone, e.g. the type used for the measurement of insertion gain in hearing aids, and a tape recorder may be used. Also equipment for phonocardiographic recording has been used with success. The impedance audiometer with a paper recorder may also be able to pick up the periodic sounds in most cases of objective tinnitus.

In subjective tinnitus, the aim is to identify an external sound that corresponds best to the tinnitus according to the patient's subjective evaluation – a so-called tinnitus analysis. A complete analysis contains three parts: identification, masking and evaluation of residual inhibition. The purpose of the *identification* is to be able to specify the tinnitus sound in acoustic terms as well as possible. In cases of monaural tinnitus, the test sound is presented by means of an earphone to the contralateral ear and, in binaural cases, to the ear affected least by tinnitus. If the patient describes the character of the tinnitus as tonal, the test sound to be used should be a pure tone of variable frequency. If the tinnitus character is noise-like, a band-pass-filtered noise with variable cut-off frequencies should be used. The level of the test sound should be balanced first and then its frequency content. After obtaining a matching acceptable to the patient, a control to avoid octave confusion should be made. In this, the listening comparison should be repeated using half and double frequency values relative to those first obtained. In particular with tonal tinnitus, octave confusion is quite common.

In the *masking* test, the purpose is to find a sound that is capable of masking the tinnitus. The test sound is presented ipsilaterally. In cases with tonal tinnitus, a narrow-band noise with a centre frequency equal to the tinnitus frequency should be the first choice. If the tinnitus character is noise, the noise band found in the identification process should be used. The minimum masking level (MML) is then determined, i.e. the lowest sound level that masks the tinnitus. If a tonal tinnitus cannot be masked completely by a noise band, the addition of a tone of frequency equal to the tinnitus frequency determined in the identification should also be tried.

In testing for *residual inhibition* (RI), the purpose is to determine whether the tinnitus can be silenced or reduced for a shorter or longer period after masking. According to Vernon (1977), the masker should be presented at a level equal to MML plus 10 dB. As a measure of degree of RI, the duration of partial or total RI after masking for 1 minute is used as well as time needed for the tinnitus to return to normal level again. If no RI is obtained at a masker level of MML + 10 dB, MML + 20 and MML + 30 dB may be tried as long as the loudness discomfort level is not exceeded.

A conventional pure-tone audiometer may be of some use, one with continuously variable pure-tone frequency being better and the best being a special tinnitus analyser where pure tones and noise bands can be added with total variability in frequency and level.

Clinical Interpretation

Audible pulse-synchronous sounds indicate a vascular source. Glomus tumours and vascular malformations in the middle ear often have a positive finding in otoscopy and pathological pulsatile activity during impedance recordings. A circulatory evaluation with determination of blood pressure and cardiac auscultation may show pathological changes there. In other cases, angiographic tests are often indicated (Harris, Brismar and Cronqvist, 1979). The disappearance of the sound at the compression of the carotid artery on the tinnitus side indicates a vascular source. Sometimes elderly patients complain about pulsatile tinnitus where in fact the tinnitus is a continuous cochlear type that is perceived as varying with the cardiac cycle. Sometimes otosclerosis patients have similar complaints at an early stage where the hearing loss is still very small. Impedance audiometry will usually give valuable information as to the correct diagnosis. The general anamnestic information, otomicroscopy and the recording of temporal changes in the acoustic impedance of the middle ear often provide important diagnostic information in cases of objective tinnitus with muscular origin. Tuba aperta gives rise to impedance variations which occur synchronously with the respiratory cycle, and sometimes otomicroscopy will also reveal this situation.

The measurements recommended are primarily for diagnostic purposes but are often found also to have a significant therapeutic value. To many patients, a careful and professional evaluation of hearing, tinnitus analysis and detailed information, preferably both oral and written, are sufficient to relieve them from their anxiety and accept the tinnitus as it is. For a few patients with significantly annoying tinnitus, the use of a tinnitus masker is of considerable help. This relief may be due to residual inhibition but also the sense of having control of the tinnitus by means of the masking sound is found valuable by many. Tinnitus maskers are typically shaped like a head-worn hearing aid, but also portable cassette recorders with recordings of suitable masking sounds have been used. Due to different criteria for the selection of patients and type of maskers used the results from studies with tinnitus maskers show large variations (McFadden, 1982; Hazell, 1987; Coles, 1988), but typically 5–20% of the patients tested have shown benefit.

References

BOECK, O. (1967). Rhinoskopischer Befund bei einem knackenden Geräusch im Ohr. *Archiv für Hals-, Nasen- und Ohrenheilkunde* **2**, 203–207.

COLES, R.R.A. (1988). Tinnitus and its management. In: Kerr, A.G. (Ed.) *Scott-Brown's Otolaryngology*, Vol. 2, 5th edn, pp. 368–414. London: Butterworths.

FELDMANN, H. (1971). Homolateral and contralateral masking of tinnitus by noise-bands and pure tones. *Audiology* **10**, 138–144.

HARRIS, S., BRISMAR, J. and CRONQVIST, S. (1979). Pulsatile tinnitus and therapeutic embolization. *Acta Oto-Laryngologica* **88**, 220–226.

HAZELL, J. (1987). *Tinnitus.* London: Churchill Livingstone.

JASTREBOFF, P.J. and SASAKI, C.T. (1986). Salicylate-induced changes in spontaneous activity of single units in the inferior colliculus of the guinea-pig. *Journal of the Acoustical Society of America* **80**, 1384–1391.

KLOCKHOFF, I. (1981). Impedance fluctuation and a tensor tympani syndrome. In: Penha, R. and Pizarro, P. (Eds.) *Proceedings of the Fourth International Symposium on Acoustic Impedance Measurements*, pp. 69–76. Lisbon: Universidade Nova de Lisboa.

KLOCKHOFF, I. and LINDBLOM, U. (1967). Menière's disease and hydrochlorothiazide (dichlotride R) – a critical analysis of symptoms and therapeutic effects. *Acta Oto-Laryngologica* **63**, 347–352.

LUNDBORG, T. (1952). Diagnostic problems concerning acoustic tumours. *Acta Oto-Laryngologica Supplementum* 99.

McFADDEN, D. (1982). *Tinnitus: Facts, Theories and Treatments.* Washington DC: National Academic Press.

SCHUCART, V.A. and TENNER, M. (1981). Tinnitus and neurosurgical disease. *Journal of Laryngology and Otology* Suppl. 4, 166–171.

VERNON, J. (1977). Attempts to relieve tinnitus. *Journal of the Acoustical Society of America* **62**, 124–131.

ZUREK, P.M. (1985). Acoustic emissions from the ear: a summary of results from humans and animals. *Journal of the Acoustical Society of America* **78**, 340–344.

Index

A/D conversion, 161
ABLB, 65
ABR, 170, 195, 197
accuracy, 24
acoustic coupler, 48
acoustic impedance, 111
acoustic neuroma, 65, 70, 74, 79, 135, 140, 177, 192
action potential, 156, 166
adaptation, 11, 32, 72
adaptive method, 16
admittance, 111
aggravation, 199
air conduction, 40
air–bone gap, 59, 189
allophone, 97
ambient sound levels, 35, 207
AMLB, 67
amplifier, 158
anechoic room, 74
artefact rejection, 182
articulation index, 21
artificial ear, 48
artificial mastoid, 57
ascending method, 43
asphyxia, 102
asymmetry, 210
audiogram classification, 53
autophony, 145, 229
averaging, 160

backward masking, 9
basic test report, 1
Békésy audiometry, 16, 61, 194, 207
binomial distribution, 28
blinking reflex, 105, 106
bone conduction, 53
bone vibrator, 53
BRA, 170, 194
brain stem, 95, 192
brain-stem lesion, 74, 100, 136
brain-stem response, 156
brain-stem response audiometry (BRA), 170, 194

calibration, 36, 89, 209
calibration signal, 89
Carhart's notch, 56, 189
carrier phrase, 87
carrier tone, 111
central lesion, 94, 100, 192
central masking, 34, 48
central nervous system, 96, 192
central tinnitus, 229
cerebellopontine angle tumour, 94, 177, 192
chopped speech, 98
chromosomal aberrations, 102
click, 162, 174
cochlear hearing loss, 62, 93, 94, 133, 191
cochlear microphonic (CM), 166
cochlear nerve, 192
cochlear nucleus, 124, 155
cochlear tinnitus, 229
combined lesion, 189
common mode rejection, 159
comparison method, 219
competing speech, 98
compliance, 112
conductance, 113
conductive lesion, 59, 93, 130, 170, 189
conductive recruitment, 131
continuous variable, 25
conversation test, 109
cortex, 155, 193
cortical lesion, 100
cortical response, 156, 179
cortical response audiometry (CRA), 179
coupler, 48, 57
CRA, 179, 194
critical bandwidth, 8, 45
critical ratio, 9
cross-hearing, 44

delayed speech, 199
descending method, 43
detection, 13
dichotic test, 97
difference limen, 10
differential amplifier, 158
differential threshold, 10
dipole, 154
discrete variable, 25
discrimination, 11, 14
distorted speech audiometry, 95, 194
distortion, 56
diversion test, 199

eardrum, 103, 113
eardrum perforation, 122, 147, 190
effective masking, 47
electric shock, 1
electrocochleography, 156, 165, 194
electrode, 154
electrode impedance, 157
electrode placement, 158
electrode polarity, 167, 173
electronystagmography (ENG), 195
embryology, 103
equivalent noise level, 209
equivalent volume, 112
ERA, 154
eustachian tube, 103, 143
evoked acoustic emission, 110
external auditory canal, 103
external ear component, 54

facial nerve, 124
facial paresis, 137
facial tics, 142
fatique, 12, 32
fifth, 7
filter, 160
fixation, 131, 189
formant, 85
forward masking, 9
frequency glide, 184, 199
frequency modulated tone, 219, 221
functional gain, 218, 221

gap detection, 10
Gellé test, 55
geniculate body, 155

habituation, 13, 32
half gain rule, 215
hearing aid, 68, 212
hearing aid fitting, 92, 212
hearing aid indication, 212
hearing aid prescription, 212
hearing handicap index, 214
hearing level (HL), 4
hearing threshold, 4
    determination of, 40
    estimation of, 138, 169, 178
hearing threshold level, 5
hemifacial spasm, 142
hereditary hearing loss, 137
heredity, 102, 188
high-frequency audiometry, 41
HL, 4
hysteresis, 62

immittance, 111
impedance, 111
impedance audiometry, 189
infectious disease, 188, 191
inferior colliculus, 155
informal tests, 109
inner-ear component, 54
insert masking, 47
insertion gain, 218
instruction, 33
isophon curves, 5, 68

JND (just noticeable difference), 10

latency, 125, 170, 174, 183
lateral lemniscus, 155
leakage current, 2
learning effects, 34
loudness, 5, 65
loudness balance, 65, 193
loudness discomfort level, 68, 88, 215
loudness level, 5

malformation, 102
masking, 9, 57, 175
masking dilemma, 47, 189
masking plateau, 46
masking test, 231
mass, 113
maximum speech recognition, 87, 93
mean value, 25
mel, 6
membranous labyrinth, 103
Menière's disease, 60, 72, 93, 169, 189
meningitis, 102
method of adjustment, 15
method of constants, 16
method of limits, 15
middle ear, 103, 111
middle-ear component, 54
middle-ear surgery, 94, 190
middle latency response (MLR), 156
minimum audible field, 5
minimum masking level, 231
monotic test, 98
most comfortable loudness level, 214, 216
multiple sclerosis (MS), 193
muscular disease, 137
muscular tinnitus, 228
myasthenia gravis, 137

NAL method, 215
needle electrode, 166

neonatal sepsis, 102
neurological diagnosis, 179
noise excluding headset, 49, 208
noise exposure, 202, 206
noise-induced hearing loss, 124, 191, 206
non-organic hearing loss, 92, 134, 179, 199
normal distribution, 25

objective tinnitus, 228
observation audiometry, 107
occlusion effect, 45, 55, 57
occupational health, 206
octave, 7
organ of Corti, 103
ossicular chain, 116, 122
otalgia, 142
otitis, 122
otomicroscopy, 188
otocyst, 103
otoneurological evaluation, 179, 184, 196
otosalpingitis, 202
otosclerosis, 59, 94, 116, 131, 142, 189
ototoxic, 188, 191
overmasking, 46

parotitis, 102
peak equivalent (SPL), 164
perilymph, 103
phase audiometry, 74, 194, 196
phon, 5
physiological noise, 31
pitch, 6
play audiometry, 108
POGO method, 214
precision, 24
presbyacusis, 191
pressure method, 219
promontory, 167
psychoacoustic tuning curve (PTC), 9
psychoacoustics, 4
psychometric function, 14
psychophysics, 4
PTC, 9
pure-tone audiometry, 40, 53, 188, 207
pure-tone average, 53

quantisation error, 28

random error, 25
reactance, 113
recruitment, 11, 67, 133, 191
redundancy, 95
reference microphone, 219
reflex decay, 125, 138
reliability, 24
residual inhibition, 229, 231
resistance, 113
resonance, 113
resonance frequency, 117
respiration audiometry, 107
respiratory tinnitus, 229
responsibility, 2
retrocochlear lesion, 62, 70, 74, 94, 134, 140, 176, 184, 192
retrocochlear tinnitus, 229
rubella, 102

safety, 1
scaling, 14
screening audiometry, 44, 202, 208
screening level, 44, 203, 208
sedation, 173
sensation level, 5
sensitivity, 28, 193
sensorineural hearing loss, 59, 133, 176, 188
signal-to-noise ratio, 162
simulation, 199
skull attenuation, 44
sone, 5
sonotubometry, 146
sound localisation, 74, 193
specificity, 28, 193
speech audiometry, 84, 192, 224
speech recognition, 84
speech recognition threshold, 85
speech transmission index, 22
spondee, 86
spontaneous activity, 31
standard deviation, 25
stapedius muscle, 124
stapedius reflex, 105, 123, 189, 194
startle reaction, 141
startle reflex, 106
step size, 43
stimulus artefact, 127, 164
subjective tinnitus, 227, 229
substitution method, 219
summation potential (SP), 166
superior olive, 155
surface electrode, 157, 173, 181
susceptance, 113
systematic error, 24

tactile stimulation, 141
temporal integration, 7, 32, 42
temporal lobe, 95, 180
temporary threshold shift, *see* TTS
tensor reflex, 141
tensor tympani muscle, 141, 228
tensor tympani syndrome, 142, 228
tensor veli palatini, 144, 228
test–retest difference, 27
threshold criterion, 43
threshold tone decay, 72, 193
time compressed speech, 98
time constant, 7
tinnitus, 32, 142, 227
tone burst, 162
topical diagnosis, 51
tracking method, 16
transtympanic electrode, 157, 167

trapezoid body, 155
trauma, 102
trigeminal nerve, 141, 228
TTS, 12
tuba aperta, 145, 229
tubal function, 143, 191
tympanometry, 115, 189, 203
tympanosclerosis, 132

validity, 24
vascular tinnitus, 228
vertex, 181
VU-meter, 89

waking audiometry, 106
Weber test, 55, 189
whispering test, 109